Perspectives on Complementary and Alternative Medicine

A Reader

Should popular complementary therapies be delivered alongside orthodox forms of medical practice? What does the future hold for complementary and alternative medicine and for western healthcare more broadly?

Complementary and alternative medicine (CAM) is an emerging and increasingly popular group of treatments, therapies and philosophies of health and wellbeing. It is a fascinating and fast-changing area of social life, which also poses an interesting challenge to current healthcare delivery and policy making.

This reader presents a lively and engaging collection of classic, controversial and new readings on complementary and alternative medicine (CAM). Issues covered throughout the collection are:

- changes in the way CAM is developing and being delivered
- holism and what this concept means to CAM practice
- changes in consumption and the health consumer that have lead to increased interest in CAM
- the safety and effectiveness of CAM treatments
- how integration is being achieved in contemporary society.

Perspectives on Complementary and Alternative Medicine: A Reader provides insight into many of the current and complex issues surrounding CAM, and will appeal to everyone who is concerned with or who has an interest in complementary and alternative healthcare. The book will be essential reading for students of CAM, health studies, nursing, medicine and allied health subjects, as well as medical sociology and modern health policy.

Open University Course: Perspectives on Complementary and Alternative Medicine (K221)

This Reader forms part of The Open University course *Perspectives on Complementary and Alternative Medicine (K221)*, a 30 points second level undergraduate course. It is an optional course for the BA/BSc (Open) and both named degrees, BA/BSc in Health Studies and BA/BSc in Health and Social Care, as well as being a core course for the Diploma in Health and Social Welfare. The readings in this book have been designed as a source for students during their study of this course. The book brings together a variety of diverse readings on how CAM is developing and being delivered, mainly in the UK, but also in other western countries.

Opinions expressed in the Reader are not necessarily those of the Course Team or of The Open University.

If you are interested in studying this course, please write to the Information Officer, School of Health and Social Welfare, The Open University, Walton Hall, Milton Keynes, MK7 6AA, UK. Details can also be reviewed on our web page http://www.open.ac.uk.

Perspectives on Complementary and Alternative Medicine

A Reader

Edited by Geraldine Lee-Treweek, Tom Heller, Susan Spurr, Hilary MacQueen and Jeanne Katz

Routledge
Taylor & Francis Group
LONDON AND NEW YORK

The Open University

First published 2005
by Routledge
2 Park Square, Milton Park, Abingdon, Oxon OX14 4RN
605 Third Avenue, New York, NY 10017

Routledge is an imprint of the Taylor & Francis Group, an informa business

British Library Cataloguing in Publication Data
A catalogue record for this book is available from the British Library

Library of Congress Cataloging in Publication Data
A catalog record for this book has been requested

Typeset in 10/12 Sabon by Scribe Design, Ashford, Kent

ISBN 13: 978-0-415-35158-4 (hbk)
ISBN 13: 978-0-415-35159-1 (pbk)

CONTENTS

SECTION 6
CAM in practice: diversity, integrations and development

INTRODUCTION
CHANGE AND DEVELOPMENT IN COMPLEMENTARY AND ALTERNATIVE MEDICINE

Geraldine Lee-Treweek and Tom Heller

This Reader brings together a range of classic and more contemporary readings about complementary and alternative medicine (CAM). It provides an essential commentary on many of the current and complex issues raised by this emerging and increasingly popular group of treatments, therapies and philosophies of health and wellbeing in Britain today and to some extent within an international context. Complementary and alternative medicine (CAM) is increasingly popular in British society and throughout the 'Western' world.

Whilst it is useful to think about the popularity of a social movement or phenomenon, it is also important to think about the levels of dynamism and change it exhibits and its potential for growth in the future. CAM certainly displays immense change and potential for development; indeed, new forms of CAM therapy are being developed all the time. Many people have heard of the five most common modalities (labelled the 'big five' in policy documents (House of Lords 2000)), chiropractic, osteopathy, herbalism, homoeopathy and acupuncture, but others such as aromatherapy, reflexology and hypnotherapy are also rapidly becoming household names. At the same time new therapies such as zone rebalancing, sedona method and reiki are also becoming more and more popular. Some of these are therapies imported from other cultures and countries, for example reiki comes from Japan. Others are totally new having been developed by people who have built upon the principles of other CAMs, or have discovered that particular healing techniques are apparently effective. It is easy to see that with more than 200 therapies currently on offer in Britain

(Stone 2001), and this number growing, that CAM is a dynamic field, both for those who are practitioners and for users of these therapies.

Such immense growth coupled with increasing public awareness and interest raises important questions about how CAM can be understood. For example; what are its key ideals and ethics, how are the relationships between CAM practitioners and the users of such services different or similar to 'orthodox' relationships, how is CAM to be used in relation to orthodox treatments, is it really safe, who is competent to be a practitioner and what kinds of tests and measures should be applied to these new forms of medicine? These are some of the questions facing the various CAM modalities as decisions are made by individual practitioners and professional bodies about what kind of 'shape' a CAM practitioner should take. Should they, for instance, follow the models provided by orthodox health care practitioners? On the other hand it could be argued that many CAM modalities have ideals, ethics and values which suggest a different model of a health professional – perhaps based upon a deeply embedded notion of holism, different views of what health, illness and disease involve, or on a view of practitioner and user as equal partners in the healing relationship? These types of fundamental issues are explored in readings that bring together a range of viewpoints.

Other issues of change involve CAM professions and occupational groups themselves as they seek public acceptance and (in some cases) medical approval. Educational and regulatory issues have come to the fore as has the issue of integration with orthodox services – whether integration between CAM and orthodox medical approaches should happen and how. However, there is little consensus on these areas with some modalities wanting highly structured and formal systems and others following a model of small informal training settings along with a laissez-faire approach to self-regulation (if any at all). Similarly CAM practitioner and professional group notions about research, evidence and efficacy differ tremendously. This spectrum spans those who are working hard to develop an evidence base in line with scientific principles, to those who refute the importance of any scientific approach. There are even those who would seek to replace 'old' notions of science with a 'new' science that emphasises, for example, the importance of energy and thought fields. There is immense difference and constant change in the attitudes to the question of evidence within CAM. And, as with other areas in this exciting emerging field, the debates are furious and ongoing. This liveliness and vigour is reflected in the selection of readings in this collection.

THE STRUCTURE OF THE BOOK

The book is divided into six sections, each with an introduction. The organisation of this collection into sections should not be seen as the creation of deep distinctions between the various issues. Indeed to understand CAM it is necessary to see the connections between concepts, ideas and beliefs; CAM is a complex area and the contrasting and challenging readings reflect this diversity.

The first section of the book acts to contextualise CAM within a contemporary context and the ways in which it is possible to understand the rise and proliferation of CAM in the UK over the last decades. The readings in the first section explore issues in relation to what CAM has to offer as a set of ideas about the world, both to individuals and to society at large. But another important issue is whether people are turning away from something (possibly orthodox health care?) in order to turn to CAM. Also, the section raises the issue of whether CAM offers something different in terms of ethics and values and to what extent it may be said to be just as ethically challenging as other forms of orthodox health care. Moreover, the readings indicate how orthodox medicine in the UK has responded to the growing public interest in CAM. They provide an overview of how CAM has become what it is in the UK and identify critical issues in its definition and development.

The collection of readings in section two addresses the fascinating area of the nature of the healing relationship, or what has become more commonly known as the therapeutic relationship. The popularity of CAM has sometimes been said to revolve around the relationship between practitioner and user/client/patient and, specifically the differences between a CAM consultation and an orthodox one in terms of length of consulting time and other indicators that might signify the quality of the relationship. This section explores the pull of CAM, emphasising the importance of culture for people's choice of healer and for their response to the healing process. Whilst the therapeutic relationship can work towards healing, it can also sometimes go wrong or have unexpected negative effects. These may include over-dependency of the user, the encouragement of greater fear or concern over health and people choosing the wrong practitioner for a particular problem. This section gives equal weight to contrasting views on the therapeutic relationship in CAM and in doing so provides a set of readings that offer an in-depth exposition of current thinking.

In section three the focus switches to issues that relate to the spatial and ecological distribution of complementary medicine and its practitioners, and the settings in which the growth of CAM has taken place. The focus on practitioners is important because attempting to understand their drives and motivations to provide services has been rather neglected in previous research literature. Readings in this section are based on research that has examined the ways that practitioners relate to the financial and business side of providing CAM services; to the different ideologies that practitioners espouse in their attempt to develop their services; the relationships between CAM ideologies and those prevalent in wider society, such as New Age movements; and the problems and opportunities relating to the development of CAMs within orthodox care services. This focus on current issues is offset by a historical examination of some of the forces that led to the development of homoeopathy services in a previous era. It is evident that understanding the current growth and development of CAM should be set within this historical context.

Section four addresses the way that CAM is under great pressure to standardise, develop education and regulatory structures, and to address the difficult problem of fraudulent practice. The general public, government and members of orthodox health care professions have for some time been pushing for safeguards and structures that would enable lay people and doctors alike to judge the competence and quality of a particular CAM practitioner or professional group. Readings in this section begin by looking at the issue of quackery and fraud and then turn to the issue of education. How should CAM practitioners be taught and how should orthodox practitioners be familiarised in these increasingly popular modalities? This issue links with the matter of regulation and three readings in this section address the ways in which regulation has been developed in the UK for osteopaths, acupuncturists and other modalities. Further questions are explored relating to how a professional community develops and changes. It is important to remember that such communities are often fraught with division and differences around philosophy and knowledge and these types of concerns also relate to the notion of fraud and who is an 'authentic' CAM practitioner. The issues raised by the readings in section four all relate to what could be termed the 'professional projects' of CAM; the ways in which they are trying to develop themselves as professional groups.

Section five considers CAM from a scientific standpoint. Whilst regulation has been a very important aim, many modalities have also viewed the issue of research as essential to their professional development. Although some CAM has embraced the idea of using science as a means by which to legitimate their practice and work towards integration with orthodoxy, it is probably fair to say that the scientific approach is a relatively new one for much of the CAM community. CAM presents a whole range of difficulties for the scientific approach. For instance, many CAM practitioners would argue that they have a holistic approach which cannot separate emotions, body energies and well-being factors, all of which are difficult to quantify or measure using 'standard' scientific techniques. However, it is important for all treatments to address the issues of efficacy and safety, both to protect the public and to provide good value for money. The readings in this section discuss the ways in which CAM may be researched and discuss some of the difficulties and benefits in applying traditional scientific methods to this field. Readings within this section also examine some popular modalities and the range of evidence available for their efficacy. In many of the readings the issue of the placebo effect is also considered.

Section six ends the collection by focusing on CAM in practice. This section allows the reader a view into some of the current uses of CAM and the way it is often being used with user groups in situations where orthodox health care has little to offer. Empowerment, change and choice are key issues that arise and are developed in these readings. The section ends by focusing explicitly on changing perspectives within the individual and changing perspectives within orthodox health care. It is clear from the diversity articulated in section six that there are diverse perspectives within CAM and a range of ways of thinking about the mind, body, emotions and illness/wellness. The challenge for society will be to harness this diversity in a way that respects the different nature of particular CAMs and in a way which provides users with the type of interventions that most help them.

SECTION 1

CAM IN CONTEXT

INTRODUCTION

Geraldine Lee-Treweek

In order to understand any social trend fully, it is necessary to understand the context in which it developed and the current issues that presently surround it. CAM did not develop in a vacuum, it arose from the myriad forms of health provision visible prior to the emergence of biomedicine. The range of CAM encompasses a very broad church of philosophies, beliefs and activities, but this section tries to discuss some of the key contextualising issues that affect the acceptance of CAM and its role in contemporary UK society.

In Stephen Fulder's reading the notion of what is different and characteristic about CAM is presented. Fulder's work presents some of the more familiar claims of CAM as a group – that these modalities are generally holistic and interested in the entirety of the person, that they often have a different ethos to orthodoxy, that they are more natural (and by implication more caring?), and that they offer some people a more spiritual way of thinking about health, illness and wellbeing.

Ted Kaptchuk and David Eisenberg begin to develop these themes further by thinking about how we can break CAM into groups or categories – whether it is possible to create a taxonomy of these modalities. This is a very important issue indeed, demonstrated by its centrality to the issues explored in the House of Lords Report (2001) and to the furore that arose from this report as various modalities complained about their respective positions in the chosen taxonomy. Dividing up CAM into various categories is a contentious and difficult exercise; however, it is a necessary task for the purposes of policy.

Janet Richardson's reading provides an absorbing commentary on some of the historical and sociological features that differentiate 'complementary' forms of medicine from those that have come to be accepted within current orthodoxy. The reading focuses on the ways that these two competing ideologies use, and possibly abuse, concepts relating to 'evidence'. Within orthodox systems the drive towards 'evidence-based medicine' has led to increasingly narrow definitions of what constitutes evidence, whereas in the world of complementary and alternative medicine the notion of evidence continues to be debated. An expansion of the concepts of evidence, she argues, should move away from rigid bioscience and embrace sociological and anthropological features as well as integrate both quantitative and qualitative methodologies.

The next two readings provide differing opinions on why people may have embraced CAM. Ray Moynihan and Richard Smith raise the issue of the omnipresence and omnipotence of modern orthodox medicine. Is it over medication that leads people to want to try something that they perceive to be more natural and more gentle? In contrast, Barry Beyerstein's reading reads as a retort to these ideas. For him, those who use CAM are confused and deluded. Whilst modern medicine has provided enormous leaps forward in lowering mortality and providing a high standard of health care, CAM is able to pander to the worried well; those for whom a misunderstood notion of science makes them more liable to misinterpret CAM as an answer to all the normal worries of life. Whilst quite an immoderate view, Beyerstein's argument is compelling in the sense that much CAM does have a leisure element to it and much of the 'science' behind many CAMs is not rigorous or (as yet) accepted by the scientific mainstream. These two pieces of work complement one another by their strikingly different analyses on the public popularity of CAM.

Two excerpts from British Medical Association (BMA) reports follow to demonstrate the growing interest in CAM from the medical establishment. Designed to be read together, excerpts of both reports are included to demonstrate the sea change in the BMA's public attitude to CAM, visible between the 1986 and 1993 reports. The impact of these cannot be underestimated when the audience that these writings were intended for is considered: doctors, managers making decisions about whether CAMs were useful to patients and policy makers. Whilst the 1986 report writes of the dangers of CAM and calls it 'alternative therapy', the 1993 report's tone is accommodative, even providing guidelines on how doctors might train in CAM modalities. It writes of 'complementary medicine' and, in particular, focuses upon standards in CAM, ensuring competence, proper training and the issue of possible routes to regulation. These two reports are pivotal historical documents when considering the change in medical attitudes around the emerging area of CAM.

Edzard Ernst, Michael Cohen and Julie Stone's reading addresses the issue of ethics in CAM. Ethics and ethical standards are increasingly important in a whole range of areas of social life – from genetics to marketing. Within CAM there are many assumptions about this form of health care. For instance, there are assumptions about it being more ethical by virtue of its notional core values, such as holism and (allegedly) a strong connection to nature and the natural world. This reading dissects the ethics of CAM and asks whether special ethical standards are needed for this type of health and wellbeing work.

Finally, Philip Harris and Rebecca Rees outline the prevalence of CAM usage in the UK. The growth of public interest is a very important contextualising factor in understanding a number of other issues in CAM. This growth impacts upon the public visibility of CAM and the number of people wanting to go into it as an occupation or profession. It also affects processes such as regulation as professional groups and umbrella bodies realise that growing public interest means increased calls for professional structures from the state, medicine and the public themselves. The issues raised by Philip Harris and Rebecca Rees frame a number of other readings within the collection by enabling readers to understand the popular context of CAM.

CHAPTER 1

THE BASIC CONCEPTS OF ALTERNATIVE MEDICINE AND THEIR IMPACT ON OUR VIEWS OF HEALTH

Stephen Fulder

INTRODUCTION

Conventional medicine can be said to have been the dominant medical system in the postindustrial world for not much more than 150 years. Prior to that, although differential diagnosis was the main diagnostic method used, physicians had to compete with traditional practitioners and bonesetters. Traditional and ancient medical concepts such as the four humours, the elements, the vix medicatrix naturae, and crasis/dyscrasis (ie, that health is based on inner and outer balance) only went out of fashion during the early part of the last century (Rosenberg, 1977). In its short history, modern medicine has proven to be so apparently effective, and so well adapted to the industrial worldview that it gave the impression that indigenous, ancient, or traditional medicine had no validity, and was nearly extinct. In fact, this was not so. It clearly existed in the East and the Third World, and was in hiding in Western culture, where it took a defensive cultic posture in the face of modern medicine's self-confidence.

However in the last 20 years, there has been a radical renewal of interest in, and use of, traditional or alternative medicine. So much so, that we are re-entering a period in which scientific medicine and its services

Edited from *Journal of Alternative and Complementary Medicine*, 1998;4(2):147–58.
Mary Ann Liebert, Inc.

share and compete for customers with alternative medicine, within a pluralistic national medicine (Pietroni, 1988; 1990). Indeed, the British Medical Association's new report acknowledges that alternative medical systems are full systems, that they are here to stay, that doctors must learn about them even at undergraduate level, and if a doctor wishes to study them, he or she must undertake a full course of instruction (British Medical Association, 1993). Alternative medicine is becoming available on the National Health Service throughout the United Kingdom (Cameron-Blackie, 1993; Richardson, 1995). The scale of the current use of alternative medicine is not always appreciated. Surveys have shown that in Europe, roughly a third of the population have used alternative medicine (Fisher and Ward, 1994), and roughly the same proportion in the United States (Eisenberg et al, 1993). Polls of doctors have shown that three-fourths of British general practitioner trainees and nearly half of those in practice want to learn one or more alternative medical techniques (Reilly, 1983), that virtually all doctors in primary care want alternative medicine to become fully part of national medicine (Perkin et al, 1984). In addition, where doctors work with complementary practitioners, complementary medicine is highly popular (Budd et al, 1990), demand outstrips supply (Himmel et al, 1990).

COMMON FEATURES OF NONCONVENTIONAL MEDICINE

Nonconventional medicine is an aggregate term for a variety of ancient or traditional medical systems in their modern forms.

Some modalities are complete medical systems with their own diagnostic and therapeutic methods based on a unique, global, and self-consistent theory of health and disease (eg, acupuncture, herbalism, homeopathy, and naturopathy). Others (such as the physical and manual therapies), are subsidiary techniques. Practitioners of these subsidiary methods do not consider themselves to be first-call primary care practitioners. Compatibility of alternative theories with conventional medical theory also varies. The physical therapies such as chiropractic, medical herbalism, and to some extent naturopathy utilize essentially conventional diagnosis together with concepts of disease that are different from, but understandable by, conventional science. For example chiropractic is based on conventional anatomy and physiology, but extends knowledge of the pathogenesis and treatment of musculoskeletal problems (such as 'adhesions' and 'subluxations') into subtle areas that are regarded as invisible and unproven by conventional medicine. Herbal medicine recognizes and uses conventional descriptions of disease such as eczema. However, it chooses medicines that affect the supposed deeper imbalances (eg, that allergies originate in part from inadequacies in the liver housekeeping functions) as well as treatments that attempt to restore proper local tissue function. On the other hand, homeopathy, naturopathy, and Oriental medicine use different concepts of disease, based on an alternative world-view that is not easily translatable or compatible with scientific medicine. It has been difficult or impossible to map these systems onto conventional medicine or vice versa. Even in China, where strenuous efforts have been made, there is still no agreement on whether acupuncture meridians or Oriental viscera such as 'kidney' correspond to any known anatomic structures (Bensoussan, 1991).

CHARACTERISTICS OF ALTERNATIVE MEDICINE RELEVANT TO DESCRIPTIONS OF HEALTH

There are certain basic features of the practice of alternative medicine that involve a view of health different from that implicit within modern medicine and modern life. Not all therapists will use these concepts. However, they represent the foundation of authentic alternative medicine, are laid out in the texts, and taught in the colleges, even if the therapy has compromised to the biomedical model during the current struggles between various competing systems. For example, many acupuncturists find themselves called on to focus on symptoms more directly at the expense of the slower restoration of energetic balance, because of the expectations of patients who are conditioned by modern medicine to expect a fast restoration of comfort.

Self-healing is paramount

The in-built natural healing process is respected and recruited during treatment, although it is not necessarily understood. Resistance is improved by preventive measures. Particularly in Oriental and Ayurvedic medicine, a considerable proportion of traditional practice is devoted to the restoration of vital force and self-healing energy. For example, in Western herbal medicine there is very frequent use of a category of herbs called 'alteratives' or 'blood purifiers.' These are herbs such as echinacea (Echinacea purpurea), cleavers (Gallium aparine), burdock (Arctium lappa), sage (Salvia spp), and myrrh (Commiphora mol-mol). They are used during the treatment of most acute and chronic infections and inflammations, along with fasting or special diets and nutrients, and other herbs to promote circulation of lymph and body fluids, all of which is intended to awaken a more powerful immune response and encourage long-term immune function. Other natural remedies such as garlic or thyme may be used as natural antimicrobials, but they are not the primary tools. This is also a fundamental position of naturopathy and homeopathy.

Working with, not against, symptoms

Symptoms are a guide in the journey to a cure. They are managed, not suppressed. For example the daily ebb and flow of a symptom such as headache may be used by an acupuncturist or homeopath as a guide to the course of treatment of deeper problems with organ function. For example a migraine-type headache could be seen by an acupuncturist as arising from overactive liver metabolism (liver 'fire' or yang). Real treatment involves an adjustment to the propensity of the liver to create inflammation, not merely relief of symptoms by analgesia. The type and location of the headaches (frequency, severity, vertigo, sharpness, one-sidedness, etc.) is constantly monitored throughout the treatment as a guide to the effectiveness of the draining of the liver's excess. Accompanying symptoms, such as nausea, may be an indication of the energetic state of other organ systems such as the spleen.

Individuality

Each person's condition is different, has arisen from different reasons against a different constitutional background, and requires a different path for treatment. Decisions are personal and individualistic, not statistical. One of the indications of the richness of the medical system is the development of a typology in which individual differences in health, disease, and response to the environment can be understood. For example, the constitutional picture in Ayurvedic medicine is a highly detailed art that integrates thousands of characteristics of body, skin, personality, habits, etc., defined in terms of Vata ('airiness'), Pitta ('fieriness') and Kapha ('wateriness'). This establishes an individual's susceptibilities, strengths, and weaknesses, and guides both prevention and treatment. By contrast, Western (Thompsonian) herbalism does not make extensive use of constitutional differences, and modern medicine ignores it completely unless there are inherited pathologies.

Integration of human facets

Individuals are regarded 'holistically' in diagnosis and treatment. There is less a priori division between mind-body-spirit or environment-society-individual. 'Holism' is just one of the approaches that may or may not be incorporated within a therapeutic modality. It is not a medical system in itself, although the term 'holistic medicine' is sometimes loosely used. Alternative medicine is essentially more holistic. In homeopathy and Oriental medicine, for example, emotional, psychological, and behavioral signs are always included in diagnosis. This is rather less so in naturopathy, herbalism, and the manual therapies, but even here, holism is often applied as an approach of an individual practitioner. For example, naturopaths may encourage relaxation and imagery along with diet and herbs to treat high blood pressure. Or osteopaths and chiropractors occasionally explore the psychosocial stresses that may give rise to a repeated musculoskeletal problem in a certain patient.

No fixed beginning or ending

There is no defined or determined state of illness where treatment must begin, and wellness where treatment must end. Such points are defined contextually. One patient may require assistance to reach a state of well-being and accommodation to his cancer. Treatment will finish when this is achieved, although in conventional terms the patient is still seriously ill. Conversely, another client may be treated so as to improve his energetic balance and condition or vitality. He may seek treatment with Oriental medicine to cope with an addiction, an energetic dullness, convalescence or even to improve Shen, ie, to bring light to his eyes. Treatment in this case, in conventional terms, is of a healthy person.

Conformity to universal principles

Remedies are discovered and used in conformity to patterns of relations (such as yin/yang) between all living creatures and their environment. These patterns are often subtle and involve energetic rather than material phenomena. For example Ch'i in Chinese medicine is a tangible but invisible vital force that operates continually as the basis of all function. In Oriental medicine it is sensed and utilized in much the same way that modern man would sense and also utilize gravity. Despite the fact that Ch'i is so universal, it is enormously elaborated as an explanatory principle to describe detailed changes in function, eg, constrained, stagnant, wild, deficient, excess, etc., of liver, spleen, kidney, etc. This is in contrast to conventional medicine, which derives from reductionist science. Therefore, processes in the body are examined as discrete entities, unconnected to basic forces and elemental qualities. Consider again the use of Ch'i in the diagnosis of 'Excess Liver "Ch'i" rising' for a migrainous headache, in contrast to the conventional medical view of 'overstimulation of local vascular serotonin receptors at the pain site.'

REFERENCES

Bensoussan A. *The Vital Meridian: A Modern Exploration of Acupuncture*, Edinburgh: Churchill Livingstone, 1991.

British Medical Association. *New Approaches to Good Practice*, Oxford: Oxford University Press, 1993.

Budd C, Fisher B, Parrinder D, Price L. A model of co-operation between complementary and allopathic medicine in a primary care setting, *Br J Gen Pract* 1990;40:376–8.

Cameron-Blackie G. *Complementary Therapies in the NHS*, Birmingham: National Association of Health Authorities, 1993.

Eisenberg DM, Kessler RC, Foster C et al. Unconventional medicine in the United States, *N Engl J Med* 1993;328:246–52.

Fisher P, Ward A. Complementary medicine in Europe, *Br Med J* 1994;309:107–11.

Himmel W, Schulte M, Kochen MM. Complementary medicine: Are patients' expectations being met by their general practitioners? *Br J Gen Pract* 1993;43:232–5.

Perkin MR, Pearcy RM, Fraser JS. A comparison of the attitudes shown by General Practitioners, hospital doctors and medical students towards alternative medicine, *J R Soc Med* 1994;87:523–5.

Pietroni P. Alternative medicine. *R Soc Arts J* 1988;136:791–801.

Pietroni P. *The Greening of Medicine*, London: Gollancz, 1990.

Reilly D. Young doctors views on alternative medicine, *Br Med J* 1983;287:337–40.

Richardson J. Complementary therapies on the NHS: The experience of a new service, *Complement Therap Med* 1995;3:153–7.

Rosenberg CE. The therapeutic revolution: medicine, meaning and social change in the nineteenth century, *Perspect Biol Med* 1977;20:485–506.

CHAPTER 2

A TAXONOMY OF UNCONVENTIONAL HEALING PRACTICES

Ted J Kaptchuk and David M Eisenberg

Defining unconventional medicine by 'what it is' does not work. *Alternative medicine* is an umbrella-like term that 'represents a heterogeneous population promoting disparate beliefs and practices that vary considerably from one movement or tradition to another and form no consistent ... body of knowledge' (Gevitz, 1995). Alternative medicine is a large residual category of health care practices generally defined by their exclusion and 'alienation from the dominant medical profession' (Gevitz, 1988).

Besides an absence of shared principles, an accurate definition of alternative medicine is further confounded because the boundary demarcating conventional and irregular medicine has always been porous and flexible (CAM Research Methodology Conference, 1997). Therapies move across that border; for example, nitroglycerin (Fye, 1986) and digitalis (Eisenberg and Kaptchuk, 2000) began as alternative drugs, just as corn flakes and graham crackers began as unconventional health foods (Whorton, 1982). Entire professions change sides. In 1903, when the American Medical Association needed both a larger referral base for specialists and new allies in its fight with osteopaths, chiropractors, and Christian Scientists, it boldly reversed its policy and declared homeopaths to be conventional MDs (Rothstein, 1972). Likewise, osteopathy ceased being a renegade profession after World War II (Albrecht and Levy, 1982; Gevitz, 1982; Wardwell, 1994).

Edited from *Complementary and Alternative Medicine Series*, David M Eisenberg and Ted J Kaptchuk (eds).

The first of two essays in this issue (pp 189–195) demonstrated that the United States has had a rich history of medical pluralism. This essay offers an overview of alternative medicine. Because of the inherent problems in defining a flexible residual category, we present a taxonomy of what is currently considered unconventional healing in the United States.

The number of named alternative therapies available in the United States easily soars into the hundreds (Burroughs and Kastner, 1993; Hafner et al, 1992; Hafner et al, 1993; McGuire, 1983; National Institutes of Health on Alternative Medical Systems and Practices in the United States, 1994; Segen, 1998). Many classification systems have been proposed (British Medical Association, 1992; English-Lueck, 1990; Furnham, 2000; Kemper, 1996; Lancet, 2000; McGuire, 1988; Newman Turner, 1998; Pietroni, 1992). In an effort to further discussion, we offer a new taxonomy that we believe configures the domains of unconventional medicine across a broader spectrum of health practices. We do not expect that our attempt will be definitive (nor do we necessarily believe a perfect schema is possible). Any classification system is limited because such human phenomena resist discreteness as well as being fixed in time. As we point out, overlap often occurs. Inevitably, subjectivity affects the categorization and perceptions of 'affinities.' A summary of our schema is presented in Figure 2.1.

Unconventional healing practices can be divided into two types: one that appeals to the general public and another that confines itself to specific ethnic or religious groups. The broadest category of unconventional medicine is easily recognized because its health care claims to be independent of any sectarian belief or faith and is said to depend on universal and even 'scientific' laws (Kaptchuk and Eisenberg, 1998). It is the best-known variety of unconventional medicine in the United States and recently, in a loose alliance, has become known as complementary and alternative medicine (CAM) (Kaptchuk and Eisenberg, 1998).

The second kind of unconventional practice is typically confined to narrow groups, such as members of particular religions (for example, Pentecostal Christians), ethnic groups (for example, Puerto-Rican spiritism), or regions (for example, southern Appalachian folk beliefs). These practices are culturally self-contained, function outside any broader coalition, often lack the markings of a health delivery system, and in this essay are referred to as parochial unconventional medicine.

COMPLEMENTARY AND ALTERNATIVE MEDICINE

The wide-ranging category of CAM can be divided into five main sectors, which are described below.

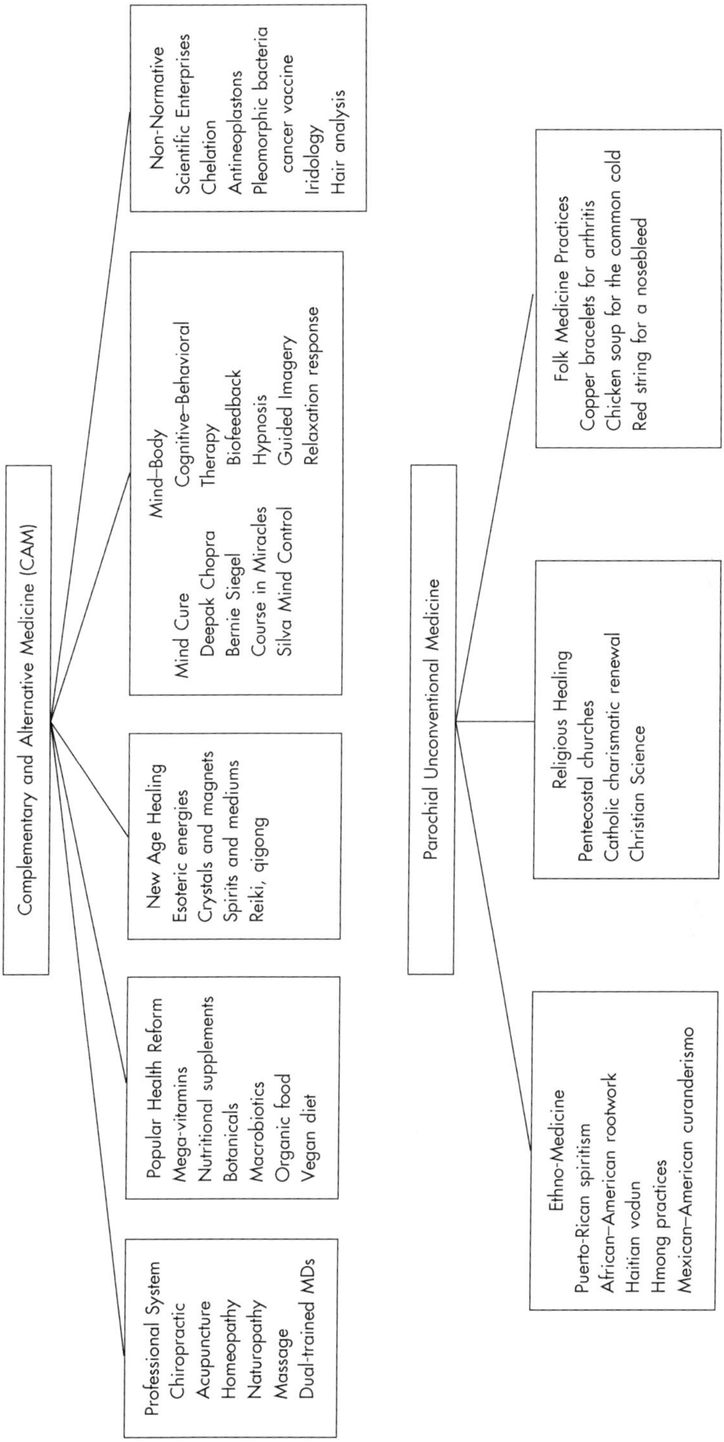

Figure 2.1 Unconventional healing practices: taxonomy with examples

Professionalized or distinct medical systems

Probably the most recognizable alternative healing practices are those that are organized into medical movements with distinct theories, practices, and institutions. Licensure as an independent profession is a goal if not always an actuality. Medical institutions, such as schools, professional associations, and offices with secretaries and billing procedures, are readily visible. An extensive corpus of technical literature helps guide therapy and practice and sharpens distinctness. Because they are easiest to describe and define, these systems are the most prominent in discussions of CAM. The six major components of this sector of CAM are chiropractic, acupuncture, homeopathy, naturopathy, massage, and dual-functioning MDs.

Chiropractic, the largest alternative medical profession in the United States, accounts for almost a third of all visits to CAM providers (Eisenberg and Davis, 1998). The body's biomechanical structure, especially the spine, is seen as basic to health, and chiropractic emphasizes spinal manipulation as treatment (Cooter, 1987; Kaptchuk and Eisenberg, 1998). Licensed as primary health care providers in all 50 states, chiropractors especially treat musculoskeletal disorders (Wardwell, 1992; Coulehan, 1985).

Osteopathy was once a second manual therapy competing for the same patients as chiropractic. Since World War II, osteopathy has reconfigured itself and has become 'conventional'; the status of an osteopathic physician is equivalent to that of an MD. A minority of patients (<17%) visiting DOs receives the kind of manipulative therapy that would still be considered unconventional by orthodox MDs (National Center for Health Statistics, 1975; Johnson, Kurtz and Kurtz, 1997).

Acupuncture relies on the insertion of fine needles at well-defined specific sites to regulate and balance humoral forces and 'energy' (*qi*) and to promote health (Kaptchuk, 2000). As a component of East Asian medicine, acupuncture is often complemented with herbal treatment. Since the 1970s, acupuncture has spread throughout the United States and is independently licensed as a health care profession in 37 states (Mitchell, 1997).

Homeopathy uses the principle of 'like cures like': A substance that produces a set of symptoms in a healthy person is used to treat an identical symptom complex in a sick person (Ernst and Kaptchuk, 1996; Kaufman, 1971). The substance, however, is extremely diluted, often to the extent that none of the original substance is likely to remain. Currently, homeopaths can be independently licensed in only three states, but other licensed practitioners also prescribe these remedies.

Naturopathy uses a wide assortment of therapies that its practitioners call 'natural.' Herbs, nutritional supplements, dietary and lifestyle advice, homeopathy, manipulation, and counseling can all be components of the repertoire (Gort and Coburn, 1988). The term *naturopathy* was adopted in 1902 to replace the old word *hydropathy*, which denoted water-cure therapy.

Currently, naturopaths can be licensed as primary care providers in 11 states: naturopathy is most common in the Pacific Northwest (Baer, 1992).

Massage therapists can be professionally licensed in more than 25 states (Eisenberg, 1997). Although massage therapists (also called 'body-workers' or 'hands-on therapists') clearly perform unorthodox interventions (Good and Good 1981; Knapp and Antonucci, 1990; Tappen, 1988), they overlap with recognized biomedical professions, such as physical therapy, or simple attempts at relaxation. Complementary alternative medicine techniques that address body alignment and awareness (such as the Feldenkrais method [Rywerant, 1983] and the Alexander technique [Leibowitz and Connington, 1990]) are often classified as massage therapy because they involve 'body-work.'

Medical doctors who have opted to deliver, supervise, or advocate CAM are a significant force in alternative medicine (Goldstein et al, 1987; Yahn, 1979). These dual-trained practitioners lend enormous prestige and legitimacy to alternative medicine and can be prominent spokespersons (Chopra, 1989; Dossey, 1991; Gordon, 1996; Weil, 1995). Providing what is sometimes called 'integrative' medicine, these physicians can deliver a broad range of CAM services or can focus on a single therapy.

Popular health reform (alternative dietary and lifestyle practices)

The health food movement, also known as alternative dietary and lifestyle practices, is an important component of CAM. Depending on how one calculates, it may in fact dwarf the professional sector (Kaptchuk and Eisenberg, 1998). In the scholarly literature, this type of healing is labeled 'popular health reform' because these practices are often advocated by untrained laypersons who often claim knowledge superior to that of expert scientists (Whorton, 1982).

Popular health reform is delivered by a melange of resources, such as health food stores, popular books and journals, charismatic leaders, alternative provider recommendations, mass media attention, and a considerable amount of neighborly advice. This popular movement usually espouses a vegetarian or near-vegetarian diet, or avoidance of chemically treated and, more recently, radiated or genetically altered food. Details of particular programs tend to have enormous heterogeneity. Recommendations might range from eating only cooked food (for example, macrobiotics [Kandel, 1976]) to eating only raw food (for example, fruitarianism) (Kirschner, 1991), or from heavy reliance on nutritional and botanical supplements or aromatherapy to their absolute prohibition. Recent shifts in biomedicine's understanding of nutrition and its role in pathophysiology have also encouraged a general social movement toward behaviors that were once thought to belong to health food 'nuts'

(Deutsch, 1977). This, in turn, has caused a blurring of the distinction between orthodox and unorthodox lifestyles and has helped increase the awareness of CAM in society (Kaptchuk and Eisenberg, 1998).

New Age healing

The New Age is the source of many extremely disparate beliefs and practices that can describe overlapping religious and healing movements (Ellwood, 1979; Melton, 1990). Furthermore, confounding discussion, the term *New Age* may not be 'adopted by a given individual (indeed, may be rejected), even though to outsiders the practice appears to fall into this category' (Barnes, 1998). As a religious movement, the New Age is about a 'new dispensation': less about law and limitation and more about unrestricted self-expression and unlimited abundance. Instead of any fixed religious doctrine, the movement emphases a fluid 'spirituality.' It is not uncommon to see an iconography that is a grab bag of Hindu, Christian, Buddhist, Rosicrucian, and pagan motifs (English-Lueck, 1990).

The New Age is also a health care category because spiritual equanimity and physical health are considered to be linked. In fact, New Age beliefs resist any separation between spirituality and physical health or faith and medicine. Scholars point out that the New Age seeks a 'third way,' 'a spiritual science,' between revealed biblical religion and 'atheistic–materialist' science (Oppenheim, 1988).

A key New Age connection between the spiritual and physical realms involves esoteric energies that resemble a veritable 'electromagnetic' dimension of wellness (Fuller, 1982; Glik, 1988). The names of the energies change – life force, universal innate intelligence, psychic, parapsychological, psi, astral, spiritual vital force – but they inevitably elude scientific detection (Kaptchuk, 2001). Healers can transmit these forces. Devices and substances that emit them, such as radionic machines, magnetic devices, pyramids, crystals, and other electromagnetic gadgets, are constantly being incarnated. The health influence of planets and stars and some medical astrology could be considered another type of such energy (Feher, 1992). Healing energy therapies not explicitly connected to the New Age, such as 'therapeutic touch' (often applied by nurses) (Krieger, Peper and Ancoli, 1979) and 'laying-on of hands' (Zefron, 1975), can ultimately be traced here. New 'energy' forces are being recruited from Asia. Chinese qigong (Miura, 1989) and Japanese Reiki (Yasuo, 1993), while obviously not originally New Age, find it a hospitable environment for cross-cultural migration (Kaptchuk, 2001).

Sometimes the religious and health domains are bridged through 'clairvoyant physicians' or the healing presence of the spirits, religious icons, or leaders (Easthope, 1986; Johnson, 1998; Kerr and Crow, 1983; Levin and Coreil, 1986). Best-selling books by spirit mediums who describe spiritual healing for 'incurable diseases and maladies' help keep the phenomena in prominent view (Van Praag, 1997). A third type of New Age healing connection between the cosmos and human health operates through 'mind' forces and can also be considered a subcategory of CAM psychological intervention (see following discussion).

Psychological interventions: mind cure and 'mind–body' medicine

Psychotherapeutics in CAM has two sources: one that is purely CAM and one that overlaps with conventional psychological interventions. In the scholarly literature, the exclusively CAM psychological tradition is referred to as Mind Cure or New Thought (Braden, 1963; Judah, 1967; McGuire, 1988; Parker, 1973). These therapies, which can include a myriad assortment of visualizations, affirmations, intentions, medications, and emotional release techniques, all share a single point: mental forces are the preeminent arbiters of health. Psychotherapists affiliated with CAM believe that the mind is the most dominant agency for restoring well-being and maintaining health. The notions that 'What you think is what is real' and that 'Your emotions determine cancer or other major disease' are dogma repeated over and over like mantras. Such bestsellers as Bernie Siegel's *Love, Medicine and Miracles* and Deepak Chopra's *Ageless Body, Timeless Mind: The Quantum Alternative to Growing Old* testify to the appeal of these beliefs.

The other sector of CAM 'mind–body' therapies merges into conventional psychotherapy and cognitive–behavioral interventions. The relationship can be confusing or can produce gray areas. Generally speaking, in conventional medicine, psychotherapeutics is conceded only limited agency and is primarily used to treat psychological problems or to help patients cope when conventional treatments are not available or are insufficient. Psychotherapeutics remains a subordinate component of the conventional medical system (Kirmayer, 1988; Osherson and AmaraSingham, 1981).

However, whenever too much power or efficacy is attributed to regular psychological therapies and they are used 'off-label,' they 'transgress' and can become CAM. For example, most MDs would consider psychotherapy appropriate for reactive depression after a cancer diagnosis, but psychotherapy used to cure a metastatic tumor would be considered unconventional (Cassileth, 1996). The same holds true for various cognitive–behavioral therapies that use 'passive nonvolitional intention,' such as biofeedback, stress management, relaxation response, meditation, guided imagery, and hypnosis. When practitioners of these techniques make modest claims limited to small physiologic changes, the techniques are acceptable as subordinate components of conventional medicine. For example, biofeedback for fecal incontinence (Ko et al, 1997) or, more debatably, relaxation response for mild hypertension (Eisenberg et al, 1993; Linden and Chambers, 1994) can seem legitimate or can at least achieve borderline acceptability, but both would be considered distinctly alternative if used to treat diabetes.

Another source of CAM psychotherapeutics involves the fact that between 250 (Herink, 1980) and 400 (Karasu, 1986) named types of psychological treatments are thought to exist. Any therapy deemed unacceptable by the mainstream can find a receptive home in CAM. Also, whether self-help groups, such as Alcoholics Anonymous, are CAM is highly debatable, but to the extent that they are not conventional they can automatically be described as alternative (Jones, 1970; Uva, 1991).

Non-normative scientific enterprises

Non-normative scientific enterprises typically appeal to patients with potentially catastrophic illnesses, such as cancer. These therapies can include sophisticated pharmacologic agents and often revolve around a well-known proponent who can have legitimate and even impressive scientific or medical credentials but advocates theories and practices unacceptable to the general scientific community. Examples include Dr Stanislaw Burzynski's 'antineoplastons' and Dr Virginia Livingston-Wheeler's 'pleomorphic bacteria cancer vaccine' (Lerner, 1994; U.S. Congress Office of Technology Assessment, 1990). Non-normative interventions can sometimes blur into the conventional practice of prescribing recognized pharmaceuticals for off-label uses (Cohen, Shevitz and Mayer, 1992; Laetz T, Silberman, 1991; O'Connor, 1995). Unvalidated diagnostic methods and unconventional technological devices that diagnose or heal can be considered part of the non-normative science category. Representative examples are hair analysis, which purportedly detects a wide variety of diseases and nutrient imbalances (Barrett, 1985); iridology, in which illness is diagnosed through a detailed examination of the iris (Ernst, 1999); and chelation therapy to reverse the processes of arteriosclerotic disease (Ernst, 1997).

PAROCHIAL UNCONVENTIONAL MEDICINE

Unlike CAM, parochial unconventional practices appeal to a more narrowly defined constituency. Three main parochial categories exist.

Ethno-medicine

The healing practices of specific ethnic populations make up a critical component of US community health care (Harwood, 1981). These practices are rooted in the widely differing medical or religious traditions of various cultures. Well-known examples include Puerto-Rican spiritism (Fisch, 1968; Harwood, 1977), Mexican–American curanderismo (Martinez and Martin, 1966; Trotter and Chavira, 1981), Haitian vodun (Brown, 1991; Scott, 1974), Native American traditional medicine (Fuchs and Bashshur, 1975), Hmong folk practices (Fadiman, 1997), African–American 'rootwork' (Mathews, 1987), and African–American spiritual church healing (Jacobs, 1990; Snow, 1978). Occasionally, a culture-bound medical system ventures outside its historical sphere of influence and becomes another option available to the general US population. This is true of acupuncture and seems to be coming true for India's Ayurvedic medicine as it follows in the footsteps of yoga, its pioneering offspring (Goldman, 1991). Partly because of New Age affinities, this may also happen with Tibetan medicine and Native American ceremonies (Albanese, 1990; Anderson, 1997). Nonetheless, as a general taxonomic statement, consistent with stubborn racist prejudices, one could say that medical practices of ethnic communities are described as ethno-medicine while the 'ethno-medicine' of mainstream white Americans is generally classified as CAM.

Folk medicine practices

Folk healing practices form a deeply embedded, unorganized, and seemingly spontaneous response to illness. Many of these practices are confined to specific geographic areas, such as southern Appalachia (Cavender, 1992) or rural New Hampshire (Levine, 1941). Sometimes they can be traced back to remnants of ethnic (including Anglo-Saxon) magical traditions or earlier lay forms of self-care and home remedies. Common practices include wearing copper bracelets for arthritis, covering a wart with a penny and then burying the penny, stopping a nosebleed by placing a red string around the neck, and curing a cold with chicken soup (Cook and Baisden, 1986; Hand, 1971; Rinzler, 1991; Saketkhoo, Januszkiewicz and Sackner, 1978). Besides cures, folk beliefs can also generate culture-bound diseases, symptoms, and treatment-seeking behaviors (Hufford, 1997; Pachter, 1994). Some folk practices have a more widespread currency and are derived from earlier layers of premodern medicine (for example, humoral Hippocratic medicine) or medieval medical schools (for example, astrological medicine) (Curry, 1987; Dick, 1946). Examples of remnants of Hippocratic ideas include such folk wisdom as 'Bundle up to prevent a cold' or 'Feed a cold and starve a fever' (Gebhard, 1976; Helman, 1978; Hufford, 1997).

Religious healing

Many Americans rely on religion for salutary effects on their health (Koenig, Moberg and Kvale, 1988; Yates et al, 1981). Generally, normative mainstream religious institutions have seen their role as supporting the 'spiritual' dimension and avoid direct overlap or competition with the biomedical system (Numbers and Amundsen, 1986). This division of labor has weakened somewhat lately; 'healing' services of one kind or another have appeared even in liberal churches and synagogues (Johnson, 1986; King, Sobal and DeForge, 1988).

The most salient forms of religious healing for physical disease can be found in Christian churches that see their ministry as replicating the miraculous healings recorded in the Bible (Amundsen, 1982; Ferngren, 1992). This is especially true of the Pentecostal and charismatic churches, which seek to encounter and affirm the divine as manifest in both physical and mental healing (Csordas, 1994; Harrell, 1975). People rising from wheelchairs or discarding crutches can be convincing signs of God's power (Dowling, 1984; Kelsey, 1973). Christian Science, whose origins may be closer to Mind Cure than to Christianity, also continues to be an important non-normative source of healing in the United States (Fox, 1984; Schoepflin, 1988). Some religious denominations are also known for nonadherence to normative procedures (for example, Jehovah's Witnesses, who routinely decline blood transfusions) (Mann et al, 1992; Singelenberg, 1990). For any of these religious approaches, genuine 'faith' is required in exchange for the promised effectiveness. Also, these approaches sharply distinguish themselves from participation in any professed coalition with the CAM movement (Hexham, 1992).

OVERVIEW

Unconventional healing is a far-flung landscape of diverse practices. A taxonomy balances distinction with commonality. Other perspectives that emphasize interconnection and common themes are possible. Healing behaviors can be grouped into those that focus on the primacy of substances to be taken orally (herbs, homeopathy, dietary supplements, or food), those that rely on the human hand (manipulation, needles, or anointing the sick), or those that emphasize words (ritual or psychotherapy) (Kemper, 1996; Kaptchuk and Crocher, 1986). One could also discuss CAM approaches on the basis of shared common themes (for example, belief in nature, vitalism, and spirituality), as has been done extensively elsewhere (Kaptchuk and Eisenberg, 1998). No matter how it is classified, however, this entire domain provides concrete practices and 'pathways of words, feelings, values, expectations [and] beliefs' that reorder and organize the illness experience (Kleinman, 1973). Because patients include unconventional healing as an important component of their response to illness, physicians must understand this complex spectrum of health care practices.

CONCLUSION

A single definition of alternative medicine that tries to state 'what it is' inevitably is not satisfying, since alternative healing includes a wide assortment of heterogeneous therapies and beliefs. A taxonomy of unconventional health care practices can help define alternative medicine and provide a conceptual framework for it. Such a model can help physicians understand and participate in the current discussion on unconventional healing practices as it rapidly unfolds.

REFERENCES

Albanese CL. *Nature Religion in America: From the Algonkian Indians to the New Age*. Chicago: Univ of Chicago Pr; 1990.

Albrecht GL, Levy JA. The professionalization of osteopathy: adaptation in the medical marketplace. In: Roth JA, ed. *Research in the Sociology of Health Care*. v 2. Greenwich. CT: JAI Pr; 1982.

Alternative Medicine Expanding Medical Horizons. A Report to the National Institutes of Health on Alternative Medical Systems and Practices in the United States. Washington. DC: U.S. Government Printing Office; 1994.

Amundsen DW. Medicine and faith in early Christianity. *Bull Hist Med*. 1982;56:326–50. [PMID: 0006753984]

Anderson J. Far side of faith: Tibetan medicine's miracle cures. *Newsday*, 5 Nov 1997:B10.

Baer HA. The potential rejuvenation of American naturopathy as a consequence of the holistic health movement. *Med Anthropol*. 1992;13:369–83. [PMID: 0001545694]

Barnes LL. The psychologizing of Chinese healing practices in the United States. *Cult Med Psychiatry*. 1998;22:413–43. [PMID: 0010063466]

Barrett S. Commercial hair analysis Science or scam? *JAMA*. 1985;254:1041–5. [PMID: 0004021042]

Braden CS. *Spirits in Rebellion: The Rise and Development of New Thought*. Dallas: Southern Methodist Univ Pr; 1963.

Brown KM. *Mama Lola: A Vodou Priestess in Brooklyn*. Berkeley, CA: Univ of California Pr; 1991.

Burroughs H, Kastner M. *Alternative Healing: The Complete A-Z Guide to over 160 Different Alternative Therapies*. La Mesa, CA: Halcyon; 1993.

Cassileth BR, Chapman CC. Alternative cancer medicine: a ten-year update. *Cancer Invest*. 1996;14:396–404. [PMID: 0008689436]

Cavender AP. Theoretic orientations and folk medicine research in the Appalachian South. *South Med J*. 1992;85:170–8. [PMID: 0001738884]

Chopra D. *Quantum Healing: Exploring the Frontiers of Mind/Body Medicine*. New York: Bantam; 1989.

Cohen C, Shevitz A, Mayer K. Expanding access to investigational new therapies. *Prim Care*. 1992;19:87–96. [PMID: 0001594704]

Complementary medicine time for critical engagement [Editorial]. *Lancet* 2000;356:2023. [PMID: 0011145481]

Cook C, Baisden D. Ancillary use of folk medicine by patients in primary care clinics in southwestern West Virginia. *South Med J.* 1986;79:1098–101. [PMID: 0003749993]

Cooter R. Bones of contention? Orthodox medicine and the mystery of the bone-setter's craft. In: Bynum WF, Porter R, eds. *Medical Fringe & Medical Orthodoxy*, 1750–1850. London: Croom Helm; 1987.

Coulehan JL. Chiropractic and the clinical art. *Soc Sci Med.* 1985;21:383–90. [PMID: 0002931804]

Csordas TJ. *The Sacred Self: A Cultural Phenomenology of Charismatic Healing.* Berkeley, CA: Univ of California Pr; 1994.

Curry P, ed. *Astrology, Science and Society: Historical Essays.* Woodbridge, Suffolk, England: Boydell Pr; 1987.

Defining and describing complementary and alternative medicine. Panel on Definition and Description, CAM Research Methodology Conference. April 1995. *Altern Ther Health Med.* 1997;3:49–57. [PMID: 0009061989]

Deutsch RM. *The New Nuts among the Berries.* Palo Alto. CA: Deutsch; 1977.

Dick HG. Students of physic and astrology: a survey of astrological medicine in the age of science. *Journal of the History of Medicine.* 1946;13:300–15.

Dossey L. *Meaning & Medicine.* New York: Bantam; 1991.

Dowling SJ. Lourdes cures and their medical assessment. *J R Soc Med.* 1984;77:634–8. [PMID: 0006384509]

Easthope G. *Healers and Alternative Medicine: A Sociological Examination.* Hants, England: Alderson; 1986.

Eisenberg DM. Advising patients who seek alternative medical therapies. *Ann Intern Med.* 1997;127:61–9. [PMID: 0009214254]

Eisenberg DM, Davis RB, Ettner SL, Appel S, Wilkey S, Van Rompay M, et al. Trends in alternative medicine use in the United States, 1990–1997: results of a follow-up national survey. *JAMA.* 1998;280:1569–75. [PMID: 0009820257]

Eisenberg DM, Delbanco TL, Berkey CS, Kaptchuk TJ, Kepelnick B, Kuhl J, et al. Cognitive behavioral techniques for hypertension: are they effective? *Ann Intern Med.* 1993;118:964–72. [PMID: 0008489111]

Eisenberg DM, Kaptchuk TJ. The herbal history of digitalis: lessons for alternative medicine [Letter]. *JAMA.* 2000;283:884–6. [PMID: 0010685707]

Ellwood RS. *Alternative Altars: Unconventional and Eastern Spirituality in America.* Chicago: Univ of Chicago Pr; 1979.

English-Lueck JA. *Health in the New Age: A Study in California Holistic Practices.* Albuquerque, NM: Univ of New Mexico Pr; 1990.

Ernst E. Chelation therapy for peripheral arterial occlusive disease a systematic review. *Circulation.* 1997;96:1031–3. [PMID: 0009264515]

Ernst E. Iridology: a systematic review. *Forsch Komplementärmed.* 1999;6:7–9. [PMID: 0010213874]

Ernst E, Kaptchuk TJ. Homeopathy revisited. *Arch Intern Med.* 1996;156: 2162–4. [PMID: 0008885813]

Fadiman A. *The Spirit Catches You and You Fall Down. A Hmong Child. Her American Doctors, and the Collision of Two Cultures.* New York: Farrar, Straus, and Giroux; 1997.

Feher S. Who holds the cards? Women and new age astrology. In: Lewis JR, Melton JG. eds. *Perspectives on the New Age*. Albany, NY: State Univ of New York Pr; 1992.

Ferngren GB. Early Christianity as a religion of healing. *Bull Hist Med*. 1992;66:1–15. [PMID: 0001559026]

Fisch S. Botanicas and spiritualism in a metropolis. *Milbank Mem Fund Q*. 1968;46:377–88. [PMID: 0005672031]

Fox M. Conflict to coexistence: Christian Science and medicine. *Med Anthropol*. 1984;8:292–301. [PMID: 0006399347]

Fuchs M, Bashshur R. Use of traditional Indian medicine among urban native *Americans. Med Care*. 1975;13:915–27. [PMID: 0001195900]

Fuller RC. *Mesmerism and the American Cure of Souls*. Philadelphia: Univ of Pennsylvania Pr; 1982.

Furnham A. How the public classify complementary medicine: a factor analytic study. *Complement Ther Med*. 2000;8:82–7. [PMID: 0010859600]

Fye WB. Nitroglycerin: a homeopathic remedy. *Circulation*. 1986:73:21–9. [PMID: 0002866851]

Gebhard B. The interrelationship of scientific and folk medicine in the United States of America since 1850. In Hand WD, ed. *American Folk Medicine*. Berkeley, CA: Univ of California Pr; 1976.

Gevitz N. *The D.O.'s: Osteopathic Medicine in America*. Baltimore: Johns Hopkins Univ Pr; 1982. [PMID: 0006362988]

Gevitz N. Three perspectives on unorthodox medicine. In: Gevitz N, ed. *Other Healers: Unorthodox Medicine in America*. Baltimore: Johns Hopkins Univ Pr; 1988.

Gevitz N. Alternative medicine and the orthodox canon. *Mt Sinai J Med*. 1995;62:127–31. [PMID: 0007753079]

Glik DC. Symbolic, ritual and social dynamics of spiritual healing. *Soc Sci Med*. 1988;27:1197–206. [PMID: 0002462751]

Goldman B. Ayurvedism: eastern medicine moves west. *CMAJ*. 1991;144:218–21. [PMID: 0001986838]

Goldstein MS, Jaffe DT, Sutherland C, Wilson J. Holistic physicians: implications for the study of the medical profession. *J Health Soc Behav*. 1987;28: 103–19. [PMID: 0005611700]

Good BJ, Good MJ. *Alternative Health Care in a California Community*. Report No. 8. A Study Conducted for the California Board of Medical Quality Assurance by the Public Affairs Research Group. Sacramento: Public Regulation of Health Care Occupations in California; 1981.

Gordon JS. *Manifesto for a New Medicine*. Reading MA: Addison-Wesley; 1996.

Gort EH, Coburn D. Naturopathy in Canada: changing relationships to medicine, chiropractic and the state. *Soc Sci Med*. 1988;26:1061–72. [PMID: 0003293229]

Hafner AW, Carson JG, Zwicky JF, eds. *Guide to the American Medical Association Historical Health Fraud and Alternative Medicine Collection*. Chicago: American Medical Assoc; 1992.

Hafner AW, Zwicky JF, Barret S, Jarvis WT. *Reader's Guide to Alternative Health Methods*. Chicago: American Medical Assoc; 1993.

Hand WD. The folk healer: calling and endowment. *J Hist Med Allied Sci*. 1971;26:263–75. [PMID: 0004938939]

Harrell DE. *All Things Are Possible. The Healing and Charismatic Revivals in Modern America*. Bloomington, IN: Indiana Univ Pr; 1975.

Harwood A. Puerto Rican spiritism. Part I–Description and analysis of an alternative psychotherapeutic approach. *Cult Med Psychiatry*. 1977;1:69–95 [PMID: 0000756355]

Harwood A, ed. *Ethnicity and Medical Care*. Cambridge, MA: Harvard Univ Pr; 1981.

Hexham I. The evangelical response to the New Age. In: Lewis JR, Melton JG, eds. *Perspectives on the New Age*. Albany, NY: State Univ of New York Pr; 1992.

Helman CG. "Feed a cold, starve a fever" – folk models of infection in an English suburban community, and their relation to medical treatment. *Cult Med Psychiatry*. 1978:2:107–37. [PMID: 0000081735]

Herink R, ed. *The Psychotherapy Handbook*. New York: New American Library; 1980.

Hufford DJ. Folk medicine and health culture in contemporary society. *Prim Care*. 1997;24:723–41. [PMID: 0009386255]

Jacobs CF. Healing and prophecy in the black Spiritual churches: a need for re-examination. *Med Anthropol*. 1990;12:349–70. [PMID: 0002287192]

Johnson DM. Religion, health and healing: findings from a southern city. *Sociological Analysis*. 1986;47:66–73.

Johnson KP. *Edgar Cayce in Context*. Albany. NY: State Univ of New York Pr; 1998.

Johnson SM, Kurtz ME, Kurtz JC. Variables influencing the use of osteopathic manipulative treatment in family practice. *J Am Osteopath Assoc*. 1997; 97:80–7. [PMID: 0009059002]

Jones RK. Sectarian characteristics of Alcoholics Anonymous. *Sociology*. 1970;4:181–95.

Judah JS. *The History and Philosophy of the Metaphysical Movements in America*. Philadelphia: Westminster Pr; 1967.

Kandel RF. Rice, ice cream, and the guru: decision-making and innovation in a macrobiotic community [Dissertation]. New York: State Univ of New York; 1976.

Kaptchuk TJ. *The Web That Has No Weaver: Understanding Chinese Medicine*. Chicago: Contemporary Books; 2000.

Kaptchuk TJ. History of vitalism. In: Micozri MS, ed. *Fundamentals of Complementary and Alternative Medicine*. New York: Churchill Livingstone; 2001.

Kaptchuk TJ, Crocher M. *The Healing Arts: A Journey through the Faces of Medicine*. London: British Broadcasting, 1986.

Kaptchuk TJ, Eisenberg DM. Chiropractic: origins, controversies, and contributions. *Arch Intern Med*. 1998;158:2215–24. [PMID: 0009818801]

Kaptchuk TJ, Eisenberg DM. The persuasive appeal of alternative medicine. *Ann Intern Med*. 1998;129:1061–5. [PMID: 0009867762]

Kaptchuk TJ, Eisenberg DM. The health food movement [Editorial]. *Nutrition*. 1998;14:471–3. [PMID: 0009614517]

Karasu TB. The specificity versus nonspecificity dilemma: toward identifying therapeutic change agents. *Am J Psychiatry*. 1986;143:687–95. [PMID: 0003717390]

Kaufman M. *Homeopathy in America: The Rise and Fall of a Medical Heresy*. Baltimore: Johns Hopkins Univ Pr; 1971.

Kelsey MT. *Healing and Christianity*. New York: Harper & Row; 1973.

Kemper KJ. Separation or synthesis: a holistic approach to therapeutics. *Pediatr Rev*. 1996;17:279–83. [PMID: 0008758669]

Kerr H. Crow CL, eds. *The Occult in America: New Historical Perspectives*. Urbana, IL.: Univ of Illinois Pr; 1983.

King DE, Sobal J, DeForge BR. Family practice patients' experiences and beliefs in faith healing. *J Fam Pract*. 1988;27:505–8. [PMID: 0003264015]

Kirmayer LJ. Mind and body as metaphors: hidden values in biomedicine. In: Lock M, Gordon D, eds. *Biomedicine Examined*. Boston: Kluwer Academic Publishers; 1988.

Kirschner HE. *Live Food Juices*. Monrovia, CA: Kirscher; 1991.

Kleinman AM. Medicine's symbolic reality. On a central problem in the philosophy of medicine. *Inquiry*. 1973;16:206–13.

Knapp JE, Antonucci EJ. *A National Study of the Profession of Massage Therapy/Bodywork*. Princeton, NJ: Knapp and Assoc; 1990.

Ko CY, Tong J, Lehman RE, Shelton AA, Schrock TR, Welton ML. Biofeedback is effective therapy for fecal incontinence and constipation. *Arch Surg*. 1997;132:829–34. [PMID: 0009267265]

Koenig HG, Moberg DO, Kvale JN. Religious activities and attitudes of older adults in a geriatric assessment clinic. *J Am Med Soc*. 1988;36:362–74. [PMID: 0003351176]

Krieger D, Peper E, Ancoli S. Therapeutic touch: searching for evidence of physiological change. *Am J Nurs*. 1979;79:660–2. [PMID: 0000373441]

Laetz T, Silberman G. Reimbursement policies constrain the practice of oncology. *JAMA*. 1991;266:2996–9. [PMID: 0001820471]

Leibowitz J, Connington B. *The Alexander Technique*. New York: Harper & Row; 1990.

Lerner M. *Choices in Healing: Integrating the Best of Conventional and Complementary Approaches to Cancer*. Cambridge, MA: MIT Pr; 1994.

Levin JS, Coreil J. 'New age' healing in the U.S. *Soc Sci Med*. 1986;23:889–97. [PMID: 0003798167]

Levine HD. Folk medicine in New Hampshire. *N Engl J Med*. 1941;224:487–92.

Linden W, Chambers L. Clinical effectiveness of non-drug treatment for hypertension: a meta-analysis. *Ann Behav Med*. 1994;16:35–45.

Mann MC, Votto J, Kambe J, McNamee MJ. Management of the severely anemic patient who refuses transfusion: lessons learned during the care of a Jehovah's Witness. *Ann Intern Med*. 1992;117:1042–8. [PMID: 0001307705]

Martinez C, Martin HW. Folk diseases among urban Mexican–Americans. Etiology, symptoms, and treatment. *JAMA*. 1966;196:161–4. [PMID: 0005952114]

Mathews HF. Rootwork: description of an ethnomedical system in the American South. *South Med J*. 1987;80:885–91. [PMID: 0003603109]

McGuire MB. Words of power: personal empowerment and healing. *Cult Med Psychiatry*. 1983;7:221–40. [PMID: 0006362988]

McGuire MB. *Ritual Healing in Suburban America*. New Brunswick, NJ: Rutgers Univ Pr; 1988.

Melton JG. *New Age Encyclopedia*. Detroit: Gale Research; 1990.

Mitchell BB. *Acupuncture and Oriental Medicine Laws.* Washington, DC: National Acupuncture Foundation; 1997.

Miura K. The revival of qi: qigong in contemporary China. In: Kohn L, ed. *Taoist Meditation and Longevity Techniques.* Ann Arbor, MI: Center for Chinese Studies, Univ of Michigan; 1989.

National Center for Health Statistics. Office Visits to Osteopathic Physicians. Jan.-Dec. 1974: Provisional Data from the National Ambulatory Medical Care Survey. Washington. DC: U.S. Government Printing Office; 1975.

Newman Turner R. A proposal for classifying complementary therapies. *Complement Ther Med.* 1998;6:141–3.

Numbers RI, Amundsen DW. *Caring and Curing: Health and Medicine in the Western Religious Traditions.* New York: Macmillan; 1986.

O'Connor BB. *Healing Traditions: Alternative Medicine and the Health Professions.* Philadelphia: Univ of Pennsylvania Pr; 1995.

Oppenheim J. *The Other World: Spiritualism and Psychical Research in England. 1850–1914.* Cambridge: Cambridge Univ Pr; 1988.

Osherson S, AmaraSingham L. The machine metaphor in medicine. In: Mishler EG, AmaraSingham L. Osherson SD, Hauser ST, Waxler NE, Liem R. *Social Contexts of Health, Illness and Patient Care.* New York: Cambridge Univ Pr; 1981.

Pachter LM. Culture and clinical care. Folk illness beliefs and behaviors and their implications for health care delivery. *JAMA.* 1994;271:690–4. [PMID: 0008309032]

Parker GT. *Mind Cure in New England from the Civil War to World War I.* Hanover, NH: Univ Pr of New England; 1973.

Pietroni PC. Beyond the boundaries: relationship between general practice and complementary medicine. *BMJ.* 1992;305:564–6. [PMID: 0001393039]

Report on alternative medicine. British Medical Association. In: Saks M, ed. *Alternative Medicine in Britain.* Oxford: Clarendon Pr; 1992.

Rinzler CA. *Feed a Cold, Starve a Fever: A Dictionary of Medical Folklore.* New York: Facts on File; 1991.

Rothstein WG. *American Physicians in the 19th Century: From Sects to Science.* Baltimore: Johns Hopkins Univ Pr; 1972.

Rywerant Y. *The Feldenkrais Method.* San Francisco: Harper & Row; 1983.

Saketkhoo K, Januszkiewicz A, Sackner MA. Effects of drinking hot water, cold water, and chicken soup on nasal mucus velocity and nasal airflow resistance. *Chest.* 1978;74:408–10. [PMID: 0000359266]

Schoepflin RB. Christian Science healing in America. In: Gevitz N, ed. *Other Healers: Unorthodox Medicine in America.* Baltimore: Johns Hopkins Univ Pr; 1988.

Scott CS. Health and healing practices among five ethnic groups in Miami, Florida. *Public Health Rep.* 1974;89:524–32. [PMID: 0004218901]

Segen JC. *Dictionary of Alternative Medicine.* Stamford, CT: Appleton & Lange; 1998.

Singelenberg R. The blood transfusion taboo of Jehovah's Witnesses: origin, development and function of a controversial doctrine. *Soc Sci Med.* 1990;31:515–23. [PMID: 0002218633]

Snow LF. Sorcerers, saints and charlatans: black folk healers in urban America. *Cult Med Psychiatry.* 1978:2:69–106. [PMID: 0000699623]

Tappen FM. *Healing Massage Techniques: Holistic, Classic and Emerging Methods.* Norwalk, CT: Appleton & Lange; 1988.

Trotter RT II, Chavira JA. *Curanderismo: Mexican American Folk Healing.* Athens, GA: Univ of Georgia Pr; 1981.

U.S. Congress Office of Technology Assessment. *Unconventional Cancer Treatments.* Washington, DC: U.S Government Printing Office; 1990.

Uva JL. Alcoholics anonymous: medical recovery through a higher power. *JAMA.* 1991;266:3065–7. [PMID: 0001820486]

Van Praag J. *Talking to Heaven: A Medium's Message of Life after Death.* New York: Dutton; 1997.

Wardwell WI. *Chiropractic: History and Evolution of a New Profession.* St. Louis: Mosby–Year Book; 1992.

Wardwell WI. Differential evolution of the osteopathic and chiropractic professions in the United States. *Perspect Biol Med.* 1994;37:595–608. [PMID: 0008084743]

Weil A. *Spontaneous Healing.* New York: Knopf; 1995.

Whorton JC. *Crusaders for Fitness: The History of American Health Reformers.* Princeton. NJ: Princeton Univ Pr; 1982.

Yahn G. The impact of holistic medicine, medical groups, and health concepts. *JAMA.* 1979;242:2202–5. [PMID: 0000490807]

Yasuo Y. *The Body. Self-Cultivation and Ki-Energy.* Albany, NY: State Univ of New York Pr; 1993.

Yates JW, Chalmer BJ, St. James P, Follansbee M, McKegney FP. Religion in patients with advanced cancer. *Med Pediatr Oncol.* 1981;9:121–8. [PMID: 0007231358]

Zefron LJ. The history of the laying-on of hands in nursing. *Nurs Forum.* 1975;14:350–63. [PMID: 0000772630]

CHAPTER 3

COMPLEMENTARY AND ALTERNATIVE MEDICINE: SOCIALLY CONSTRUCTED OR EVIDENCE-BASED?

Janet Richardson

The field of complementary medicine is moving and developing at a great pace. Many important milestones have been achieved. However, there is still work to be done to address evidence and policy issues. Medicine does not develop in isolation. Healthcare practices are often driven by cultural context, economics, politics and power. Recently a great emphasis has been placed on 'evidence-based practice' and discussion about the role of evidence-based practice is topical (Wilson et al, 2002a, 2002b). Kelner and Wellman's sociological perspective (2003) provides important insights into the evolution and acceptance by the 'establishment' of a range of therapies that currently, to varying degrees, fall outside the Western medical establishment. It is clear from the definition of complementary and alternative medicine (CAM) used in Kelner and Wellman's paper that a semi-permeable membrane exists between CAM and the 'dominant health system of a particular culture or society.' It is interesting to see from a sociological perspective what factors influence the movement across this membrane from the alternative to the dominant health system. Kelner and Wellman appear to suggest a number of factors that can broadly be defined as historical (political), evidential and integrative.

Edited from *Healthcare Papers* 2003;3(5):30–6.

THE SOCIAL CONSTRUCTION OF MEDICINE

In order to understand the current state and status of CAM, some historical context is required. Key moments in the development of complementary medicine in the West and an understanding of the social construction of medical knowledge provide insight into the present state of this fascinating area. Scheid (1993) speaks of different discourses in medicine and suggests that these discourses are interwoven into different institutional arrangements and their associated privileges. Alternative discourses threaten the hierarchical structures and the privileged within those structures. In order to assert their own discourse and way of life (or medical practices), people adopt different strategies: (1) they may annihilate the alternatives; (2) they may acknowledge alternatives but systematically exclude them; (3) they may assimilate them; or (4) a genuine new discourse may emerge from the meeting of two traditions (Scheid 1993). By examining the development of medicine it is possible to see how these different strategies manifest in the establishment's reaction to alternative systems of medicine.

Graham (1999) provides a clear account of ancient healing perspectives and the development of healing in the Western world. In ancient times mysticism was inextricably linked with medicine. A shaman, for example, would go on a journey for the purpose of diagnosing or treating illness. In 'The Yellow Emperor's Treatise on Internal Medicine,' man was thought to be inherently attuned to nature, not separate from it. In ancient Greece the concept of harmony was of central importance. Hippocrates, who established a medical school on the island of Kos in the fifth century BC, viewed health in terms of the equivalence of basic elements. Galen developed the theory of 'humours' and a system of medicine that dominated the Western world until the Middle Ages. During the Middle Ages, those who possessed the most superior of medical knowledge (mostly herb lore) were known as witches. Many of their practices were shamanic in origin. In the 15th century Paracelsus was one of the most enduring influences in the development of medicine, pioneering treatments to remedy particular diseases by using the distilled essence of herbs and chemical compounds. Much of this work was based on folk medicine and the knowledge of 'wise women' (witches). However, with the rise of Christianity as the established orthodoxy, many of these women were purged relentlessly by the church as heretics. The theory advanced by the Church was that disease was caused by Satan, and therefore pagan (folk) medicine could have no role: midwives were burned at the stake. This period exemplified the annihilation of the alternative as described by Scheid (1993) as a policy of genocide and ethnic cleansing. According to Graham (1999), the Church expunged the surgical and herbal skills of the Greeks and substituted instead brutal practices such as mortifying the flesh, bringing the practice of medicine to an all-time low.

THE AGE OF QUACKERY AND SYSTEMATIC EXCLUSION

This led to a period where the alternative was acknowledged but excluded, and might be described as the age of quackery, where a policy of apartheid existed. The development of science and the scientific method replaced the Church as the orthodoxy, and thus began the professionalization of medicine. In the 17th century astrology and herb lore were fundamental to the practice of medicine and were used by both licensed and unlicensed practitioners. Treatments were varied and had little to do with proof of effectiveness (Wright, 1992). It was possible to claim the title of 'doctor' and obtain an official licence to practise – often with no medical training. The licensed practitioners (physicians, surgeons and apothecaries whose practice was to some extent regulated and based on an apprenticeship) at first sight resembled modem 'professional' doctors. However, only a minority of the sick consulted the licensed practitioners. Others, in particular the poor, went to semi-professional healers such as midwives, wise women and bone setters. What differentiated the licensed practitioners from the rest was the fact that they were members of an organized professional group with a legal authority to exclude others (Wright, 1992). So, it was the social power, not the characteristics of these licensed practitioners and the therapies they practised, that separated them from the unlicensed. A major factor that determines which practices are orthodox and which are unorthodox is professional power – the power to determine the conceptual framework used to describe different forms of treatment, and the power to protect the interests of the professional group.

It was during this time that the 'quack' began to occupy some of the highest positions in the social hierarchy (Maple, 1992). One of the best known was William Read, an illiterate tailor, who, in the words of his critics: 'Having failed as a mender of garments became a mender of eyes' (Maple, 1992: 55). The reaction of the licensed practitioners was hostile. However, the quacks continued to find status in the social community because the 'orthodox' physicians had nothing better to offer (Maple, 1992).

By the mid-19th century homeopathy was winning converts from doctors and surgeons. By the end of 1866 the London Homeopathic Hospital had received over 59,000 patients (Nicholls, 1992). However, there was much opposition to homeopathy from orthodox physicians. The universities of Edinburgh and St. Andrews refused to grant diplomas to practitioners of homeopathy, and only very rarely were homeopaths allowed to defend themselves or their system in regular medical journals (Nicholls, 1992). The policy of apartheid therefore extended to publication. The rubbishing of homeopathic principles in the medical literature resulted in homeopathy going into decline (Nicholls, 1992).

More recently, interest in Chinese medicine was stimulated by President Richard Nixon's visit to China during the Cultural Revolution. British doctors, including Medical Research Council representatives, visited the People's Republic of China in the 1970s to examine the use of acupuncture in anaesthesia (Saks, 1992). However, the orthodox medical establishment resisted much of this, and Chinese medicine was mostly practised outside the orthodox system by non-medically qualified and unregulated practitioners (Saks, 1992).

THE QUESTION OF EVIDENCE: ASSIMILATION LEAVING THE ORTHODOXY INTACT

The establishment of the Cochrane Centre in the United Kingdom in 1992 and the new emphasis on evidence-based medicine threatened to continue the policy of apartheid and the entrenchment of orthodox medicine as the establishment. But this was not to be the case. Public interest continued to develop, and people consulted complementary practitioners in ever-increasing numbers in the West, as Kelner and Wellman (2003) have described. A number of key events moved the discourse from exclusion to that of assimilation, leading to minor changes but leaving the orthodoxy intact. For example, in the United Kingdom bodies such as the British Holistic Medicine Association and the Research Council for Complementary Medicine continued to work toward shared dialogue between orthodox and alternative medicine. The language began to change, and 'complementary medicine' (rather than alternative) became the preferred term. The second British Medical Association report on complementary medicine published in 1993 was more supportive. Rather than suggesting exclusion in support of science, it recommended establishing good practice through training and research.

In 1994 the first complementary therapy outpatient department to be established within a general NHS hospital was opened. An important aspect of this development was a detailed evaluation that examined the effect of the treatment on the health of patients visiting the department (Richardson, 2001a, 2001b). The House of Lords Select Committee on complementary and alternative medicine reported in November 2000. The report made clear recommendations, and the government response was prompt, with three main areas of focus: regulation, training and research. It was clear from this report that, in an evidence-based culture, it would be the publication of evidence for the effectiveness of complementary medicine that would determine its future acceptance as a form of treatment within a publicly funded healthcare system.

Kelner and Wellman (2003) discuss at length the question of what constitutes evidence in CAM, and in particular the thorny issue of the 'levels' of evidence. The applicability of the randomized control trial (RCT) to evaluating CAM is a debate that has been well rehearsed, and many CAM treatments have been evaluated using an RCT approach (Richardson, 2000a). Kelner and Wellman suggest that the individualized nature of CAM treatments mitigate against the use of RCTs. However, pragmatic approaches that capitalize on individualized approaches and the subtle (placebo) effects of treatments have been suggested (Richardson, 2000a, 2001b). Yet, even very sophisticated RCTs may fail to detect the complexity of factors that lurk in the swampy lowlands of the consultation and contribute to the therapeutic outcome (Richardson, 2000b, 2002; Verhoef et al, 2002).

The challenge of research methodology on CAM is real, but it is also exciting and provides an opportunity for diverse research disciplines to engage. The research questions in CAM are not simply about 'evidence' in a narrowly defined biosciences definition. When development of CAM is considered in a cultural context it is obvious that it is not only professionals who socially construct medicine and define the orthodoxy. Kelner and Wellman highlight the role of the 'consumer' in the development of CAM. This points to a different level of evidence from that proposed by our evidence-based professional colleagues. This is 'first-person evidence' constructed by the consumer and based on personal experience. It is only by examining the first-person experience as well as using complex RCTs to assess evidence for effectiveness that we will reach a fuller understanding of the effects of CAM. Inevitably this requires a multidisciplinary approach and a combination of quantitative and qualitative methods. Further, if reality is socially constructed (as Kelner and Wellman suggest), then the 'reality' of what is orthodox and what is not orthodox is also socially constructed. Sociological and anthropological research in CAM is essential as it provides a living history of professionalization and struggles between those who are part of the establishment and those who are not. This will be of particular importance as CAM professions move toward regulation and the question of 'integration' takes greater prominence.

INTEGRATION: ASSIMILATION LEAVING THE ORTHODOXY INTACT OR A NEW DISCOURSE?

The development of medicine is embedded in culture, context and economics. The power, influences and importance of profit in the pharmaceutical industry cannot be ignored. There is increasing pressure to control herbal medicine in the same way that the drug industry is controlled. Safety, of course, is important, but this raises important issues. The first is the cost of licensing: the wealthy pharmaceutical companies are in a position to fund the development, testing and licensing costs, but other small-scale producers of herbal products are not. This means that any attempt to license herbal medicines will produce products that are selected and controlled by the pharmaceutical industry. This could be disastrous, as their approach is often one of reducing the plant to a very specific component. However, plant-based medicine often works on very different principles, using the whole of the plant in the treatment process. If the pharmaceutical companies control the licensing, they will control what is licensed and the nature of the products that are available. This also has implications for the practice of herbal medicine. Herbal products that are licensed may only be available on prescription, thereby taking herbal medicine away from herbal medicine practitioners and putting it in the hands of orthodox doctors.

'Integrated (integrative) medicine' is a term fast replacing that of 'complementary medicine.' For some, 'integration' means taking components of complementary medicine and delivering them within the orthodox system, keeping orthodox practitioners in control. This fits neatly into Scheid's concept of assimilation, where the orthodoxy remains intact and continues to hold the power. When this happens, the dialogue of the 'alternative' is replaced by the discourse of the establishment. This can also affect the way the medicine is practised. For example, conventional RCTs may show specific acupuncture points to be effective for specific conditions. This might lead to the 'integration' of the technique into orthodox-practice 'cherry-picking,' replacing the concepts and theoretical underpinnings of the therapy with Western explanations and reductionist practices. Does this matter? Unless social and anthropological research investigates such questions we will not know the answer. The different concepts of health and illness provided by CAM approaches have the potential to expand our knowledge and approach to helping patients toward wellness and well-being.

This is an interesting time in the development of complementary medicine in the West. Investment in CAM research development is varied, but the concept of evidence needs to be broadened, as Kelner and Wellman suggest. Safety and competence are important, as is the regulation of different therapies. However, product licensing and regulation could equate to control and exclusion. Integrative medicine seems to be the utopia – the system of medicine most desired. But who seeks this utopia? Is it the establishment or the alternative? Is integration about the selective assimilation of aspects of the alternative, or is it about the creation of something new out of the meeting of different discourses? Perhaps the latter is too difficult as there are many different discourses within complementary medicine and, to some extent, within orthodox medicine. Genuine understanding may be more difficult than we may wish to imagine (Scheid, 1993).

Complementary medicine is a popular form of healthcare used by increasing numbers of the population. Access through government-funded healthcare will require evidence for effectiveness, assurances of safety and regulation of the professions. Kelner and Wellman make a number of policy recommendations that would support a balanced strategy for regulation, research and funding. The culture is indeed changing – in support of more access to complementary therapies. However, there will inevitably be some resistance from those who see a threat to their own construction of medical knowledge and the power that it holds.

REFERENCES

Graham H. *Complementary Therapies in Context: The Psychology of Healing*. London: Jessica Kingsley Publishers, 1999.

Kelner M, Wellman B. 'Complementary and Alternative Medicine: How do we know if it works?' *Healthcare Papers*, 2003;3(5):10–29.

Maple E. 'The Great Age of Quakery.' In M Saks, ed, *Alternative Medicine in Britain*. New York: Oxford University Press, 1992.

Nicholls P. 'Homeopathy in Britain after the Mid-Nineteenth Century.' In M Saks, ed, *Alternative Medicine in Britain*. New York: Oxford University Press, 1992.

Richardson J. 'The Use of Randomized Control Trials in Complementary Therapy: Exploring the Methodological Issues.' *Journal of Advanced Nursing* 2000a;32(2):398–406.

Richardson J. 'Clinical Implications of an Intersubjective Science.' In M Velmans, ed, *Investigating Phenomenal Consciousness: New Methodologies and Maps*. Amsterdam: John Benjamins, 2000b.

Richardson J. 'Developing and Evaluating Complementary Therapy Services. Part 1. Establishing Service Provision through the use of Evidence and Consensus Development.' *Journal of Alternative and Complementary Medicine: Research on Paradigm, Practice, and Policy* 2001a;7(3):253–60.

Richardson J. 'Developing and Evaluating Complementary Therapy Services. Part 2. Examining the Effect of Treatment on Health Status.' *Journal of Alternative and Complementary Medicine: Research on Paradigm, Practice, and Policy* 2001b;8(3):221–23.

Saks M. 'The Paradox of Incorporation: Acupuncture and the Medical Professional in Modern Britain.' In M Saks, ed, *Alternative Medicine in Britain*. New York: Oxford University Press, 1992.

Verhoef MJ, Casebeer AL, Hilsden RJ. 'Assessing Efficacy of Complementary Medicine: Adding Qualitative Research Methods to the 'Gold Standard'.' *Journal of Alternative and Complementary Medicine: Research on Paradigm, Practice, and Policy* 2002;8(3):275–81.

Wilson K, Mills EJ, Hollyer T et al. 'Teaching Evidence-Based Complementary and Alternative Medicine: A Conceptual Approach to Causation – Part I.' *Journal of Alternative and Complementary Medicine: Research on Paradigm, Practice, and Policy* 2002a;8(3):379–83.

Wilson K, Mills EJ, Hollyer T et al. 'Teaching Evidence-Based Complementary and Alternative Medicine: A Conceptual Approach to Causation – Part 2. *Journal of Alternative and Complementary Medicine: Research on Paradigm, Practice, and Policy* 2002b;8(3):385–9.

Wright P. 'Astrology in Seventeenth-Century England.' In M Saks, ed, *Alternative Medicine in Britain*. New York: Oxford University Press, 1992.

CHAPTER 4

TOO MUCH MEDICINE? ALMOST CERTAINLY

Ray Moynihan and Richard Smith

Most doctors believe medicine to be a force for good. Why else would they have become doctors? Yet while all know medicine's power to harm individual patients and whole populations, presumably few would agree with Ivan Illich that 'The medical establishment has become a major threat to health' (Illich, 1976). Many might, however, accept the concept of the health economist Alain Enthoven that increasing medical inputs will at some point become counterproductive and produce more harm than good. So where is that point, and might we have reached it already?

Readers of the *BMJ* voted in a poll to explore these questions in a theme issue of the *BMJ*. Unsurprisingly, we reach no clear answers, but the questions deserve far more intense debate in a world where many countries are steadily increasing their investment in health care. Presumably no one wants to keep cutting back on education, the arts, scientific research, good food, travel, and much else as we spend more and more of our resources on an unwinnable battle against death, pain, and sickness – particularly if Illich is right that in doing so we destroy our humanity. And do we in the rich world want to keep developing increasingly expensive treatments that achieve marginal benefits when most in the developing world do not have the undoubted benefits that come with simple measures like sanitation, clean water, and immunisation?

Any consideration of the limits of medicine has to begin a quarter of a century ago with Illich, who has so far produced the most radical critique of modern – or industrialised – medicine (Illich, 1976). His argument is in some ways simple. Death, pain, and sickness are part of being human.

Edited from *British Medical Journal* 2002;324:859–60.

All cultures have developed means to help people cope with all three. Indeed, health can even be defined as being successful in coping with these realities. Modern medicine has unfortunately destroyed these cultural and individual capacities, launching instead an inhuman attempt to defeat death, pain, and sickness. It has sapped the will of the people to suffer reality. 'People are conditioned to *get* things rather than to *do* them ... They want to be taught, moved, treated, or guided rather than to learn, to heal, and to find their own way.' The analysis is supported by Amartya Sen's data showing that the more a society spends on health care the more likely are its inhabitants to regard themselves as sick (Sen, 2002).

Illich's critique may seem laughable, even offensive, to the doctor standing at the end of the bed of a seriously ill person. Should the patient be thrown out and told to cope? It is of course much easier to offer a critique of cultures than to create new ones – and Illich (like doctors, ironically) is much stronger on diagnosis than cure. But he does write about recovering the ability for mutual self care and then learning to combine this with the use of modem technology. Though his polemic was published long before the internet, this most contemporary of technologies – combined with the move to patient partnership – is shifting power from doctors back to people. People may increasingly take charge, more consciously weighing the costs and benefits of the 'medicalisation' of their lives. Armed with better information about the natural course of common conditions, they may more judiciously assess the real value of medicine's never ending regimen of tests and treatments.

Although some forces – the internet and patients' empowerment – might offer opportunities for 'demedicalisation,' many others encourage greater medicalisation. Patients and their professional advocacy groups can gain moral and financial benefit from having their condition defined as a disease (Leibovici and Lièvre, 2002). Doctors, particularly some specialists, may welcome the boost to status, influence, and income that comes when new territory is defined as medical Advances in genetics open up the possibility of defining almost all of us as sick, by diagnosing the 'deficient' genes that predispose us to disease (Melzer and Zimmern, 2002). Global pharmaceutical companies have a clear interest in medicalising life's problems (Freemantle, 2002; Moynihan et al, 2002), and there is now an ill for every pill (Mintzes, 2002). Likewise companies manufacturing mammography equipment or tests for prostate specific antigen can grow rich on the medicalisation of risk (Gotzsche, 2002). Many journalists and editors still delight in mindless medical formulas, where fear mongering about the latest killer disease is accompanied by news of the latest wonder drug (Sweet, 2002). Governments may even welcome some of society's problems – within, for example, criminal justice – being redefined as medical, with the possibility of new solutions.

As the *BMJ*'s debate over 'non-diseases' has shown, the concept of what is and what is not a disease is extremely slippery (Smith, 2002; BMJ,

2002). It is easy to create new diseases and new treatments, and many of life's normal processes – birth (Johanson, Newburn and Macfarlane, 2002), ageing (Ebrahim, 2002), sexuality (Hart and Wellings, 2002), unhappiness (Double, 2002), and death (Clark, 2002) – can be medicalised. However, there is also much undertreatment, suggesting a need for more medicalisation (Ebrahim, 2002; Bonaccorso and Sturchio, 2002). The challenge is to get the balance right.

It is those who pay for health care who might be expected to resist medicalisation, and governments, insurers, and employers have tried to restrain the rapid and unceasing growth in healthcare budgets. They have had little or no success, and Britain's government now plans to raise taxes to pay for more health care. Labour, the party in power, will have calculated that the risk of trying to bottle up demand is greater than the – substantial – risk of raising taxes. But while increased resources will be widely welcomed, the cost of trying to defeat death, pain, and sickness is unlimited, and beyond a certain point every penny spent may make the problem worse, eroding still further the human capacity to cope with reality.

Ivan Illich did not want the wholesale dismantling of medicine. He favoured 'sanitation, inoculation, and vector control, well-distributed health education, healthy architecture, and safe machinery, general competence in first aid, equally distributed access to dental and primary medical care, as well as judiciously selected complex services' (Illich, 1976). These should be embedded within 'a truly modern culture that fostered self-care and autonomy.' This is a package that many doctors would find acceptable, particularly if available to everybody everywhere.

Doctors and their organisations understandably argue for increased spending – because they are otherwise left paying a personal price, trying to cope with increasing demand with inadequate resources. Indeed this is one of the sources of worldwide unhappiness among doctors (Smith, 2001; Edwards, Kornacki and Silversin, 2002; Ham and Alberti, 2002). Although seen by many as the perpetrators of medicalisation, doctors may actually be some of its most prominent victims (Leibovici and Lièvre, 2002).

Perhaps some doctors will now become the pioneers of de-medicalisation. They can hand back power to patients, encourage self care and autonomy, call for better worldwide distribution of simple effective health care, resist the categorisation of life's problem as medical, promote the de-professionalisation of primary care, and help decide which complex services should be available. This is no longer a radical agenda.

REFERENCES

Bonaccorso SN, Sturchio JL. Direct to consumer advertising is medicalising normal human experience [against]. *BMJ* 2002;324:910–11.

Clark D. Between hope and acceptance: the medicalisation of dying. *BMJ* 2002;324:905–7.

Correspondence. What do you think is a non-disease? *BMJ* 2002;324:912–4.

Double D. The limits of psychiatry. *BMJ* 2002;324:900–4.

Ebrahim S. The medicalisation of old age. *BMJ* 2002;324:861–3.

Edwards N, Kornacki MJ, Silversin J. Unhappy doctors: what are the causes and what can be done? *BMJ* 2002;324:835–8.

Freemantle N. Medicalisation; limits to medicine, or never enough money to go around? *BMJ* 2002;324:864–5.

Gotzsche PC. The medicalisation of risk factors [commentary]. *BMJ* 2002;324:890–1.

Ham C, Alberti KGMM. The medical profession, the public, and the government. *BMJ* 2002;324:838–42.

Hart G, Wellings K. Sexual behaviour and its medicalisation: in sickness and in health. *BMJ* 2002;324:896–900.

Illich I. *Limits to Medicine*. London: Marion Boyars, 1976.

Johanson R, Newburn M, Macfarlane A. Has the medicalisation of childbirth gone too far? *BMJ* 2002;324:892–5.

Leibovici I, Lièvre M. Medicalisation: peering from inside a department of medicine. *BMJ* 2002;324:866.

Melzer D, Zimmern R. Genetics and medicalisation. *BMJ* 2002;324:863–4.

Mintzes B. Direct to consumer advertising is medicalising normal human experience. *BMJ* 2002;324:908–9.

Moynihan R, Heath I, Henry D. Selling sickness: the pharmaceutical industry and disease mongering. *BMJ* 2002;324:886–90.

Smith R. Why are doctors so unhappy? *BMJ* 2001; 23:1073–4.

Smith R. In search of 'non-disease'. *BMJ* 2002;324:883–5.

Sweet M. How medicine sells the media. *BMJ* 2002;324:924.

Sen A. Health: perception versus observation. *BMJ* 2002;324:859–60.

CHAPTER 5

ALTERNATIVE MEDICINE AND COMMON ERRORS OF REASONING

Barry L Beyerstein

If only the ignorant and gullible were swayed by far-fetched claims, little else would be needed to explain the abundance of folly in modern society. But oddly enough, many people who are neither foolish nor ill-educated cling to beliefs repudiated by science. For example, college graduates, and even some physicians, accept certain aspects of complementary and alternative medicine (CAM), including therapeutic touch, iridology, ear candling, and homeopathy. Even highly trained experts can be misled when they rely on personal experience and informal reasoning to infer the causes of complex events (Gilovich, 1991; Levy, 1997; Nisbett and Ross, 1980; Schick and Vaughn, 1995). This is especially true if they are evaluating situations to which they have an emotional, doctrinal, or monetary attachment. Indeed, it was the realization that shortcomings of perception, reasoning, and memory incline us toward comforting, rather than true, conclusions that led the pioneers of modern science to substitute controlled observations and formal logic for the anecdotes and surmises that can so easily lead us astray. This lesson seems to have been largely lost on proponents of CAM. Some, such as Andrew Weil, reject it explicitly, advocating instead what Weil calls 'stoned thinking,' a melange of mystical intuition and emotional satisfaction, for determining the validity of a therapy (Relman, 1998).

Those who advocate therapies of any kind have an obligation to prove that their products are both safe and effective. The latter is the more difficult task because there are many subtle ways that honest, intelligent

Edited from *Academic Medicine* 2001:76(3).

patients and therapists can be led into thinking that a useless treatment has produced a cure. CAM remains 'alternative' because its practitioners depend on subjective testimonials rather than randomized clinical trials (RCTs) for support, and because most of their hypothesized mechanisms are at variance with those accepted by basic science. It is my intent here to draw attention to several social, psychologic, and cognitive factors that have helped convince many well-educated people that scientifically discredited or unproven treatments have merit.

In the last century, objective procedures have been developed that test the effectiveness of putative remedies and help distinguish therapeutically induced changes in an underlying pathologic condition from the subjective relief that might follow any intervention. These procedures form the basis of so-called 'evidence-based medicine,' and without such a demonstration that a treatment is safe and effective, it is ethically questionable to offer that treatment to the public. Since most 'alternative,' 'complementary,' or 'integrative' therapies lack this kind of support, one must ask why so many otherwise savvy consumers trustingly pay out considerable sums for unproven, and possibly dangerous, health products. We must also wonder why claims of alternative practitioners remain so refractory to contrary data.

If an unorthodox therapy: (1) is implausible on a priori grounds (because its implied mechanisms or putative effects run afoul of well-established laws or empirical findings in physics, chemistry, or biology); (2) lacks a scientifically acceptable rationale of its own; (3) has insufficient supporting evidence derived from controlled clinical trials; (4) has failed in well-controlled clinical studies conducted by impartial evaluators and has been unable to rule out competing explanations for why it might *seem* to work in everyday settings; and (5) should seem improbable, even to the layperson, on 'common sense' grounds, then why would so many well-educated people continue to purchase such a treatment?

Consumers of unscientific treatments can be classified broadly into two groups. Once a buyer from either group tries an unconventional treatment, the judgmental biases discussed below have a tendency to make even the most worthless interventions seem valid. Patrons of one type often gravitate to CAM because they suffer from chronic conditions that orthodox medicine does not handle to their satisfaction or because they live in morbid fear that they will lose their 'wellness.' They assume, erroneously, that competent authorities have validated CAM's wares. The other type of user chooses alternative treatments out of a philosophical commitment to the animistic, vitalistic cosmology of CAM, which rejects the mechanistic–empiricist underpinnings of scientific biomedicine (Beyerstein and Downie, 1998). CAM embraces subjective, emotive truth criteria, whereas its detractors demand objective evidence. Because one's concept of health is entwined with one's fundamental assumptions about reality, an attack on someone's belief in unorthodox healing becomes a threat to his or her entire metaphysical outlook. Understandably, this will be resisted fervently.

The ability to defend one's basic world-view is abetted by a number of cognitive biases that filter and distort contrary information. I shall return to these processes that incline supporters to misconstrue their experiences to bolster their belief in CAM. But first let us examine the cultural milieu that has fostered a widespread desire to espouse such practices.

SOCIAL AND CULTURAL REASONS FOR THE POPULARITY OF UNPROVEN THERAPIES

Several trends have contributed to today's popularity of CAM, in spite of (and to some degree, because of) its rejection by mainstream science. The resurgence of folk medicine can be traced, in large part, to nostalgic holdovers from the neo-romantic search for simplicity and spirituality that permeated the 'counterculture' of the 1960s and 1970s (Frankel, 1973). The flower children of that generation now form the backbone of the 'New Age' movement, which enthusiastically promotes unorthodox healing (Basil, 1988). CAM suits the iconoclasm, mystical longings, desire for simpler times, and naive trust in the beneficence of 'Nature' absorbed during those tumultuous earlier times. How, then, has this history benefited non-scientific medicine?

Poor scientific literacy. Surveys consistently find that, despite our overwhelming dependence on technology, the average citizen of the industrialized world is shockingly ignorant of even the rudiments of science (Kiernan, 1995). Consequently, most people lack the knowledge to make an informed choice when they must decide whether a highly-touted health care product is sensible or not.

Anti-intellectualism and anti-scientific attitudes piggybacking on New Age mysticism. As a major New Age industry, CAM shares the movement's magical world-view (Beyerstein and Downie, 1998). In advocating emotional criteria for truth over criteria based on empirical data and logic, New Age medical gurus such as Andrew Weil and Deepak Chopra have convinced many that 'anything goes' (Relman, 1998). Even in elite academic institutions today, there are strong proponents (mostly in humanities departments) of the notion that objectivity is an illusion and one's feeling about something determines its truth value (Gross and Levitt, 1994; Sokal and Bricmont, 1998). By denigrating science, these detractors have enlarged the potential following for magical and pseudoscientific health products (Barrett and Jarvis, 1993; Stalker and Glymour, 1985).

Mind–body dualism permeates New Age thought, including CAM, though ironically, it is CAM's disciples who accuse their scientific critics of being dualists (Beyerstein, 1987, 1999). That CAM devotees are the real mystics and dualists can be seen by their constant appeal to undetectable spiritual interveners to confer 'wellness' on those who deserve it. This obfuscation is needed to sell the oft-heard canard that scientific medicine undervalues the effects of mental processes on health (Beyerstein and Downie, 1998). Admittedly, there are psychologic effects on disease, but their importance has been grossly exaggerated by CAM promoters such as Herbert Benson (Benson, 1996). Overstatements of this kind have prompted a resurgence of ancient 'mind cures' that assert that the real causes and cures for disease lie in the mind, conceived by New Agers to be equivalent to the soul (Meyer, 1965). Several good critiques have appeared recently, which expose the confusion and artifacts that dog the literature on spirituality and health (Sloan, Bagiella and Powell, 1999; Tessman and Tessman, 1997a, b)

Another troubling supposition in New Age health propaganda is that one's moral standing alters the impact of natural forces on one's body. In accepting this anthropocentric, vitalistic worldview, alternative healers are reverting to the pre-scientific view of disease as supernatural retribution. Sad to say, it also amounts to blaming the victim, for implicitly, patients must have done something bad to 'deserve' their afflictions.

Vigorous marketing and extravagant claims. According to a recent survey (Eisenberg, 1998), in the United States alone, 'total 1997 out-of-pocket expenditures relating to alternative therapies were conservatively estimated at $27.0 billion, which is comparable to the projected 1997 out-of-pocket expenditures for all U.S. physician services.' The annual number of visits to alternative healers now exceeds the total number of visits to all U.S. primary care physicians combined. With riches of this magnitude for the taking, it is not surprising that alternative healers have promoted themselves through aggressive marketing and intense legislative lobbying (Beyerstein and Sampson, 1996). Routinely, promises are made that no ethical, scientifically trained practitioner could or would make. Unfortunately, the citizenry facing this slick promotional barrage is poorly equipped with the skills or information for evaluating such hyperbole (Kiernan, 1995).

Inadequate media scrutiny and attacks on critics. With some notable exceptions, the mass media have tended to give CAM a free ride. Its enthusiastic claims make enchanting stories that are rarely disputed by the media, whose leaders know that challenging their audience's fond hopes hurts ratings. Another disturbing factor that deters some would-be critics of unscientific treatments is the realization that many of CAM's practices have been imported from non-European cultures and are championed by women. Thus self-promoters often sidestep valid criticisms by accusing detractors of racism and sexism. For example, scientifically rejected practices such as 'therapeutic touch' are being embraced by many nursing schools. Because these are still institutions largely attended by women, doubters are often tarred with accusations of sexism. Likewise, when a collegue and I criticized aspects of traditional Chinese medicine (TCM) (Beyerstein and Sampson, 1996), we were accused of cultural insensitivity and racism (Hui, 1997). We were chided for presuming to criticize TCM when we were not steeped in the philosophy that spawned it. To accept this absurd rebuke would be to concede that no one but gourmet cooks can tell when they've been served a bad meal. The truly racist and sexist attitude would be to hold empirically testable claims from other cultures or female proponents to a lower standard of proof. This *would* be an assertion of intellectual inferiority. Fortunately, there are many scientific critics from within these communities who find archaic, unproven practices just as dubious as do their white male colleagues (Knauer, 1997; Thadani, 1999).

Social malaise and mistrust of traditional authority figures – the anti-doctor backlash. Growing cultural disillusionment has nurtured the belief that society's shortcomings must be due to active connivance by powerful, secret cabals, rather than merely the cumulative mistakes of well-intentioned planners. As these grand conspiracy theories flourish, so does sniping at those suspected of plotting against the common good (Robins and Post, 1997). Many have come to view government and the scientific and medical professions as parties to the plot. These conspiratorial musings have been reinforced by two other, not entirely unjustified, undercurrents to promote an anti-doctor backlash that CAM has exploited. One is disappointment arising from the failure of certain overly optimistic predictions of medical breakthroughs to materialize. The other is the realization that medicine, as a self-regulating profession, has not always held the public good at the top of its political agenda (Starr, 1982). This has enhanced the social envy of many regarding the status, political clout, and wealth of the medical profession. The inability of many detractors to separate self-serving political actions by certain medical associations from the debate over whether scientific medicine's treatments are genuinely better than those of CAM has enriched the 'alternatives.' CAM also benefited by painting itself as the defender of the democratic ideal of 'choice.' This would be commendable if consumers had the wherewithal to make an *informed* choice.

Dislike of the delivery of scientific biomedicine. CAM has played on a widespread but exaggerated fear that modern medicine has become excessively technocratic, bureaucratic, and impersonal. The narrowing of medical specialties, the need to maximize the cost-efficient utilization of expensive facilities, the advent of third-party payment and managed care, and the staggering workloads of physicians have led some patients to long nostalgically for the simpler days of the kindly country doctor with ample time and a soothing bedside manner. They tend to forget, however, that this was often all a doctor of that era could offer.

Safety and side effects. A quaint bit of romanticism that promotes 'holistic' health care is the belief that 'natural' remedies are necessarily safer, gentler, and more efficacious than scientific ones (Beyerstein and Downie, 1998). Web sites such as (www.quackwatch.com) readily dispel such myths, however. For example, it is often claimed that herbal concoctions have no side effects, whereas, in fact, some popular herbal products can be far from benign – reports of allergic, toxic, and even lethal reactions are accumulating (Betz, n.d.; Ernst, 1998; Sutter, 1995; Winslow and Kroll, 1998). Mislabeling and serious contaminations have been discovered (Ko, 1998), while the potential for adverse interactions with prescribed pharmaceuticals is also becoming more widely recognized.

Public awareness of these perils remains spotty, however, because centralized reporting of ill effects of alternative treatments is not required. Unfortunately, under current U.S. law, the government must show that herb or supplement is unsafe before vendors can be forced to desist (Winslow and Kroll, 1998). And when harmful effects do occur, users are likely to attribute them to other causes because of their touching belief that benevolent 'Nature' would never pull such dirty tricks. Boosters of 'natural' products should be reminded that tobacco is also quite natural and that plants produce some of the most deadly poisons known. On the other hand, they should know that several common drugs in scientific biomedicine were originally derived from plants (Thadani, 1999; Winslow and Kroll, 1998). The difference, of course, is that the active ingredients in plants that led to drugs approved by the Food and Drug Administration were identified, synthesized, and rigorously tested for efficacy and safety. Thus, unlike herbal concoctions, their purity and dosages can be closely regulated.

PSYCHOLOGICAL REASONS FOR THE POPULARITY OF CAM

Psychologists have long been aware that people generally strive to make their attitudes, beliefs, and behaviors conform to a harmonious whole. When disquieting information cannot easily be ignored, individuals have a great ability to distort or sequester it to reduce the inevitable friction. It is to these mental gyrations that we now turn.

The will to believe. We all exhibit a willingness to endorse comforting beliefs and to accept, uncritically, information that reinforces our core attitudes and self-esteem (Alcock, 1995). Because it would be nice if the hopeful shibboleths of CAM were true, it is not surprising that they are often seized upon with little demand for evidence. Once adopted, such beliefs will be defended strongly, by misconstruing contrary input if need be (Beyerstein and Hadaway, 1991; Zusne and Jones, 1989).

Logical errors, shortcomings of judgment, and missing control groups. One of the most prevalent pitfalls in everyday decision making is the mistaking of correlation for causation. We are all prone to assume that if two things occur together one must cause the other, although, obviously, this need not be the case. This logical error underlies most superstitions. Testimonials for the ministrations of alternative healers commit the same blunder in assuming that when improvement follows a treatment, the treatment must have been responsible. The value of CAM's personal endorsements is limited by what Gilovich (Gilovich, 1997) has called the 'compared to what?' problem. It cannot be known that any vaunted treatment is effective without blinded comparisons with placebo-treated controls. Although this makes user testimonials all but worthless, promoters of CAM such as Andrew Weil offer little else (Relman, 1998).

Those who impugn fringe treatments are frequently dismissed by practitioners with the rejoinder, 'I don't care what your research says. I have seen my treatments work hundreds of times.' Unfortunately, this kind of intuitive judgment is also conducive to false conclusions (Gilovich, 1991; Gilovich, 1997; Levy, 1997; Nisbett and Ross, 1980; Schick and Vaughn, 1995). These therapists ignore much research in the area of 'cognitive heuristics' (Gilovich, 1997; Tversky and Kahneman, 1974) that shows how mistaken causal attributions can arise when we rely on informal observations to determine what causes or alleviates symptoms. It is especially difficult to determine cause and effect when evaluating therapies because many relevant variables are interacting simultaneously – determinations that casual observation cannot reliably tease apart.

For example, Redelmeier and Tversky (Redelmeier and Tversky, 1996) showed how people are likely to perceive illusory correlations in random events. They then demonstrated how these 'hunches' lead to false but widespread beliefs, including the concept that arthritis pain is influenced by the weather. Because CAM derives its diagnoses and treatments from just this kind of unreliable folklore, potential patrons should demand that all alternative treatments be held to the same standards of proof as those in scientific biomedicine. By introducing controlled clinical trials and epidemiologic methods, the pioneers of scientific medicine hoped to reduce the kind of false ascriptions of cause that these frailties of human reasoning can produce. A recent critique of studies purporting to show that various religious practices enhance health (Sloan, Bagiella and Powell, 1999) offers good examples of how dubious causal attributions arise when the need for the simple control group is ignored.

Wishful thinking and 'demand characteristics.' Warping perceived reality in the service of dogma is commonplace (Alcock, 1995; Zusne and Jones, 1989). According to cognitive dissonance theory (Festinger, 1957), mental distress is produced when new information contradicts existing attitudes, feelings, or beliefs. To alleviate the unease, we tend to distort the offending input, our memories, or both. For example, dissonance would be created if an individual received no benefit from an alternative treatment after committing time, money, and 'face.' Therefore, there would be strong pressure to find some redeeming value in the treatment rather than accept the psychologic implications of admitting that it had been a waste. Thus, CAM patients and therapists often remember things as they wish they had happened, rather than as they really occurred. And since CAM practitioners scorn careful record keeping and randomized clinical trials, they can be selective in what they recall, leading to an overestimation of their success rates while ignoring or explaining away their failures.

Likewise, there are many self-serving biases that help maintain self-esteem and promote harmonious social interchange. An illusory feeling that one's symptoms have abated could also be due to a number of so-called 'demand characteristics' found in any therapeutic setting. In all societies there exists a 'norm of reciprocity,' an implicit rule that obliges people to respond in kind when someone does them a good turn. Most therapists sincerely want to help their patients, and it is only natural that patients want to please them in return. Without clients necessarily realizing it, such obligations (in the form of implicit social demands) are sufficient to inflate their perceptions on how much benefit they have received. Thus, controls for these compliance effects must also be built into clinical trials (Adair, 1973).

WHY MIGHT THERAPISTS AND CLIENTS CONCLUDE THAT INEFFECTIVE THERAPIES WORK?

Although the terms 'disease' and 'illness' are often used interchangeably, it is worthwhile to distinguish between the two. I use 'disease' to refer to a pathologic state of an organism. By the term 'illness' I will mean subjective *feelings* of malaise, pain, disorientation, or dysfunctionality, which might accompany a disease state. Our subjective reaction to the raw sensations we call symptoms is, like all other perceptions, a complex cognitive construction. As such, it is molded by factors such as attitudes, suggestions, expectations, demand characteristics, self-serving biases, and self-deception. The experience of illness is also affected (often unconsciously) by a host of social, monetary, and psychologic payoffs that accrue to those admitted to the 'sick role' in society (Alcock, 1986). For certain individuals, these privileges and benefits are sufficient to perpetuate the experience of illness after a disease has abated, or even to create feelings of illness in the absence of disease. Unless we can tease apart these factors that contribute to one's perception of being ill, personal testimonials are a poor basis on which to judge whether a putative therapy has, in fact, cured anyone. Why, then, might someone mistakenly believe that he or she had been helped by an inert treatment?

The disease may have run its natural course. Many diseases are self-limiting. Thus, before the curative powers of a putative therapy can be acknowledged, it must be shown that the percentage of patients who improve following treatment exceeds the proportion expected to recover without any intervention at all (or that they consistently recover faster). Unless unconventional therapists release detailed records of successes *and failures* over a sufficiently large number of patients with the same complaint, they cannot claim to have exceeded the norms for unaided recovery.

Many diseases are cyclic. For example, arthritis, multiple sclerosis, asthma, allergies, migraines, and many dermatologic, gynecologic, and gastrointestinal complaints normally 'have their ups and downs.' Not surprisingly, sufferers tend to seek therapy during the downturn of any given cycle. Thus a bogus treatment will have repeated opportunities to coincide with upturns that would have happened anyway. Without randomized controlled trials, consumers and vendors alike are prone to misinterpret improvement due to normal cyclic variation as a valid therapeutic effect.

The placebo effect. *The major reason for doubtful remedies' being credited with subjective, and occasionally objective, improvements is the ubiquitous placebo effect* (Roberts, Kewman and Hovell, 1993; Shapiro and Shapiro, 1997). The history of medicine is strewn with examples of what, with hindsight, seem like crackpot procedures that were once enthusiastically endorsed by physicians and patients alike (Hamilton, 1986; Skrabanek and McCormick, 1990). These misconceptions arose from the false assumption that changes in symptoms following treatment must have been a specific consequence of that procedure. Through a combination of suggestion, expectancy, and cognitive reinterpretation, patients given biologically useless treatments often can experience subjective relief; thus, the need for placebo controls that CAM practitioners steadfastly refuse to institute in place of their customer satisfaction surveys.

Many of CAM's treatments, while unable to affect the disease itself, do make the illness more bearable, but for psychologic reasons. Pain is one example. Modern pain clinics show that suffering can often be reduced by psychologic means, even if the underlying pathology is untouched (Brose and Spiegel, 1992; Melzack, 1993). Anything that can allay anxiety, redirect attention, reduce arousal, foster a sense of control, or lead to cognitive reinterpretation of symptoms can alleviate the agony component of pain (Smith, Merskey and Gross, 1980). It is obviously beneficial if patients suffer less, but we must be careful that purely symptomatic relief does not divert people from proven remedies for the underlying condition until it is too late for them to be effective. Importantly, procedures aimed purely at relieving symptoms should never precede the appropriate diagnostic tests and at least a reasonable provisional differential diagnosis.

Because the power of expectancy and compliance effects is so strong, both therapists and recipients must be 'blind' with respect to active treatment versus placebo status (Rosenthal, 1966). Such precautions are necessary because barely perceptible cues, unintentionally conveyed by unblinded treatment providers, can bias trial results. Likewise, those who assess the treatment's effects must also be blind, for there is a large literature on 'experimenter bias' showing that scrupulous, well-trained professionals can unconsciously 'read in' the outcomes they expect when they evaluate complex outcomes (Chapman and Chapman, 1967; Rosenthal, 1966).

Defenders of CAM often complain that conventional medicine itself continues to use many treatments that have not been adequately vetted by these standards. This may be so in some instances, but the percentage of such holdovers is grossly exaggerated by the 'alternatives' (Ellis et al, 1995). At any rate, this criticism does nothing to enhance the credibility of CAM, for merely arguing that 'they're as bad as we are' offers no positive evidence in favor of one's own pet belief. The crucial difference between scientific biomedicine and CAM is that, unlike the 'alternatives,' scientific medicine is institutionally committed to weeding out treatments that fail to pass muster, and it does not cling to procedures and theories contradicted by the basic sciences.

Spontaneous remission. Any anecdotally reported cure can be due to a rare but possible 'spontaneous remission.' Even with cancers that are nearly always lethal, tumors occasionally disappear without further treatment. One experienced oncologist reports that he has seen 12 such events in about 6,000 cases he has treated (Silverman, 1987). Alternative therapists can receive unearned acclaim for such remissions because many desperate patients turn to them out of a feeling that they have nothing left to lose. When the 'alternatives' publicize such events, they rarely reveal what percentage of their apparently terminal clientele is represented by these happy exceptions. The exact mechanisms responsible for spontaneous remissions are not well understood, but much research is being devoted to revealing and possibly harnessing the mechanisms that are responsible for these unexpected turnarounds,

Somatization and fear of losing 'wellness.' Many people can be induced to think they suffer from diseases they do not have. When these healthy folk receive from orthodox physicians the oddly unwelcome news that they have no sign of disease, they often gravitate to alternative practitioners, who can always find something to treat. If 'recovery' should follow, another convert is born. Alternative healers also cater to the 'worried well' who dwell on minor symptoms and believe they must take elaborate precautions to avoid losing their good health.

There are many physical complaints that can both arise from psychosocial distress and be alleviated by support and reassurance. At first glance, these symptoms (at various times called 'psychosomatic,' 'hysterical,' or 'neurasthenic') resemble those of recognized medical syndromes (Merskey, 1995; Stewart, 1990). They are, however, examples of somatization, the tendency to express psychologic concerns in a language of bodily symptoms (McWhinney, Epstein and Freeman, 1997; Shorter, 1992).

Although there are many 'secondary gains' (i.e., psychologic, social, and economic payoffs) that accrue to those who slip into 'the sick role' in this way, we need not accuse them of conscious malingering to point out that their symptoms are nonetheless engendered and relieved by subtle psychosocial processes (Alcock, 1986; Shorter, 1992). CAM offers comfort to these individuals who need to believe their symptoms have medical rather than psychologic causes (although, paradoxically, CAM teaches that all diseases stem from mental/spiritual lapses). With the aid of pseudo-scientific diagnostic devices, fringe practitioners reinforce the somatizer's conviction that the cold-hearted, narrow-minded medical establishment, which can find nothing physically amiss, is both incompetent and unfair in refusing to acknowledge a very real organic condition. It is obviously worthwhile when unscientific 'healers' supply the reassurance, sense of belonging, and existential support that their clients are really seeking, but these provisions need not be foreign to scientific practitioners, who have much more to offer.

CAM customers hedging their bets. In an attempt to appeal to a wider clientele, many unorthodox healers have begun to refer to themselves as 'complementary' or 'integrative,' rather than 'alternative' providers. Instead of ministering primarily to the ideologically committed or to those who have been told that conventional medicine has no further treatment, the 'alternatives' have begun to advertise their ability to enhance scientific treatments. They accept that orthodox practitioners can alleviate specific symptoms but contend that alternative medicine treats the *real* causes of disease – dubious dietary imbalances and environmental sensitivities, disrupted energy fields, or even unresolved conflicts from previous incarnations (Beyerstein and Downie, 1998). If improvement follows the combined delivery of 'complementary' and scientifically based treatments, the fringe practice demands, and often gets, a disproportionate share of the credit.

Misdiagnosis. Scientifically trained physicians do not claim infallibility, and a mistaken diagnosis, followed by a trip to a shrine, alternative healer, or herbalist, can lead to a glowing testimonial for the cure of a grave condition that never existed. At other times, the diagnosis may have been correct but the predicted time course might have proved inaccurate. If a patient with a terminal condition undergoes alternative treatments and succumbs at a later time than that predicted by the conventional doctor, the alternative procedure may receive credit for prolonging life when, in fact, the discrepancy was merely due to an unduly pessimistic prognosis.

Derivative benefits. Alternative healers often have enthusiastic, charismatic personalities (Nolen, 1974; O'Connor, 1987; Randi, 1989). Patients swept up by the messianic aspects of CAM can experience a psychologic uplift that can enhance placebo effects and engender other beneficial spinoffs. Elevating patients' mood and expectations can motivate greater compliance with, and hence effectiveness of, concurrent orthodox treatments. These secondary effects also can lead patients to improve their eating and sleeping habits and to exercise and socialize more. These changes, by themselves, could help speed natural recovery, or at the very least, make the recuperative interval easier to tolerate. Psychologic spinoffs of this kind also can reduce the stress that has been shown to have deleterious effects on the immune system (Ader and Cohen, 1993). Removing this added burden may speed recovery, even if it is not a specific effect of the therapy.

CONCLUSIONS

Potential clients should ask whether any alternative treatment they are considering is supported by research published in biomedical journals whose peer-review processes strive to eliminate experimental artifacts that lead to false impressions of cures. Even then, because any single finding could always be due to an undetected confounding variable or a statistical fluke, independent replication is essential. If a supporting publication meets the foregoing criteria, clients should nevertheless always review the size of the reported treatment effect, for there are many 'true but trivial effects' that are statistically significant but too small to be clinically useful.

One should be suspicious if, instead of randomized controlled trials, the 'evidence' consists of anecdotes, testimonials, or self-published pamphlets or books. Supportive documentation should come from impartial scientific periodicals rather than from journals owned by promoters of the questionable practice or the 'vanity press,' which accepts virtually all submissions and charges a fee to the authors for publication.

Clients should be dubious of any practitioner who (1) is ignorant of or hostile to mainstream science; (2) cannot supply a reasonable rationale for his or her methods; (3) uses promotional patter laced with allusions to spiritual forces and vital energies or to vague planes, vibrations, imbalances, and sensitivities; (4) claims to possess secret ingredients or processes; (5) appeals to ancient wisdom and 'other ways of knowing'; (6) claims to 'treat the whole person' rather than organ-specific diseases; or (7) claims to be persecuted by the establishment and encourages political action on his or her behalf, or is prone to attack or sue critics rather than responding with valid research. Practitioners with degrees from unaccredited institutions or who sell their own proprietary concoctions in their offices and stress the need for frequent return visits 'in order to stay well' are also a cause for concern. The presence of pseudoscientific or conspiracy-laden literature in the waiting room ought to set a clear thinker looking for the exit. And, above all, if the promised results go well beyond those offered by conventional therapists and it is claimed that there are no side effects, the probability is that one is dealing with a quack. In short, if it sounds too good to be true, it probably is.

When people become sick, any promise of a cure is beguiling. As a result, common sense and the willingness to demand evidence are easily supplanted by false hope. In this vulnerable state, the need for critical appraisal of treatment options is more – rather than less – necessary. Those who still think they can afford to take a chance on the hawkers of untested remedies should bear in mind Goethe's wise advice: 'Nothing is more dangerous than active ignorance.'

REFERENCES

Adair J. *The Human Subject.* Boston, MA: Little, Brown, 1973.

Ader R, Cohen N. Psychoneuroimmunology: conditioning and stress. *Annu Rev Psychol.* 1993;4:53–85.

Alcock J. Chronic pain and the injured worker. *Can Psychol.* 1986;27:196–203.

Alcock J. The belief engine. *The Skeptical Inquirer.* 1995;19:14–8.

Barrett S, Jarvis W. *The Health Robbers: A Close Look at Quackery in America.* Amherst, NY: Prometheus Books, 1993.

Basil R (ed). *Not Necessarily the New Age.* Amherst, NY: Prometheus Books, 1988.

Benson H. *Timeless Healing; The Power and Biology of Belief.* New York: Simon and Schuster, 1996.

Betz W. *Herbal crisis in Europe. The Scientific Review of Alternative Medicine* [in press].

Beyerstein B. The brain and consciousness – implications for psi phenomena. *The Skeptical Inquirer.* 1987;12:163–73.

Beyerstein B. Pseudoscience and the brain: tuners and tonics for aspiring super-humans. In: Delia Sala S. (ed). *Mind Myths: Exploring Popular Misconceptions about the Mind and Brain.* Chichester, U.K.: J. Wiley and Sons, 1999:59–82,

Beyerstein B, Downie S. Naturopathy. *The Scientific Review of Alternative Medicine.* 1998;2:20–8.

Beyerstein B, Hadaway P. On avoiding folly. *J Drug Issues.* 1991;20:689–700.

Beyerstein B, Sampson W. Traditional medicine and pseudoscience in China (Part 1). *The Skeptical Inquirer.* 1996;20:18–26. Sampson W, Beyerstein B. Traditional medicine and pseudoscience in China (Part 2). *The Skeptical Inquirer.* 1996;20:27–34.

Brose WG, Spiegel D. Neuropsychiatric aspects of pain management. In: *The American Psychiatric Press Textbook of Neuropsychiatry.* Washington, DC: American Psychiatric Press, 1992:245–75.

Chapman L, Chapman J. Genesis of popular but erroneous diagnostic observations, *J Abnorm Psychol.* 1967;72:193–204.

Eisenberg DM, et al. Trends in alternative medicine use in the United States, 1990–1997: results of a follow-up national survey. *JAMA.* 1998;280:1569–75.

Ellis J, Mulligan I, Rowe J, Sackett D. Inpatient general medicine is evidence based. *Lancet.* 1995;346:407–10.

Ernst E. Harmless herbs? A review of the recent literature. *Am J Med.* 1998;104:170–8.

Festinger L. *A Theory of Cognitive Dissonance*. Stanford, CA: Stanford University Press, 1957.

Frankel C. The nature and sources of irrationalism. *Science*. 1973;180:927–31.

Gilovich T. *How We Know What Isn't So: The Fallibility of Human Reason in Everyday Life*. New York: Free Press/Macmillan, 1991.

Gilovich T. Some systematic biases of everyday judgment. *The Skeptical Inquirer*. 1997;21:31–5.

Gross P, Levitt N. *Higher Superstition*. Baltimore, MD: Johns Hopkins University Press, 1994.

Hamilton D. *The Monkey Gland Affair*. London, U.K.: Chatto and Windus, 1986.

Hui KK. Is there a role for traditional Chinese medicine? *JAMA*. 1997;277:714. [A reply by W. Sampson and B. Beyerstein follows.]

Kiernan V. Survey plumbs the depths of international ignorance. *The New Scientist*. 1995;146 (29 April):7.

Knauer D. Therapeutic touch on the hot-seat. *The Canadian Nurse*. 1997;X:10.

Ko RJ. Adulterants in Asian patient medicines. *N Engl J Med*. 1998;339:847.

Levy D. *Tools of Critical Thinking*. Needam Heights, MA: Allyn and Bacon, 1997.

McWhinney IR, Epstein RM, Freeman TR. Rethinking somatization. *Ann Intern Med*. 1997;126:747–50.

Melzack R. Pain: past, present and future. *Can J Psychol*. 1993;47:615–29.

Merskey H. *The Analysis of Hysteria: Understanding Conversion and Dissociation*. 2nd ed. London, U.K.: Royal College of Psychiatrists, 1995.

Meyer D. *The Positive Thinkers: A Study of the American Quest for Health, Wealth, and Personal Power from Mary Baker Eddy to Norman Vincent Peale*. New York: Doubleday–Anchor, 1965.

Nisbett R, Ross L. *Human Inference: Strategies and Shortcomings of Social Judgment*. Engelwood Cliffs, NJ: Prentice-Hall, 1980.

Nolen WA. *Healing: A Doctor in Search of a Miracle*. New York: Fawcett Crest, 1974.

O'Connor G. Confidence trick. *Med J Aust* 1987;147:456–9.

Randi J. *The Faith Healers*. Amherst, NY: Prometheus Books, 1989.

Redelmeier D, Tversky A. On the belief that arthritis pain is related to the weather. *Proc Natl Acad Sci USA*. 1996;93:2895–6.

Relman A. A trip to Stonesville. *The New Republic*. 1998;378:28–37.

Roberts A, Kewman D, Hovell L. The power of nonspecific effects in healing: implications for psychosocial and biological treatments. *Clin Psychol Rev* 1993;13:375–91.

Robins R, Post J. *Political Paranoia: The Psychopathology of Hatred*. New Haven, CT: Yale University Press, 1997.

Rosenthal R. *Experimenter Effects in Behavioral Research*. New York: Appleton–Century–Crofts, 1966.

Schick T, Vaughn L. *How to Think About Weird Things: Critical Thinking for a New Age*. Mountain View, CA: Mayfield Publishing, 1995.

Shapiro AK, Shapiro E. *The Powerful Placebo*. Baltimore, MD: Johns Hopkins University Press, 1997.

Shorter E. *From Paralysis to Fatigue: A History of Psychosomatic Medicine in the Modem Era*. New York: Free Press/Macmillan, 1992.

Silverman S. Medical 'miracles': still mysterious despite claims of believers. *Psientific American*. July 1987:5–7. (Newsletter of the Sacramento Skeptics Society, Sacramento, CA)

Skrabanek P, McCormick J. *Follies and Fallacies in Medicine.* Amherst, NY: Prometheus Books, 1990.

Sloan RP, Bagiella E, Powell T. Religion, spirituality and medicine. *Lancet.* 1999;353:664–7.

Smith W, Merskey H, Gross S (eds). *Pain: Meaning and Management.* New York: SP Medical and Scientific Books, 1980.

Sokal A, Bricmont J. *Intellectual Impostures.* London, England: Profile Books, 1998.

Stalker D, Glymour C (eds). *Examining Holistic Medicine.* Amherst, NY: Prometheus Books, 1985.

Starr P. *The Social Transformation of American Medicine.* New York: Basic Books, 1982.

Stewart D. Emotional disorders misdiagnosed as physical illness: environmental hypersensitivity, candidiasis hypersensitivity, and chronic fatigue syndrome. *Int J Mental Health.* 1990;19:56–68.

Sutter MC. Therapeutic effectiveness and adverse effects of herbs and herbal extracts. *British Columbia Med J.* 1995;37:766–70.

Tessman I, Tessman J. Mind and body. *Science.* 1997a;276:369–70.

Tessman I, Tessman J. Troubling matters. *Science.* 1997b;278:561.

Thadani M. *Herbal Remedies: Weeding Fact from Fiction.* Winnipeg, Manitoba, Canada: Context Publications, 1999.

Tversky A, Kahneman, D. Judgement under uncertainty: heuristics and biases. *Science.* 1974;185:1124–31.

Winslow L, Kroll D. Herbs as medicines. *Arch Intern Med.* 1998;158:2192–9.

Zusne L, Jones W. *Anomalistic Psychology: A Study of Magical Thinking.* 2nd ed. Hillsdale, NJ: Lawrence Erlbaum Associates, 1989.

CHAPTER 6

ORTHODOX MEDICINE OR ALTERNATIVE THERAPY: A PERSPECTIVE

British Medical Association Board of Science and Education

A notable feature of society in the 1980s is the interest now taken by all in what, but a generation ago, was the preoccupation of the few. The origins of this interest are to be found in part in the remarkable developments in the physical sciences, for which the current achievements of Voyager II, the space-probe that met with the planet Uranus, provides an apt example, in the biological sciences with the developments in genetic engineering, and not least in the advances made in medicine. But the reasons for the widespread development of this interest lie with the prominent role played in the field of communication by the written word, the popular press, the specialised magazines, and perhaps predominantly by television and radio.

One effect of this spread of awareness, and this a wholly desirable one, is the awakening of a sense of enquiry, and of involvement in these developments. With this has developed the exercise of the right to question and to criticise the significance and outcome of these astonishing advances. That these critical attitudes have been applied to the craft of medicine is hardly surprising, for modern medicine – preventive, curative or palliative – impinges on the lives of everyone and this critical attitude is to be welcomed.

That additional and basic changes are at work in society at large is the current theme of the social historian. The thesis that we have become a

Edited from *Alternative Therapy*: report of the board of science and education.

more materialistic, less law-observing, less caring society is perhaps a too sweeping generalisation. Yet, it is one the city-dweller would recognise. With this development is an identifiable growth of an underlying hostility to technology and science, allied to a distrust of innovation. Compounding this development is that acceleration of social, political and material change, together with the progressive intrusion of bureaucracy into our lives, combining to produce that which is commonly identified as 'progress'. Together, these two facets appear to lie at the root of a quite general criticism of governance and from which orthodox medicine is itself not immune.

Should this prove to be so, as we are inclined to accept, then we can identify in particular criticisms a real lack of understanding on the part of the public. The making good of this deficit, and the elimination of confusion and its associated loss of perspective, is a duty involving society as a whole, and of the medical profession in particular.

It is particularly interesting that these criticisms of medicine should appear at a time when the great modern developments in rational therapeutics and in diagnostic techniques have revolutionised the effective treatment of many diseases, and since the 1950s have greatly enhanced our expectations of medical science.

These changes have altered also in significant and subtle ways the relation between patient and doctor. Relatively few years ago, when little therapeutic help could be offered, the physician devoted much time to counsel and to support the patient. Now therapeutic intervention, often life-saving, is quickly and skilfully available, and has become so commonplace that the swiftness of the changes is forgotten and the significance of the consequences passes unnoticed.

One of the consequences of the changed nature of the relation of the doctor to the patient is that the current pressures and the technical demands of modern medicine do not allow him the opportunities formerly devoted to counselling, sympathetic contact, and support. This change is largely regretted by doctors and is perceived as the product of the increased effectiveness and intricate requirements of modern treatment, together with the restrictions imposed by current financial stringency.

An additional consequence of the advances in medicine in the latter part of this century is the impact of these far-reaching changes on the nature of the doctor's training, with increasing emphasis on the scientific aspects of the curriculum, and a growth of specialisation at the postgraduate stages. This new professionalism is evident in the quality of the primary care exercised by the general practitioner and is reflected in the expectations of his patients.

Yet this new orientation and attitude of doctors trained in the last 30 years has not been matched in the provision of support services to meet the novel and still-growing demand from the modern patient for communication, information and instruction. Not all of this essential provision is lacking; some, foreseen in the development of health centres are flourishing, but more usually these services have lagged behind expectation and perhaps need.

An additional aspect should be mentioned. The growth and dependence on new diagnostic aids of all kinds, the nature of the haematological and pathological services, and their matter-of-fact and impersonal nature are identified by the patient, the physician and the medical technologist alike as an intrusion juxtaposed between patient and physician.

Almost as a consequence of a widespread appreciation of the above developments, there has grown up a demand which is hardly rational for instant cures for the currently incurable diseases of mankind. There is also the ill-founded suspicion that nothing is being done to attack these problems, and little perception of the great difficulty of these essential researches, and their very long time course. In noting the need for information about this problem, we also have to note that a consequence of ignoring these factors is the turning back to primitive beliefs and outmoded practices, almost all purposeless and without a sound base, however well-meaning. Some can be dangerous in their effects and others appear to be promoted for less than laudable purposes.

In attempting to identify the basis of the current, but in no sense novel, preoccupation with alternative kinds of therapy, we have sought to identify those facets which appear to lie at the root of a general criticism of governance which is directed to orthodox medicine as it is to the other scientific disciplines. Should this analysis prove to be valid, as we believe it is, then we can recognise in particular criticisms a need for general information about the recent advances in medicine and of its immediate prospectives.

While the cultivation of sane attitudes to the preservation of good health and of the nature of common illness is clearly an obligation of society as a whole, the need to define the many areas in which orthodox medicine can provide effective treatment, and to indicate those areas where support can be offered for conditions as yet not amenable to current therapy, is a duty devolving particularly upon the craft of medicine.

CHAPTER 7

COMPLEMENTARY MEDICINE: NEW APPROACHES TO GOOD PRACTICE: SUMMARY AND RECOMMENDATIONS

British Medical Association

The term 'non-conventional therapies' covers a wide and diverse range of practices. Some treat particular parts of the body or conditions and others aim to provide complete treatment or therapy for the generality of diseases and patients. It is apparent that different therapies have little in common in the way of aspirations, practice, and tradition. The means of control over these therapies varies widely from country to country within Europe. The Commission of the European Communities has stated emphatically that legislation at EC level is unlikely in coming years in the area of non-conventional therapies. With the possible exception of medicinal products, a uniform system of regulation across Europe is only a remote possibility. The most important influence on the regulation of non-conventional therapies will continue to be national law.

While no attempt has been made to evaluate different therapies in this report, it is clear that the key to enhancing the credibility of different practices, whether in orthodox medicine or non-conventional therapies, is research. Good-quality research is essential in order to maximize the benefits and minimize the harms of different treatments. There is at present a paucity of systematically collected data on the use and recorded adverse effects of non-conventional therapies. There are areas of orthodox medicine where such information is similarly unavailable. Such evidence, obtained

Edited from BMA (1993) *Complementary Medicine: New Approaches to Good Practice.* London: BMA.

by carefully designed research investigations, is necessary in order to make informed decisions on the risks and benefits of different treatments.

Much of this report is focused on those practices which we have labelled as *discrete clinical disciplines*. These are the therapies which have established foundations of training and have the potential for greatest use alongside orthodox medical care. Our category of discrete clinical disciplines covers the practices of acupuncture, chiropractic, herbalism, homoeopathy, and osteopathy which appear to be the five most common therapies in use in the UK today.

Given the wide diversity in non-conventional therapies, from discrete clinical disciplines through to healing and self-help therapies such as yoga, it is not possible to set out a single model for regulation which would be appropriate for all practices. However, it is hoped that this report will make a positive contribution by highlighting areas of good practice in disciplines which may be emerging or lacking the support of more established therapies. The development of more rigorous means of control and regulation for different therapies can only benefit the patient, which must be the goal for doctors and therapists alike.

GOOD PRACTICE

It is difficult at present for individuals to be certain that the therapist whom they are consulting is competent to practise. Similarly, it is not easy for doctors to ensure that the therapists to whom they transfer care of patients are competent. The present situation, in which anybody is free to practise, irrespective of their training or experience, is unacceptable. Where individuals undergo courses of training designed to equip them for the practice of particular therapies, these should conform to minimum standards appropriate to the responsibilities and demands of that therapy.

The BMA recommends that a *single* regulating body be established for each therapy. Such organizations should follow best practice in adopting all of the following features:

Registration

- A single register of members, open to public scrutiny, entry to which is limited to competent practitioners.

Professional standards

- A defined protocol for communicating with medical practitioners and other therapists both within and without their own discipline and a system for maintaining case records of patients/clients;

- clearly understood areas of competence, including limits of competence and contra-indications to treatment;
- enforceable ethical code governing all aspects of professional conduct, linked to effective disciplinary mechanism;
- well-publicized and accessible complaints procedure.

Training

- Training structure appropriate to the task and of a credible duration at accredited and externally monitored educational establishments;
- all practices claiming to have a therapeutic influence should include in their training courses a foundation in the basic medical sciences;
- consideration should be given to a core curriculum for the training schedule of each therapy including appropriate clinical and medical input;
- limits of competence must be established for each therapy during the training process. Patients suffering from conditions not amenable to treatment must be identified and referred to the appropriate agency. This is particularly important in cases where medical attention is needed;
- provision should be made for continuing education for qualified members, and for refresher courses;
- training in clinical audit, so that practice and management of patients are evaluated rigorously at regular intervals.

Research

- Encouragement of professional development and research.

REGULATION

The criteria above represent best practice which should be the aim of all therapies. However, in order to protect patients, some therapies should be regulated by statute. Those therapies in which the diagnostic process is integral to the application of the therapy, and whose practice involves invasive or potentially harmful techniques, should be subject to regulation by law. The BMA therefore recommends that:

- the case for the statutory self-regulation of each discrete clinical discipline should be considered by an appropriate independent body and, where applicable, appropriate legislation introduced.

DOCTORS AND THERAPISTS

Increasing numbers of doctors wish to make use of non-conventional therapies for their patients. A distinction has been made between the powers of referral and of delegation. The doctor refers a patient to another individual to use his or her professional judgement to assess the patient and decide if (and what) treatment is necessary and, where appropriate, to provide that treatment. In the referral model, the general practitioner refers care of the patient to a specialist for the duration of a particular episode of treatment, but will retain clinical responsibility for the overall care of the patient. In delegating care, by contrast, tasks which are routinely performed by the doctor are transferred to another health-care professional, such as a nurse. The doctor remains clinically accountable for the patient during that treatment.

The question arises as to how appropriate the model of delegation is for non-conventional therapies, in particular the discrete clinical disciplines, when the treatment may be outside the scope of the doctor's skill and experience. It may be difficult at present for the doctor to be confident that the practitioner is competent in this area. In the case of therapies which are subject to statutory regulation, such as osteopathy, the onus for determining the clinical competence of the therapist is to a large extent removed from the doctor. The BMA therefore recommends that:

- the General Medical Council be asked to consider whether doctors should be permitted to *refer* patients for specific treatments to registered practitioners in those therapies which are subject to statutory self-regulation.

DOCTOR–THERAPIST COMMUNICATION

Responsibility for complete medical diagnosis and overall management of the patient rests with the patient's general medical practitioner. Paragraph 92 of the current General Medical Council guide-lines states that 'it is in the best interests of patients for one doctor to be fully informed about and responsible for the comprehensive management of a patient's medical care'. The situation where a patient is given advice by a therapist which conflicts with the drug regimen or treatment given by their registered medical practitioner is detrimental to the best interests of the patient. It is essential that proper channels of communication be established between non-conventional therapists and doctors to prevent the occurrence of such a situation. In addition, the doctor should be fully informed of any non-conventional treatment which the patient is receiving. The BMA therefore recommends that:

- therapists should not alter the instructions or prescriptions given by a patient's medical practitioner without prior consultation and agreement with that doctor;
- doctors should ask about their patients' use of non-conventional therapies whenever they obtain a medical history.

RESEARCH

Research is extremely valuable in advancing knowledge in a given discipline and in evaluating the benefits and harms of different practices. Research in non-conventional therapies has to date been of inconsistent quality. It is recognized that this is due in part to difficulties in attracting appropriate resources to fund good-quality research. In addition to problems in funding research studies, there have been more general difficulties in inculcating a culture that recognizes research as an essential activity. Recent research initiatives in various non-conventional therapies, such as the national randomized trial of chiropractic, are welcome as an important step in ensuring public and professional confidence in particular modalities. The BMA recommends that:

- Priority should be given to research into acupuncture, chiropractic, herbalism, homoeopathy, and osteopathy as the therapies most commonly used in this country;
- in the absence of research foundations for specific therapeutic disciplines, support be given to organizations such as the Research Council for Complementary Medicine (RCCM) to raise awareness of the need for more research in non-conventional therapies;
- core curricula for undergraduate training establishments should include components on research methodology, information technology, and statistics;
- experienced practitioners in different therapies should be encouraged to undertake practice surveys measuring work-load and patient characteristics. Such research could be facilitated by postgraduate training and on-call advice on research protocols from organizations such as the RCCM.

MONITORING AND SURVEILLANCE

In order to minimize the potential harms of treatments and maximize the benefits of different treatments, it is important to record any adverse reactions occurring after an intervention. Surveillance schemes are necessary to collate information on incidents which may be used to test the safety and quality of different preparations. The BMA therefore recommends that:

- Continued funding from the Department of Health and the Ministry of Agriculture, Fisheries, and Food be made available for the investigation into adverse reactions to herbal medicines and other preparations at the National Poisons Unit;
- the Council of Europe Co-operation in Science and Technology (COST) project on non-conventional therapies be approved by the UK government.

MEDICAL UNDERSTANDING OF NON-CONVENTIONAL THERAPIES

Recent surveys suggest that doctors increasingly require more information on non-conventional therapies. Doctors need to know more about different therapies in order to delegate care appropriately, and to advise patients as to the likely benefits and hazards of treatments. Some doctors may even wish to undertake more detailed training in order to practise as a therapist. The BMA in particular recommends that:

- accredited postgraduate sessions be set up to inform clinicians on the techniques used by different therapists and the possible benefits for patients;
- consideration should be given to the inclusion of a familiarization course on non-conventional therapies within the medical undergraduate curriculum.

MEDICALLY QUALIFIED THERAPISTS

It is recognized that particular skills need to be acquired in order to achieve competence in different therapies. The General Medical Council has stated that a question of serious professional misconduct may arise by 'a doctor persisting in unsupervised practice of a branch of medicine without having the appropriate knowledge and skill or having acquired the experience which is necessary'. The BMA therefore recommends that:

- medically qualified practitioners wishing to practise any form of non-conventional therapy should undertake recognized training in that field approved by the appropriate regulatory body, and should only practise the therapy after registration.

CHAPTER 8

ETHICAL PROBLEMS ARISING IN EVIDENCE-BASED COMPLEMENTARY AND ALTERNATIVE MEDICINE

Edzard Ernst, Michael H Cohen and Julie Stone

As it turns out, at first glimpse, there are very few differences between the ethics of conventional medicine and those of CAM (Cohen, 2000; Ernst, 1996; Stone, 2002). In fact, many of the ethical rules applicable to conventional medicine – such as requirements of informed consent, practice boundaries (i.e., the duty to practice within one's scope of competence or else to appropriately refer), and duties involving confidentiality and privacy – translate across to the arena of CAM (Cohen, 2003). In addition, much of the regulatory framework governing conventional medicine – which incorporates many ethical obligations – also translates to CAM practice; this includes, for example, licensure, malpractice liability rules, and legal rules governing professional discipline (Cohen, 1998). The focus of this article is therefore on ethical aspects in areas of overt variations between CAM and conventional medicine. Because considerable national differences may exist, our article primarily focuses on CAM in the United Kingdom (UK).

DIFFERENCES BETWEEN CAM AND CONVENTIONAL MEDICINE

For the purpose of this article, it may be helpful to highlight some of the major, current conceptual and pragmatic differences between CAM and

Edited from an original article in *Journal of Medical Ethics* (2004) forthcoming.

conventional medicine, particularly those with implications concerning ethical obligations. In doing so, a degree of simplification and dichotomization may be necessary, recognizing that CAM research and practice both are evolving, that definitions embrace legal, social, and political (as well as medical and scientific) realities (Kaptchuk and Eisenberg, 2001), and that the lines between conventional medicine and CAM become blurred when CAM therapies are incorporated into routine medical practice.

CAM IS PRIVATE MEDICINE

Virtually all surveys on this topic demonstrate that, in industrialized countries, CAM-users tend to belong to the affluent, well-educated classes (Eisenberg et al, 1998; Ernst and White, 2000). CAM is by and large private medicine for which consumers pay substantial amounts out of their own pockets (Eisenberg et al, 1998). Assuming that CAM does more good than harm, this situation is far from equitable. The unequal distribution of CAM within the population violates the fundamental ethical principle of justice. Stone and Matthews put it succinctly: '...the benefits of CAM should be freely available to all...' (Stone and Matthews, 1996).

The obvious way to remedy this problem is to render the distribution of CAM more even across all socioeconomic classes. However, this is likely to fail for at least two reasons: firstly the already tight resources in healthcare are not sufficient to allow everyone free access to CAM. Secondly, permitting such general access within an evidence-based healthcare system would require that the evidence for the safety and efficacy of CAM be more solid than is presently the case (see below) (Ernst et al, 2001). As long as efficacy and safety of CAM are uncertain (i.e. significantly more uncertain than in conventional medicine), the principle of justice may be in conflict with the principles of beneficence and non-maleficence (Ernst, 1996; Stone and Matthews, 1996). There is no easy solution to this dilemma – other than swiftly conducting the research that is necessary to establish efficacy and safety.

PROVIDERS OF CAM ARE OFTEN NOT MEDICALLY TRAINED

The vast majority of CAM providers in the UK are non-doctors. Most CAM providers, one would hope, have adequate training in the methods they practice but their understanding of anatomy, physiology, pathology, and other disciplines of Western medical science, may be limited, and many may adhere to views or philosophies or perspectives (for example, the notion of acupuncture 'meridians' in Traditional Chinese Medicine) which are in overt contradiction to the concepts, principles and accepted facts of conventional medicine and science. These differences of view create several ethically relevant questions: How can practitioners of CAM meaningfully communicate with practitioners of conventional medicine and vice versa? If communication is sub-optimal, does that have the potential to put patients at risk? From the perspective of mainstream medicine, do CAM providers view the potential limitations of their own methods realistically? The ethical principle that may be at stake here is that of non-maleficence (Ernst, 1996; Stone and Matthews, 1996). Currently there is little research into the questions raised above. Allegations of violations of principle of non-maleficence obviously run on both sides of the debate.

CAM (AT LEAST IN THE UK) IS NOT REGULATED AS RIGOROUSLY AS CONVENTIONAL MEDICINE

Stone and Matthews point out that the aims of professional self-regulation are to ensure: i) high, uniform standards of practice, ii) identification of competent practitioners, and iii) accountability (Stone and Matthews, 1996). Essentially they relate to the ethical principle of non-maleficence. Unlike the situation of widespread licensure in the US for chiropractors, acupuncturists, massage therapists, and to some extent, naturopathic physicians (Cohen, 1998), most CAM professions in the UK are not statutorily regulated (the only two exceptions in the UK are chiropractors and osteopaths). In the UK, several professional bodies of acupuncture, homeopathy, medical herbalism etc exist. Yet it is not obligatory to belong to them, and essentially anyone could set up as an acupuncturist, homeopath, herbalist etc.

This situation creates serious ethical questions similar to the ones mentioned previously. If someone practices acupuncture, homeopathy, herbalism, etc with insufficient training, to what extent are they likely to put patients at risk? If a CAM provider does not belong to a professional organization, to whom do their patients complain to if they feel badly treated? How far do unregulated CAM providers adhere to essential ethical issues such as informed consent, confidentiality and maintaining appropriate boundaries?

Stone and Matthews discuss the strengths and weaknesses of statutory self-regulation and voluntary self-regulation (Stone and Matthews, 1996). They conclude that for therapies unlikely to cause direct physical harm, the latter is a 'cheaper and more flexible means of achieving the same regulatory aims'. Perhaps it is less important *how* these aims are reached than the fact *that* they are reached.

THE EFFECTIVENESS AND SAFETY OF CAM ARE OFTEN CONSIDERED UNPROVEN

Many consumers may be attracted to CAM because they assume that CAM is effective and almost free of risk. For some types of CAM this may well be true. However, in many areas of CAM we have so far insufficient evidence to state with confidence that more good than harm is being done.

Obviously this means that more research is required to define both risk and benefit more accurately. But until it is available, clinical CAM practice operates in the presence of uncertainty. Uncertainty is not an unusual factor in medicine. The point, however, is that the level of uncertainty in CAM is considerably greater than that of conventional medicine. This means that CAM-users might not experience the benefit they were led to believe. In other words, the ethical principles of beneficence and nonmaleficence could be violated in a unpredictable way and with unknown frequency. One solution to this quandary is the application of legal sanction to cases of excessive claims, exaggerated promises, and deception and fraud (Cohen, 1995).

And how can more research be done within CAM? It seems that changes are required on several levels. The need for CAM research requires widespread recognition, not least by CAM practitioners. Career scientists should be attracted to CAM research to provide scientific expertise where it presently is underdeveloped. Adequate research funds must be made available to fuel this process. From a UK perspective, it is interesting to observe how the availability of research funds in the US has driven the process towards more and methodologically sounder research in that country. Rigorous research is certainly not confined to randomized clinical trials. For defining the safety of CAM, for instance, other methodologies (e.g. post-marketing surveillance studies) are much more adequate.

RESEARCH FUNDS ARE SCARCE

Funds are scarce for CAM research compared to most areas of medical research (Ernst, 1999). Governments and other funding bodies usually allocate health resources on the basis of existing evidence (Eddy, 1996). Because the evidence for CAM is fragmentary and evolving, research applications in CAM – other than to government agencies specifically created to fund CAM research, such as the (rather unique) National Center for Complementary and Alternative Medicine (NCCAM) at the NIH in the US – have a lower chance of receiving funding than those in conventional medicine. This situation creates a systemic bias, which results in allocation of resources to those areas of (conventional) medicine for which reasonably good evidence already exists. The resulting funding stream is at the expense of areas in which no or less such evidence currently exists, e.g. CAM (Kerridge, Lowe and Henry, 1998). This impinges on the ethical principle of justice. In principle, it also perpetuates the under-researched status of CAM.

CAM HAS AN UNDERDEVELOPED RESEARCH CULTURE

Because CAM historically has lacked the established, research infrastructure of conventional medicine, it has attracted relatively few high-caliber researchers. As a consequence, the field suffers from a general lack of research expertise (potentiated and perpetuated by lack of funds). This, in turn, has resulted in a situation where many of the relatively few scientific investigations in CAM are methodologically weak, or outright flawed (Linde et al, 2001). Yet flawed science is unlikely to be ethical (Freedman, 1987) – expressed in the words of the BMA: 'Studies which are unscientific are also unethical' (Stone and Matthews, 1996).

In recent years the Cochrane Collaboration has established a 'field' in CAM (Ezzo et al, 1998). Essentially this facilitates systematic reviews of clinical trials in a diverse range of medical disciplines. Some 50 such reviews are now available on the Cochran database. Thus the Cochrane Collaboration has made an important contribution to a research culture in CAM. What seems to be missing at present is that the CAM community at large takes these advances on board. Today, research ethics committees have the remit to watch over medical research including that in CAM. Some of the core points they must consider include (Stone and Matthews, 1996):

- scientific quality of proposal
- competence of investigators
- risks for study participants
- informed consent
- indemnity cover
- financial rewards to subjects or investigators
- data protection

Because of the lack of a vibrant research culture in CAM, many CAM researchers find it difficult or even impossible to compose research applications that would pass the scrutiny of a research ethics committee. Anecdotally, we also suspect that some ethics committees have in the past been biased against CAM research. This further hinders an active research culture from emerging. Ethics committees often have insufficient knowledge about CAM which renders a fair judgement on such research proposals difficult and further impedes CAM research.

In order to promote the growth of a CAM research culture, the attitudes among CAM practitioners and the skepticism of research ethics committees both need to be overcome. This will involve a process of learning and education. CAM practitioners have to understand the value of science and the fact that without scientific proof CAM is unlikely to survive.

CAM IS HOLISTIC

Many proponents of CAM are keen to point out the holistic nature of CAM and claim that some of its therapeutic benefits may occur on levels not readily accessible by quantitative measurements. The whole ethos of evidence-based medicine, however, crucially depends on reproducible, quantifiable outcomes. This situation may create an ethically questionable bias within mainstream medicine against areas of medicine in which outcomes cannot be adequately quantified or defined (Kerridge, Lowe and Henry, 1998). Moreover, the so-called clash in paradigms makes it difficult to compare 'evidence' across conventional and CAM therapies, since CAM providers may have notions of efficacy that operate on different principles and spiritual, rather than solely physical levels.

COMMENT

The ethical problems encountered in CAM rarely differ significantly from those of other areas of medicine. Principles from which positive duties emerge include beneficence, a duty to promote good and act in the best interest of the patient and the health of society, and non-maleficence, the duty to protect and to do no harm to patients. Also included is respect for patient autonomy – the duty to foster a patient's pre-informed, uncoerced choices (Beauchamp and Childress, 2002). From the principle of respect for autonomy are derived the rules for truth-telling, disclosure, and informed consent. On one hand, the relative weight granted to these principles and the conflicts among them often account for the ethical problems that CAM practitioners (as well as conventional health practitioners) face. Moreover, as research demonstrates safety and/or efficacy of one or more CAM therapies, such therapies become incorporated into conventional practice and could thus cease being seen as CAM.

On the other hand, some of the cultural, legal, and political factors presently differentiating mainstream medical from CAM practice create unique ethical issues that current research has only begun to address. Furthermore, many CAM therapies have philosophical underpinnings that challenge orthodox medical perspectives, and thus hinder attempts at scientific validation with conventional methodologies. It is, however, quite clear that such challenges are not a complete block to good CAM research. There are no reasons in principle why rigorous CAM research cannot be undertaken. Ultimately, political questions – such as who should have access to therapies and under what circumstances, values – such as autonomy and medical pluralism, and developments in clinical practice – based on increasing communication between conventional and CAM providers, may shape the ethical landscape as much as scientific research and evolving legal rules.

REFERENCES

Beauchamp TL, Childress JF. *Principles of Biomedical Ethics*. 4th ed. New York: Oxford University Press, 2002.

Cohen MH. A fixed star in health care reform: the emerging paradigm of holistic healing. *Ariz State L J* 1995;27:79–173.

Cohen MH. *Complementary and Alternative Medicine: Legal Boundaries and Regulatory Perspectives*. Baltimore, MD: Johns Hopkins University Press, 1998.

Cohen MH. *Beyond Complementary Medicine*. Ann Arbor, MI: University of Michigan Press, 2000.

Cohen MH. *Future Medicine: Ethical Dilemmas, Regulatory Challenges, and Therapeutic Pathways to Health and Healing in Human Transformation*. Ann Arbor, MI: University of Michigan Press, 2003.

Eddy DK. Benefit language; criteria that will improve quality while reducing cost. *JAMA* 1996;27:650–7.

Eisenberg DM, David RB, Ettner SL et al. Trends in Alternative Medicine Use in the United States. *JAMA* 1998;280:1569–75.

Ernst E. The ethics of complementary medicine. *J Med Ethics* 1996;22:197–8.

Ernst E. Funding research into complementary medicine: the situation in Britain. *Compl Ther Med* 1999;7:250–3.

Ernst E, Pittler MH, Stevinson C, White AR. *The Desktop Guide to Complementary and Alternative Medicine*. Edinburgh: Mosby, 2001.

Ernst E, White AR. The BBC survey of complementary medicine use in the UK. *Complement Ther Med* 2000;8:32–6.

Ezzo J, Berman BM, Vickers AJ, Linde K. Complementary medicine and the Cochrane Collaboration. *JAMA* 1998;280:1628–30.

Freedman B. Scientific value and validity as ethical requirements for research: a proposed explanation. *IRB: A review of human subjects* 1987;17:7–10.

Kaptchuk TJ, Eisenberg DM. Varieties of healing. 1: medical pluralism in the United States. *Ann Intern Med* 2001;135:189–95.

Kerridge J, Lowe M, Henry D. Ethics and evidence based medicine. *BMJ* 1998;316:1151–3.

Linde K, Jonas WB, Melchart D, Willich S. The methodological quality of randomised controlled trials of homeopathy, herbal medicine and acupuncture. *Int J Epidemiol* 2001;30:S26–31.

Stone J. *An Ethical Framework for Complementary and Alternative Therapies*. London: Routledge, 2002.

Stone J, Matthews J. *Complementary Medicine and the Law*. Oxford: Oxford University Press, 1996.

CHAPTER 9

THE PREVALENCE OF COMPLEMENTARY AND ALTERNATIVE MEDICINE USE AMONG THE GENERAL POPULATION: A SYSTEMATIC REVIEW OF THE LITERATURE

Philip Harris and Rebecca Rees

BACKGROUND

To assess the implications of complementary and alternative medicine (CAM) for healthcare systems it is essential to know its prevalence, or the proportion of a population using it at a given point in time. Reliable information about the use of CAM is needed to determine the requirements for research and development, education and regulation in the CAM field. While there have been a number of reviews of CAM use among clinical populations (Ernst, 1998, 1999; Ernst and Cassileth, 1998) no systematic reviews of CAM use among general populations have been published to date.

There are difficulties in systematically addressing previous surveys of CAM. These arise partly because it is difficult to define CAM. Some have attempted to define CAM in terms of concepts and models, which differentiate CAM from conventional biomedicine (e.g. Aakster, 1986). This approach suggests that conventional and unconventional medicine differ

Edited from an original article in *Complementary Therapies in Medicine* 2000;9:88–96.

in terms of the models that underlie them and in their concepts of health, disease, diagnosis, therapy and the patient. The difficulty of dichotomizing in this way is that the defining criteria do not always apply to every member of one category and none of the other. For example, the perception of the patient as an active participant in treatment may be more prevalent in CAM (although this has yet to be demonstrated), but it is by no means exclusive to it.

Others have defined CAM by categorizing together all forms of healthcare which are outside the domain of the politically dominant health system of a particular society or culture. The Office of Alternative Medicine's Panel on Definition and Description (Office of Alternative Medicine, 1997) noted that this approach engenders the problem of fuzzy and impermanent boundaries between the CAM domain and the domain of the dominant system. It also results in a mixed bag of therapies ranging from self-care, to folk remedies native to a particular culture and practices adopted from other cultures.

For the survey researcher, the way in which CAM is defined has practical implications for the conduct and outcome of a survey. The survey technique depends upon a relatively simple form of communication between researcher and respondent, to assist high response rates, questions are necessarily short and uncomplicated. In surveys of healthcare usage, respondents are commonly presented with checklists of practices and asked to select those they have used. Evidently, the type and number of practices included in the checklists will help to determine the participants' responses and subsequently the estimated prevalence rates. Although survey research in the last decade has helped to throw some light on the types of CAM therapies that are used by the general population, there remains a lack of consensus about which type and how many therapies should be examined. Furthermore, findings are often confounded by a lack of distinction between CAM involving visits to CAM practitioners and the use of over-the-counter CAM products. The decision about which CAM practices to include in a survey checklist will depend upon the research question, however, a clear rationale for their inclusion is essential.

We know of no studies that address the question of how best to review surveys that aim to estimate prevalence of a health behaviour. One issue that has to be of considerable importance is the methodological quality of the studies found. Standard survey methods texts (e.g. Crombie and Davies, 1996; Fowler, 1995; Oppenheim, 1992) describe the importance of reliable and meaningful data collecting tools and methods that attend to the possibilities of obtaining a biased selection of the population. Sample sizes are of fundamental importance, needing to be sufficiently large to achieve prevalence estimates with acceptable confidence intervals. These confidence intervals should then be presented so that readers can see from themselves the likely precision of the survey's estimates (Gardner and Altman, 1986). Methods in general need to be described in some detail for a survey's results to be appraisable. In developing the criteria necessary for assessing study quality in this review we have used these basic aspects of quality, drawn on our own experiences as survey researchers and considered criteria used in previous reviews of CAM surveys (e.g. Ernst, 1998, 1999; Ernst and Cassileth, 1998). We hope that these criteria will also help to serve as a guide to good practice in future CAM surveys.

The study described here aimed to systematically examine published surveys addressing the question, 'what proportion of the general public uses CAM?' It describes use of an explicit protocol that contained inclusion and exclusion criteria to select papers for review, and guidelines for extracting and presenting data from studies as they were found. Findings and the limitations of this approach are discussed. Recommendations are made for future studies of CAM prevalence.

METHOD

A systematic search of the literature was conducted. Simple searches were made of two bibliographic databases. Medline (OVID CD-ROM) was searched for all years up to September 1999. The search looked for all records: 1) indexed with any term from the hierarchy of controlled index terms headed 'alternative medicine' and, 2) characterized by having either 'health care surveys' as an index term or 'survey' in their abstract or title. CISCOM, a database specializing in complementary medicine (held by the Research Council for Complementary Medicine in London), was searched for all entries up to August 1999 using the index terms 'survey' and 'usage'. Further attempts to locate papers were made by examining citations in the most relevant papers.

Papers were included for review if they met all three of the following selection criteria:

1. the study used survey methods (either structured interview or self-complete questionnaire) to estimate the extent of CAM use among a target population
2. CAM use was measured among the general population, as opposed to a clinical population or other, more narrowly defined groups
3. the prevalence of CAM estimated by the study was expressed as a percentage of the population, or sufficient information was presented so that this could be calculated.

Papers were excluded if any of the following three criteria applied:

1. the study estimated the prevalence of a single therapy only, e.g. homoeopathy, traditional Chinese medicines

2. it did not describe the study methods, e.g. brief reports describing publication elsewhere, letters to journal editors
3. it was not written in English.

The following methodological details were recorded for each included paper when and if described by the papers' author(s):

1. the mode of data collection (whether face-to-face interview, telephone interview or self-complete questionnaire)
2. number of questionnaire respondents or interview participants (n)
3. the sampling methods used to select potential respondents (sampling technique and source of the individuals sampled)
4. the response rate (as presented by the paper's authors)
5. whether the author(s) performed an initial sample size calculation
6. the authors' explanation of their choice of CAM categories and/or definitions presented to respondents and/or questionnaire design (whether these were developed through pilot studies with a similar sample, via expert review or were based on previous work)
7. whether the questionnaire or interview schedule was tested for reliability as a data collection tool
8. whether adjustments were made to account for differences between respondents and the general population and/or the representativeness of survey respondents was examined.

Each paper was then examined for the following substantive information:

1. the date of survey administration
2. the target population (in terms of country of origin, population group within that country, and age group)
3. the therapies listed or referred to in questionnaires or interview schedules
4. estimated prevalence of use of CAM.

For the last of these categories, estimates were recorded separately, when possible, to account for measurement of:

1. total usage of CAM: involving visits to CAM practitioners and use of over-the-counter (OTC) products combined
2. use of visits to CAM practitioners alone
3. use of over-the-counter products alone.

Where confidence intervals were not presented by authors, these were calculated, assuming that variance arose from simple random sampling. When figures for the prevalence of use of a specific therapy were presented in at least six papers, these estimates were also tabulated.

RESULTS

A total of 638 references were found, 491 via Medline, a further 147 via CISCOM. No additional papers were found by citation tracking. Of this 638, only 12 met all of the study's inclusion criteria (Bernstein and Shuval, 1997; Burg, Hatch and Neims, 1998; Eisenberg et al, 1993; Eisenberg et al, 1998; Landmark Healthcare, 1998; MacLennan, Wilson and Taylor, 1996; Millar, 1997; Paramore, 1997; Thomas et al, 1993; Vaskilampi, Merilainen and Sinkkonen, 1993; Verhoef, Russell and Love, 1994; Yung et al, 1988). Four hundred and forty-one had not measured the extent of CAM use. A further 137 studies had surveyed people about their use of CAM but had not used samples selected from the general population. An additional 39 papers asked respondents about a single CAM therapy or approach. A total of eight papers did not describe original research or provide sufficient detail and one study (an undergraduate thesis) was unobtainable within the timeframe of the study. A list of papers excluded is available from the authors on request.

Methodological quality

The 12 surveys reviewed are listed in Table 9.1, ordered by country of origin and then by date of publication. It is evident that some authors failed to report important methodological information. Two studies did not specify the sampling method used and three simply stated that random samples were used without providing further detail of randomization. Only one (Millar, 1997) of these five studies referred to published reports for a more comprehensive description of the survey design, sample and interview procedures. The seven remaining studies gave some description of the method of randomization used.

Three of the 12 studies failed to specify their survey's response rate (Bernstein and Shuval, 1997; Landmark Healthcare, 1998; Millar, 1997) and although all the remaining studies stated crude response rates, a detailed breakdown of responses was uncommon. Survey non-responders tend to differ systematically from responders (Oppenheim, 1992). Nevertheless, only two studies (Thomas et al, 1993; Vaskilampi, Merilainen and Sinkkonen, 1993) explored reasons for non-participation.

Only three studies stated that sample size calculations were completed, before data collection, to determine the number of participants needed to produce prevalence estimates with predetermined confidence intervals. Any mention of confidence intervals was altogether missing from six of the 12 reports (Bernstein and Shuval, 1997; Burg, Hatch and Neims, 1998; Millar, 1997; Paramore, 1997; Vaskilampi, Merilainen and Sinkkonen, 1993; Verhoef, Russell and Love, 1994).

Table 9.1 **Methodological quality of surveys of complementary and alternative medicine use**

Author Place	*Survey mode*	*n*	*Sampling methods*	*Response rate (%)*
MacLennan et al, 1996 Australia	Face-to-face interview	3004	Systematic sampling of districts, random selection of households, selection of respondents not specified	73
Verhoef et al, 1994 Canada	Face-to-face interview	563	NS	78
Millar, 1997 Canada	Face-to-face interview	17626	NS (cites reports)	NS
Vaskilampi et al, 1993 Finland	Telephone interview	1618	Stratified random sample from Census Bureau	92
Bernstein and Shuval, 1997 Israel	Face-to-face interview	2030	Random sample (no detail)	NS
Yung et al, 1988 UK	Self-complete questionnaire	4268	Systematic random sample from electoral register	70
Thomas et al, 1993 UK	Self-complete questionnaire	676	Systematic random sample from electoral register	73
Eisenberg et al, 1993 USA	Telephone interview	1539	Random digit dialling to select households, random selection of respondent within household	67
Eisenberg et al. 1998 USA	Telephone interview	2055	Ditto above with further random sample of initial refusals	60
Paramore, 1997 USA	Telephone interview	3450	National probability sample (no detail)	75
Burg et al, 1998 USA	Telephone interview	1012	Random digit dialling to select households, stratified by region	54
Landmark Healthcare, 1998 USA	Telephone interview	1500	Random sample of households (no details)	NS

Sample size calculation?	*Rationale for therapy choice and question wording*	*Reliability of survey assessed*	*Data examined/adjusted for representativeness*
Sample size calculated	NS	NS	Data weighted by age, gender and geographical region to the 1991 South Australian Census
NS	NS	NS	Sample considered to be similar to rural population of Alberta (no detail)
NS	NS	NS	Data age adjusted based on estimated 1994 Canadian population (no detail)
NS	Refers to pilot studies (no detail)	NS	Compares sample with Government statistics on a range of sociodemographic variables
NS	NS	NS	Representative sample (no detail)
NS	NS	NS	Respondents do not differ from 1981 census data for same area (no detail)
NS	Describes pilot study	5% of sample checked	Compares age and gender to 1991 OPCS General Household Survey
Sample size calculated	Refers to pilot study (no details)	5% of sample checked (no results given)	Compares sample with 1989 National Health Interview Survey on a range of sociodemographic variables
Sample size calculated	Replicates 1993 study	NS	Compares sample with US Census on a range of sociodemographic variables
NS	NS	NS	Estimates weighted to US civilian, non-institutionalised population (no detail)
NS	Investigator judgement	NS	Sample representative of Florida population for sex, race and annual household income
NS	NS	NS	Compares age, ethnicity and education of sample to 1990 US Census

Only three studies referred to the use of pilot work in the development of the data collection tools (Eisenberg et al, 1993; Thomas et al, 1993; Vaskilampi, Merilainen and Sinkkonen, 1993) although little detail is given. More seriously, all of the studies failed to give a clear rationale for the type and number of CAM categories included for data collection. This is a worrying omission as there may be a tendency for prevalence estimates to increase directly with the number of CAM categories used for data collection.

The reliability of responses to the survey was checked in only two cases: MacLennan (1996) re-interviewed 5% of the sample by telephone, but results were not described; Thomas (1993) followed-up a 5% sample of respondents by interview and comparison was made of their verbal and written responses to check for accuracy of response and comprehensibility of the questionnaire, it emerged that some respondents had confused the word 'chiropractor' with 'chiropodist', leading to possible overestimates for this therapy.

Finally, and perhaps most importantly, nine studies either described their findings as representative (Bernstein and Shuval, 1997; Burg, Hatch and Neims, 1998; Eisenberg et al, 1993; Eisenberg et al, 1998; MacLennan, Wilson and Taylor, 1996; Vaskilampi, Merilainen and Sinkkonen, 1993) or generalized their results to the target population (Landmark Healthcare, 1998; Millar, 1997; Paramore, 1997). However, only six of these studies supported the claim with some evidence: MacLennan (1996) stated that the survey data were weighted by age, gender and geographical region to the 1991 census data for the South Australian population; and the remaining five studies (Burg, Hatch and Neims, 1998; Eisenberg et al, 1993; Eisenberg et al, 1998; Landmark Healthcare, 1998; Vaskilampi, Merilainen and Sinkkonen, 1993) compared their sample with the target population on a range of demographic variables.

Substantive findings

Table 9.2 shows the prevalence rates for CAM identified in each of the studies. Due to their methodological rigour, the MacLennan (1996) and two Eisenberg studies (Eisenberg et al, 1993; Eisenberg et al, 1998) have produced the most reliable prevalence figures. MacLennan reported that during 1993, almost half the population of South Australia had used non-medically prescribed alternative medicines, and about one-fifth had visited CAM practitioners. The Eisenberg studies suggested that the use of CAM products or practitioners increased significantly in the USA from 33.8% of the population in 1990 to 42.1% in 1997. Reported visits to practitioners also increased, from 12.3% to 19.5%. The second study (Eisenberg et al, 1998) stated that expenditure on CAM increased by

45.2% between surveys and was conservatively estimated at $21.2 billion in 1997.

The remaining prevalence estimates shown in Table 9.2 are less reliable due to limitations in their methods and/or study reporting. The best estimates for the UK come from Thomas (Thomas et al, 1993). This study does not claim to be representative of the UK population. It found that in 1993, 8.5% of respondents had visited a CAM practitioner. It is difficult to compare this with the prevalence rate of 2.6% obtained by Yung in 1986 (Yung et al, 1988) because of geographical and methodological differences between the two studies. In Canada, prevalence estimates for visits to CAM practitioners ranged from 19.8% for all ages in Alberta in 1992 (Verhoef, Russell and Love, 1994), to 15% in a nation-wide study of Canadians aged 15 and above in 1995 (Millar, 1997). In 1993, about 6% of Jewish adults aged 45–75 (younger adults were not represented in this study) were reported to have visited a CAM practitioner (Bernstein and Shuval, 1997).

Estimates for the prevalence of use of CAM as a whole (consultations and/or use of products) also vary. As expected, these estimates tend to be larger than those for the prevalence of consultations alone. The two Eisenberg studies suggest that the number of people using CAM more than doubles if the definition of CAM includes use of products as well as consultations with therapists.

Table 9.3 shows prevalence estimates for individual therapies named in six or more of the 12 studies. There is some consistency among the findings, notably, chiropractic was the most prevalent therapy reported by all studies cited with the exception of the Israeli survey (which did not represent adults under 45 years). Massage tended to be the second most used therapy. Interestingly, its use was found to be particularly common in the Finnish survey (Vaskilampi, Merilainen and Sinkkonen, 1993), where effort was made to ensure that respondents could distinguish between 'alternative massage' and that provided by physiotherapists. In a separate section of the Landmark survey (Landmark Healthcare, 1998), acupuncture was identified as the best known therapy. However, with the exception of the Burg study, no study showed more than 2% of respondents reporting its use. Differences in the findings are also evident, notably, in the two USA surveys collecting data about CAM use in 1997 (Eisenberg et al, 1998; Landmark Healthcare, 1998). These two studies reported markedly different prevalence estimates, both for chiropractic and massage.

Since they impact on the measurement of CAM use, the definitions (explicit and implicit) of CAM use seen in these surveys and the populations and time periods under study need to be described in some detail. Some, but not all authors distinguished between CAM consultations and over-the-counter (OTC) product use: five studies (Bernstein and Shuval, 1997; Millar, 1997; Paramore, 1997; Verhoef, Russell and Love, 1994;

Table 9.2 Prevalence of CAM use (unless specified, figures are for use in the previous 12 months for populations described in Table 9.1)

Authors	*n*	*Date*	*Target population* *Country*	*Population*	*Age (yr)*
MacLennan et al, 1996	3004	1993	Australia	South Australia	≥15
Verhoef et al, 1994	563	1992 use in previous 6 months	Canada	Rural West-Central Alberta	all ages
Millar, 1997	17626	1995	Canada	Nationwide excepting Indian reserves/ military bases/some remote areas	≥15
Vaskilampi et al, 1993	1618	1982	Finland	Nationwide	15–64
Bernstein and Shuval, 1997	2030	1993	Israel	Jewish adults in urban settings with population of ≥5000	45–75
Yung et al, 1988	4268	1986	UK	Residents of city of Cardiff, Wales	≥18
Thomas et al, 1993	676	1993	UK	Nationwide	≥18

Therapies listed		*Prevalence – % (95% CI)* *Visits or OTC*	*Visits*	*OTC use*
Acupuncture Aromatherapy Chiropractic Herbal therapy Homoeopathy Iridology	Naturopathy/Natural therapy Osteopathy Reflexology Other	Data not presented	20.3 (18.9–21.7)	48.5 (46.7–50.3)
Chiropractic plus 'other' examples given: Environmental medicine Faith healing	Herbalism Homoeopathy Hypnosis Naturopathy Reflexology	–	19.8 (16.5–23.1)	–
Acupuncture Biofeedback Chiropractic Feldenkrais/Alexander technique Herbalism Homoeopathy Massage	Naturopathy, reflexology Relaxation therapy Rolfing Self-help group Spiritual healing Religious leader	–	15 (14.5–15.5)	–
Acupuncture Cupping/blood-letting Massage Natural food/special products Natural remedies Hypnosis	Physiotherapeutic treatments Relaxing treatments Vertebrae treatment (bone-setting) Other folk healers	23 (20.9–25.1)	Data not presented	Data not presented
Therapies given as examples only: Acupuncture Biofeedback Chiropractic	Herbalism Homoeopathy Naturopathy Reflexology	–	6 (5–7)	–
Non-NHS: Acupuncture Chiropractic/Osteopathy Herbal treatment	Homoeopathy Hypnotism Other	–	2.6 (2.2–3.0)	–
Acupuncture Chiropractic Osteopathy Herbal medicine	Homoeopathy Hypnotherapy Other	Data not presented	8.5 (6.7–10.8)	25.1 (21.8–28.4)

Continued overleaf

Table 9.2 Continued

Authors	*n*	*Date*	*Target population* *Country*	*Population*	*Age (yr)*
Eisenberg et al, 1993	1539	1991	USA	Nationwide	≥18
Eisenberg et al, 1998	2055	1997	USA	Nationwide	≥18
Burg et al, 1998	1012	1996 any use prior to this date	USA	State of Florda	≥18
Paramore, 1997	3450	1994	USA	Nationwide	all ages
Landmark Healthcare, 1998	1500	1997	USA	Members of health insurance or care plans, nationwide	≥18

Yung et al, 1988) sought and presented prevalence figures for consultations only; the studies by MacLennan (1996) and Thomas (1993) estimated product use and consultation separately, but did not present a prevalence figure for their combined usage. In contrast, the two USA studies by Eisenberg (1993, 1998) presented data for: 1) consultations and product use combined; and 2) consultations alone, but no estimate for the prevalence of product use, despite this data being presumably available to them. The remaining three studies (Burg, Hatch and Neims, 1998; Landmark Healthcare, 1998; Vaskilampi, Merilainen and Sinkkonen, 1993) only presented data for the combined use of CAM.

In most of the surveys reviewed, therapies were listed as response options. In contrast, Bernstein (1997) listed six therapies simply as examples of CAM types and two studies (Landmark Healthcare, 1998; Vaskilampi, Merilainen and Sinkkonen, 1993) failed to explain how they asked respondents about their CAM use. These differences between the

Therapies listed		*Prevalence – % (95% CI)* *Visits or OTC*	*Visits*	*OTC use*
Acupuncture Biofeedback Chiropractic Commercial diet Energy healing Folk remedies Herbal medicine	Hypnosis Imagery Lifestyle diet Massage Megavitamins Relaxation techniques Self-help group	33.8 (31–37)	12.3 (10.7–13.9)	Data not presented
Ditto above		42.1 (40.0–44.2)	19.5 (17.9–21.3)	Data not presented
Acupuncture Biofeedback Energy healing Herbal medicine Homoeopathy Hypnosis	Massage Megavitamins Relaxation techniques Special diets + Home remedies	62 (59.0–65.0)	Data not presented	Data not presented
Acupuncture Chiropractic	Massage Relaxation techniques	–	9.4 (8.4–10.4)	–
Acupressure Acupuncture Biofeedback Chiropractic Herbal therapy	Homoeopathy Hypnotherapy Massage Naturopathy Vitamin therapy Yoga	42 (39.5–44.5)	Data not presented	Data not presented

authors' implicit definitions of CAM are illustrated in Table 9.2. The number of therapies identified ranged from four (Paramore, 1997) to 16 (Eisenberg et al, 1993; Eisenberg et al, 1998) with a mean of 9.8 across all 12 studies.

Studies also varied in terms of the time period and general populations under study. All but two of the 12 studies asked respondents about their use of CAM during the previous year: Verhoef (1994) only sought information about CAM use during the previous 6 months; Burg's study (1998) only asked respondents if they had 'ever' used CAM. Half of the surveys reviewed attempted to measure prevalence nationwide, others looked at a single city (Yung et al, 1988), regions (Burg, Hatch and Neims, 1998; MacLennan, Wilson and Taylor, 1996; Verhoef, Russell and Love, 1994), nation-wide members of health insurance schemes (Landmark Healthcare, 1998). One survey (Bernstein and Shuval, 1997) only included adults aged 45 to 75.

Table 9.3 Prevalence of visits to practitioners of individual therapies (unless specified, figures are for use in the previous 12 months for populations described in Table 9.1)

Source	*n*	*Country*	*% of total population visiting practitioners of specific therapies (95% CI)*					
			Acupuncture	*Chiropractic*	*Herbal therapy*	*Homoeopathy*	*Massage*	*Hypnotherapy*
MacLennan et al, 1996	3004	Australia	2.0	15.0	0.4	1.2	–	–
Verhoef et al, 1994	563	Canada	–	28.4*	–	–	–	–
Millar, 1997	17626	Canada	–	11.0	–	–	–	–
Vaskilampi et al, 1993	1618	Finland	2.0	–	–	–	11.0	0.5
Bernstein and Shuval, 1997	2030	Israel	1.2	0.4	–	2.0	–	–
Thomas et al, 1993	676	UK	0.6	2.1	1.0	1.9	–	0.4
Eisenberg et al, 1993	1539	USA	0.4	7.2	0.3	0.2	2.9	0.5
Eisenberg et al, 1998	2055	USA	0.9	9.9	1.8	0.6	6.8	0.8
Burg et al, 1998	1012	USA	4.0**	–	18.0**	5.0**	15.0**	2.0**
Paramore, 1997	3450	USA	0.4	6.8	–	–	3.1	–
Landmark Healthcare, 1998	1500	USA	1.9	15.8	2.6	1.4	11.8	0.8

*Figures are for 6 month use.
**Figures are for use 'ever'.

DISCUSSION

This review is restricted to the literature contained in two databases, both of which specialise in papers published in English. It is possible that studies conducted in countries where English is not the first language have been overlooked. The review also relies upon the assumption outlined in our introduction that it can be meaningful to measure CAM use by asking people to identify discrete behaviours such as a visit to a therapist or a purchase. People who have used such therapies may not always consider themselves to have been 'CAM users'. Furthermore, many CAM therapists are likely to use an unpredictable mixture of techniques and medications. This review's exclusion of studies that identify themselves as being interested mainly in one therapy may effectively have overlooked information about use of the components of such approaches.

The review was also made difficult by the quality of the papers found. Future CAM surveys need to pay greater attention to their survey methods. Sample size calculations (Lemeshow et al, 1990) with predetermined confidence intervals, probability sampling, and attention to sample representativeness are essential requirements. Methods need to be reported in full.

Despite these limitations, this review suggests that substantial proportions of the population in all of the countries surveyed use complementary and alternative therapies. A rigorous survey has been replicated in the USA so as to measure trends (Eisenberg et al, 1993; Eisenberg et al, 1998) and the findings support the view that the use of CAM has increased. It is evident that the best known therapies are not necessarily the most frequently used. It is also evident that prevalence estimates, both for CAM use in general as well as for individual therapies have varied considerably between studies.

There is little doubt that a comparison of prevalence data between studies is hampered by differences in the studies' definitions of CAM. The number of therapies listed may account for part of the marked variation seen, for example, between two almost concurrent US studies (Eisenberg et al, 1998; Landmark Healthcare, 1998). Differences in the time frame of CAM use also affect the comparability of surveys. The lifetime reference period used in the Burg study is the most likely explanation for the high rate of CAM use reported, as the authors pointed out their 'data are not directly comparable to studies reporting recent utilization'. Different ways of presenting data also hamper understanding. Figures need to be given for individual therapies if studies that ask about different sets of therapies are to be compared.

To improve comparability between studies we suggest the following guidelines for researchers thinking of examining the prevalence of CAM use:

- use and present a clear rationale for the type and number of CAM therapies and OTC products surveyed
- use a pretested questionnaire or structured interview to collect data or a pilot study to investigate the relevance and reliability of a new one
- choose reference periods for the use of CAM carefully – reports of recent use (past 12 months) are likely to be most reliable and this time period is used in most studies
- distinguish between CAM therapist consultations and OTC products when communicating with respondents
- request responses for each individual CAM therapy
- present separate prevalence estimates for each of the CAM therapies surveyed
- present separate estimates for CAM therapist consultations and the use of OTC products
- also present a separate estimate for the proportion of the population that has used CAM therapist consultations and/or CAM products.

As might be expected, the surveys that were the strongest methodologically were also the larger, better-funded ones. The methodological and reporting weaknesses identified in the other studies probably reflect the opportunistic nature of much CAM research. The MacLennon and the Eisenburg studies show what can be done if resources are prioritized towards a thorough and systematic investigation.

REFERENCES

Aakster CW. Concepts in alternative medicine. *Soc Sci Med* 1986; 22:265–73.

Bernstein JH, Shuval JT. Nonconventional medicine in Israel: consultation patterns of the Israeli population and attitudes of primary care physicians. *Soc Sci Med* 1997; 44:1341–8.

Burg MA, Hatch RL, Neims AH. Lifetime use of alternative therapy: a study of Florida residents. *South Med J* 1998; 91:1126–1131.

Crombie IK with Davies HTO. *Research in health care: design, conduct and interpretation of health services research*. Chichester: Wiley, 1996.

Eisenberg DM, Kessler RC, Foster C, Norlock FE, Calkins DR, Delbanco TL. Unconventional medicine in the United States: prevalence, costs and pattern use. *N Engl J Med* 1993; 328:246–52.

Eisenberg DM, Davis RB, Ettner SL, et al. Trends in alternative medicine use in the United States, 1990–1997. *JAMA* 1998; 280:1569–1575.

Ernst E. Usage of complementary therapies in rheumatology: a systematic review. *Clin Rheumatol* 1998; 17:301–5.

Ernst E. Prevalence of complementary/alternative medicine for children: a systematic review. *Eur J Pediatr* 1999; 158:7–11.

Ernst E, Cassileth BR. The prevalence of complementary/alternative medicine in cancer: a systematic review. *Cancer* 1998; 83:777–82.

Fowler, FJ. *Improving survey questions*. London: Sage, 1995.

Gardner MJ, Altman DG. Confidence intervals rather than *P* values: estimation rather than hypothesis testing. *British Medical Journal (Clin Res Ed)* 1986 Mar 15;292(6522):746–50.

Landmark Healthcare. *The Landmark Report on Public Perceptions of Alternative Care*. Sacramento: Landmark Healthcare, 1998.

Lemeshow S, Hosmer DW, Klar J, Lwanga SK. *Adequacy of sample size in health studies*. Chichester: Wiley, 1990.

MacLennan AH, Wilson DH, Taylor AW. Prevalence and cost of alternative medicine in Australia. *Lancet* 1996; 347:569–73.

Millar WJ. Use of alternative health care practitioners by Canadians. *Can J Public Health* 1997; 88:154–8.

Office of Alternative Medicine's Panel on Definition and Description, Defining and describing complementary and alternative medicine. *Altern Ther* 1997; 3:49–57.

Oppenheim AN. *Questionnaire design, interviewing and attitude measurement* (new edition). London: Printer, 1992.

Paramore LC. Use of alternative therapies; estimates from The 1994 Robert Wood Johnson Foundation National Access to Care Survey. *J Pain Sympt Management* 1997; 13:83–9.

Thomas KJ, Fall M, Nicholl J, Williams B. *Methodological study to investigate the feasibility of conducting a population-based survey of the use of complementary health care*. University of Sheffield: SCHARR, 1993.

Vaskilampi T, Merilainen P. Sinkkonen S. The use of alternative treatments in the Finnish adult population. In: GT Lewith, D Aldridge, eds *Clinical research methodology for complementary therapies*. London: Hodder & Stoughton, pp204–229, 1993.

Verhoef MJ, Russell ML, Love EJ. Alternative medicine use in rural Alberta. *Can J Public Health* 1994; 85:308–9.

Yung B, Lewis P, Charny M, Farrow S. Complementary medicine: some population-based data. *Compl Med Res* 1988; 3:23–8.

SECTION 2

USERS, PRACTITIONERS AND HEALTH BELIEFS: THE HEALING RELATIONSHIP IN CAM

INTRODUCTION

Geraldine Lee-Treweek

The readings in section two examine the fascinating issue of the relationships between CAM practitioners and the CAM user. Increasingly it is accepted that what goes on in the consultation room, with regard to social interaction as well as issues such as rapport and trust, have a profound effect upon service users. That is to say that a core component of a good CAM interaction is communication. A CAM practitioner will often have an extended therapeutic relationship with the user that may extend into some weeks or even for years. That relationship is not just about the practitioner 'healing' the user in a passive way but many CAM practitioners argue it is also about the user being empowered to take control of their own health and illness. Moreover there are important issues about the implicit messages about health that are conveyed during communication between the two. The crucial role of the therapeutic relationship in CAM is explored here through a series of both supportive and critical readings examining what really goes on when a CAM practitioner and the CAM user meet for the purposes of healing.

This set of readings begins by focusing on some of the cultural features of healing in the United Kingdom. Cecil Helman's reading presents a model of the types of healing used in the UK and notes the different settings and structures that affect the various therapeutic relationships within these. The divisions Helman espouses are controversial; bringing together a range of practices that readers may or may not agree with. However, it serves as a starting point for analysing the position of CAM.

Annie Mitchell and Maggie Cormack discuss some of the features of complementary therapy and the ramifications of these for the therapeutic relationship. A key element, they claim, is self-help and the CAM user's own responsibility for healing. This raises questions about whether complementary therapy creates distinctly different therapeutic relationships from those within orthodox health care practice. Similarly, Merrijoy Kelner's reading considers the notion that CAM therapeutic relationships cannot be understood using the concepts and ideas that have been applied to orthodox therapeutic relationships. She seems to be suggesting that in order to fully understand what goes on between the CAM practitioner and the user of the CAM service it is necessary to develop a range of new concepts and notions of what healing is really about.

Conversely, Geraldine Lee-Treweek's reading uses empirical data to examine the interior of the therapeutic relationship in osteopathy. This reading challenges the notion of the CAM therapeutic relationship as necessarily more empowering than an orthodox one. It raises questions such as what effect do the practitioner's words have on the way patients see their bodies and their understandings of their own health? Can the placing of responsibility for health upon users lead to self blame and practitioner-dependent behaviour? These are critical issues for all CAM practitioners if they seek to demonstrate the therapeutic relationship itself is a positive feature of what they have to offer.

Turning to more philosophical discussions of CAM relationships, Fritjof Capra outlines the way CAM approaches health by focusing on the individual. He also explores the way CAM approaches seek to understand stress in the individual and work to alleviate this problem. In this reading the CAM therapeutic relationship is emphasised as a support relationship. Rosalind Coward conversely directs our attention towards some of the possible negative consequences of therapeutic relationships that emphasise self-healing and responsibility for one's own health.

CHAPTER 10

HEALTH CARE PLURALISM IN THE UK

Cecil G Helman

In the UK, as in other complex industrial societies, there is a wide range of therapeutic options available for the alleviation and prevention of physical discomfort or emotional distress, and popular, folk and professional sectors of health care can be identified. This section will concentrate mainly on the popular and folk sectors. The professional sector has been examined in detail by medical sociologists such as Stacey (1976) and Levitt (1976). An overview of the three sectors of health care in the UK illustrates the full range of options available for the management of misfortune, including ill health.

THE POPULAR SECTOR

Two studies by Elliott-Binns (1973, 1986) are among the few dealing with lay therapeutic networks in the UK. Other studies have concentrated on the phenomenon of self-medication. For example in Dunnell and Cartwright's large study in 1972, the use of self-prescribed medication was twice as common as the use of prescribed medicines. Self-medication was most commonly taken for temperature, headache, indigestion and sore throats. These and other symptoms were common in the sample, but while 91 per cent of adults reported one or more abnormal symptoms during the previous 2 weeks, only 16 per cent of them had consulted a doctor

Edited from Ch 4, pp 69–78 in Helman CG. *Culture, Health and Illness.* New York: Arnold, 2001.

for this. Self-medication was often used as an alternative to consulting the doctor, who was expected to deal with more serious conditions. The idea of using a particular self-prescribed patent medicine came from a number of sources, including: spouses (7 per cent), parents and grandparents (18 per cent), other relatives (5 per cent), friends (13 per cent) and the doctor (10 per cent). Fifty-seven per cent of the sample thought the local pharmacist a good source of health advice for many conditions. This is confirmed in Sharpe's (Sharpe, 1979) study of a London pharmacy where, in a 10-day period, 72 requests for advice were received, especially for skin complaints, respiratory tract infections, dental problems, vomiting and diarrhoea. In another study by Jefferys and colleagues (1960) in a working-class housing estate, two-thirds of people interviewed were taking some self-prescribed medication, often in addition to a prescribed drug. Laxatives and aspirins were most commonly prescribed. The aspirins, and other analgesics, were used for many symptoms, including 'arthritis and anaemia, bronchitis and backache, menstrual disorders and menopausal symptoms, nerves and neuritis, influenza and insomnia, colds and catarrh, and of course for headaches and rheumatism'.

The hoarding and exchanging of medication, both patent and prescribed, is common in the UK. People who have been ill sometimes act as what Hindmarch (1981) terms 'over-the-fence physicians', sharing their prescribed drugs with a friend, relative or neighbour with similar symptoms. Warburton (1978) found that 68 per cent of young adults in his study in Reading admitted having received psychotropic drugs from friends or relatives. In his study in Leeds, Hindmarch also found that an average of 25.9 prescribed tablets or capsules *per person* were hoarded by people living in a selected street. Decisions whether to take prescribed drugs are also part of popular health culture, and lay evaluation of the drug as 'making sense' or not may, as Stimson (1974) suggests, influence non-compliance. The rate of this phenomenon has been estimated by him at 30 per cent or more.

Few studies have been done on the efficacy of popular health care in the UK. Blaxter and Paterson (1980), in their study of working-class mothers in Aberdeen, found that common children's illnesses (such as a discharging ear) were often ignored if they did not interfere with everyday functioning. However, in another study by Pattison and colleagues (1982) the findings were very different, and it was found that mothers were able to recognize their babies' illnesses and seek medical help, even with their first children.

An important component of the popular sector is the wide range of *self-help groups* that have blossomed in the UK since the Second World War. Like other parts of the popular sector, members' *experience*, not education, is important, especially experience of a specific misfortune. The total number of members of these groups is not known, though they number many thousands. The medical magazine *Pulse* (1982) has listed 335 groups loosely labelled 'self-help' in the UK or Eire, and there are several other directories of groups available.

Most self-help groups have, as Levy (1982) notes, one or more of the following aims or activities:

- information and referral
- counselling and advice
- public and professional education
- political and social activity
- fund-raising for research or services
- provision of therapeutic services, under professional guidance
- mutual supportive activities in small groups.

Robinson and Henry (1977) give a number of reasons for the growth of these groups in the popular sector, including the perceived failure of the existing medical and social services to meet people's needs, the recognition by members of the value of mutual help, and the role of the media in publicizing the extent of shared problems in the community. Other reasons might be the nostalgia for community (especially the caring community of the extended family) in an impersonal, industrialized world, as a coping mechanism for those with stigmatized conditions or marginal social status, and as a way of explaining and dealing with misfortune in a more personalized way.

THE FOLK SECTOR

In the UK, as in other Western societies, this sector is relatively small and ill defined. While local faith healers, gypsy fortune tellers, clairvoyants, psychic consultants, herbalists and 'wise women' still exist in many rural areas, the forms of diagnosis and healing characteristic of the folk sector are more likely to be found in urban areas, especially in alternative or complementary medicine. All estimates of the total number of consultations per year with alternative practitioners agree that the number is steadily rising (BMA, 1993).

As in non-Westem societies, many alternative/complementary practitioners aim at a holistic view of the patient, which includes psychological, social, moral and physical dimensions, as well as an emphasis on health as balance.

Herbalism, faith healing and midwifery probably have the deepest roots in Britain. The first description of herbal remedies dates from 1260 AD, and numerous other 'herbals' have been published in the past 400 years. In 1636, for example, a herbal compiled by John Parkinson contained details of the medicinal use of 3800 plants (Hyde, 1978). Midwifery, another traditional form of health care, has been absorbed into the professional sector, especially since their compulsory registration under the 1902 Midwives' Act. Other forms of healing have been imported from abroad, such as acupuncture, homeopathy and osteopathy.

The folk sector includes both sacred and secular healers. An example of the former is the National Federation of Spiritual Healers (NFSH), who define spiritual healing as 'all forms of healing the sick in body, mind and spirit by means of the laying-on of hands or by either prayer or meditation whether or not in the actual presence of the patient' (National Federation of Spiritual Healers).

As a form of alternative healing, *homeopathy* has a special position in the UK. The principles of homeopathy were first enunciated in Germany by Samuel Hahnemann in 1796, and the first homeopathic hospital in Britain was founded in London in 1849. There has been a long association between the British Royal Family and homeopathy; in 1937 Sir John Weir was appointed homeopathic physician to King George VI, and this link with Royalty remains. In 1948 the homeopathic hospitals were incorporated into the National Health Service. Although it ls based on different premises from orthodox medicine, homeopathy in the UK enjoys greater legitimacy than other forms of alternative healing. Like other forms of alternative/complementary medicine, it spans both folk and professional sectors of health care.

There is a two-way influence between these two sectors. Many orthodox doctors, for example, practise one or more forms of alternative healing. They are organized into collegial organizations such as the British Homeopathic Association, The British Society of Medical and Dental Hypnosis, the Chiropractic Medical Association, the Osteopathic Medical Association, the Psionic Medical Society, and the British Association for the Medical Application of Transcendental Meditation. Similarly, alternative healers have been influenced, to a variable degree, by the training, organization, techniques, credentials and self-presentation of orthodox doctors, and are increasingly becoming 'professionalized' – forming professional organizations with an educational structure, and registers of accredited members. Some are organized on a collegial basis, like other British professions – for example, the British Acupuncture Association, the National Institute of Medical Herbalists, the Society of Homeopaths, and the General Council and Register of Osteopaths.

At the other end of the spectrum are the more individual forms of folk healing, including clairvoyants, astrologers, psychic healers, clairaudientes, palmists, Celtic mediums, Tarot readers, Gypsy fortune tellers and Irish seers, whose advertisements appear in the popular press, magazines, handouts and such publications as *Prediction*, *Horoscope* and *Old Moore's Almanack*. Many of these act as lay counsellors or psychotherapists: 'Do you have a health worry that you cannot get help on? Have you a personal or family worry you need advice on? Then maybe I can help you with both. I was born the 7th Son of a 7th Son' (*Horoscope*, 1981). The majority of this group utilize some form of *divination*, using coins, dice, tea leaves, crystal balls or Tarot cards to decipher supernatural and cosmic influences on the individual and reveal the causes of unhappiness, ill health or other misfortune. From the patient's perspective, this approach may have the advantage of placing responsibility for misfortune beyond the individual's control; fate, bad luck or birth sign, not the patient's behaviour, are the causes of misfortune. Some of these healers are also undergoing professionalization. For example, since it was founded in 1976, the British Astrological and Psychic Society has promoted a variety of esoteric, spiritual and New Age teachings, and its members offer a wide range of 'interpretive and divinatory arts' (British Astrological and Psychic Society, 1998). The forms of divination they offer include astrology, palmistry, numerology, aura readings, graphology, trance mediumship, I Ching, Tarot cards, clairvoyance, clairaudience, clairsentience and psychic art. It publishes a National Register of Consultants, has defined criteria for entry, has a Code of Ethics and Conduct, and offers courses and certificates in different forms of divination. Its booklet states that its 'consultants are competent in several disciplines and can move between them in order to fulfil a client's given needs' (British Astrological and Psychic Society, 1998).

Many ethnic minorities and immigrants in Britain continue to consult their own traditional healers, at least under certain circumstances. These include Muslim *hakims* and Hindu *vaids* from the Indian subcontinent (one estimate is that there are about 300 of them in the UK) (Qureshi, 1990), practitioners of traditional Chinese medicine (including herbalism and acupuncture), African *marabouts* and *obeah men*, and West Indian spiritual healers.

One fairly new group of healers – in the broadest sense of the word – are those involved primarily in improving their client's physical appearance, and thereby their psychological state. Throughout the UK there has been a proliferation of 'beauty clinics', staffed by 'beauty therapists'. Both the setting and atmosphere of these clinics is quasi-medical, with consultations, white coats, rows of bottles, complex machines and impressive diplomas on the wall. They are all part of a much wider phenomenon; the gradual 'medicalization' of all aspects of the human body, including its appearance.

In recent years, as there has been growing criticism of conventional medicine in some quarters, so has there been a parallel increase in all forms of complementary and alternative medicine – and a burgeoning of organizations connected with it. The British Holistic Medical Association, one of the oldest of these organizations, has 1159 members, both medical and lay, about two-thirds of whom are practising health professionals (such as doctors, nurses, social workers and complementary practitioners). The BHMA sees the emergence of holistic medicine as representing 'an attempt to heal medical science itself by re-integrating psychological and spiritual dimensions into healthcare' (Anon, 1989).

No precise statistics exist about the total numbers of non-orthodox healers in the UK and the total number of consultations with them.

In 1989, The Institute for Complementary Medicine estimated that there were about 15 000 alternative practitioners in the UK in professional practice. They defined a 'practitioner' as an individual who is 'in full time practice, who is a member of a professional organization with a code of ethics and practice and a disciplinary committee to enforce them, and who is covered by personal indemnity and a third party liability'. On this basis, their figures included 7000 spiritual healers, 1500 osteopaths, 1500 acupuncturists, 1000 massage practitioners, 500 hypnotherapists, 350 nutritionists, 350 chiropractors, 300 reflexologists and 250 aromatherapists.

Training schools and professional associations for non-medically qualified healers continue to proliferate. For example, by 1996 the (non-medically qualified) homeopaths had two professional associations and 21 training schools, while the reflexologists had 13 professional organizations and over 100 schools (Cant and Sharma, 1996).

In 1993 The British Medical Association published a detailed report into alternative medicine in the UK (BMA, 1993), and their conclusions were cautiously positive: 'It is clear that there are many encouraging initiatives currently taking place in the field of non-conventional therapy, and it is to be hoped that good practice can be extrapolated for general use'. However, they recommended that, before making use of it, potential clients should inquire:

1. Whether the therapist is registered with a professional organization
2. Whether that body has a public register of members, a code of practice, effective disciplinary procedures and sanctions and a complaints mechanism
3. The type of qualifications the therapist has, and where they were obtained
4. How long he or she has been practising
5. Whether the therapist is covered by any form of malpractice insurance.

Also in 1993, by virtue of the Osteopaths Act, osteopathy joined the ranks of the recognized health care and paramedical professions for the first time – just as the pharmacists had done in 1852 and 1868, the dentists in 1878, and the midwives in 1902.

However, not all alternative healers want to become 'professions', under the direct or indirect control of the government or the medical system. Many are ideologically opposed to all aspects of the medical model and what they see as its limitations and dangers; thus they see themselves as truly *alternative*, rather than complementary, to it. Nevertheless, many forms of alternative medicine in the UK besides osteopathy – especially chiropractic, homeopathy, herbalism and acupuncture – are gradually undergoing the same process of professionalization as is happening to traditional folk healers in parts of the developing world (Cant and Sharma, 1996; Thomas et al, 1991).

THE PROFESSIONAL SECTOR

This includes the wide range of medical and paramedical professionals, each with their own perceptions of ill health, forms of treatment, defined areas of competence, internal hierarchy, technical jargon and professional organizations. The Office of Health Economics (1981) estimated the numbers of all health professionals within the NHS in 1980 as 23 674 general practitioners, 31 421 hospital medical staff, 301 081 hospital nursing staff, 17 375 hospital midwives, 32 990 community health nurses and 2949 community health midwives. In 1981 the community nurses included 9244 health visitors (DHSS, 1982). By 1990 the total number of nurses and midwives had risen to 505 250, over 50 per cent of the total staff employed by the NHS (Merry, 1993). In addition there are a large number of chiropodists, physiotherapists, occupational therapists, pharmacists and hospital technicians. Each of these categories offers some form of defined professional care, but they may also be called upon for informal advice about illness as part of the popular sector.

Despite its large size, it has been estimated (Wadsworth et al, 1971) that about 75 per cent of abnormal symptoms are treated *outside* the professional sector – which sees only the tip of the 'iceberg of illness' – and the rest are dealt with in the popular and folk sectors of health care.

In the UK, there are two complementary forms of professional medical care, the National Health Service and private medical care, though there is an overlap of personnel between the two.

The NHS and private sectors are not watertight; as with other areas of the health care system there is a considerable flow of ill people between them, and many doctors work within both systems.

THE HEALTH CARE SYSTEM IN THE UK

To view the UK health care system in perspective, most of the available sources of health care or advice are listed in Table 10.1.

'Healer" here refers to all those who, either formally or informally, offer advice and care for those suffering from physical discomfort and/or

Table 10.1 Professional, folk and popular healers in the UK

Hospital doctors (NHS)
General practitioners (NHS)
Private doctors (hospital or GP)
Nurses (hospital, school and community)
Midwives
Health visitors
Social workers
Physiotherapists
Occupational therapists
Pharmacists
Dieticians
Opticians
Dentists
Hospital technicians
Nursing auxiliaries
Medical receptionists
Local authority health clinics
Clinical psychologists and psychoanalysts
Counsellors (marriage, child guidance, pregnancy, contraception)
Alternative psychotherapists (Gestalt, bioenergetics, primal therapy etc.)
Group therapists
Samaritans and other 'phone-in' counsellors
Self-help groups
Yoga and meditation groups
Health food shops salespeople
Media healers (advice columnists in newspapers and magazines, TV and radio doctors)
Ethnic minority healers
Muslim *hakims*
Hindu *vaids*
Chinese acupuncturists and herbalists
West Indian healing churches
African *marabouts*
Healing churches and cults
Christian healing guilds
Church counselling services
Hospital and other chaplains
Probation officers
Citizens' Advice Bureaux
Alternative healers (lay and medical)
Acupuncture
Homeopathy
Osteopathy
Chiropractic
Radionics
Herbalism
Spiritual healing
Hypnotherapy
Naturopathy
Massage etc. Diviners
Astrologers
Tarot readers
Clairvoyants
Clairaudientes
Mediums
Psychic consultants
Palmists
Fortune tellers etc.
Lay health advisers (family, friends, neighbours, acquaintances, voluntary or charitable workers, salespeople, hairdressers, etc.)

psychological distress, or who advise on how to maintain health and a feeling of wellbeing. This list therefore spans all three sectors of health care in Britain – popular, folk and professional.

Case study: Sources of lay health advice in Northampton, UK

Elliott-Binns (1973) studied 1000 patients attending a general practice in Northampton, UK. The patients were asked whether they had previously received any advice or treatment for their symptoms. The source, type and soundness of the advice were noted, as well as whether the patient had accepted it. It was found that 96 per cent of the patients had received some advice or treatment before consulting their GP. Each patient had had an average of 2.3 sources of advice, or 1.8 excluding self-treatment; that is, 2285 sources of which 1764 were outside sources and 521 self-advice. Thirty-five patients received advice from five or more sources; one boy with acne received it from 11 sources. The outside sources of advice for the sample were: friend, 499; spouse, 466; relative, 387; magazines or books, 162; pharmacists, 108; nurses giving informal advice, 102; nurses giving professional advice, 52. Among relatives and friends, wives' advice was evaluated as being among the best and that from mothers and mothers-in-law the worst. Male relatives usually said 'go to the doctor', without offering practical advice, and rarely gave advice to other men. Advice from impersonal sources, such as women's magazines, home doctor books, newspapers and television was evaluated as the least sound. Pharmacists, consulted by 11 per cent of the sample, gave the soundest advice. Home remedies accounted for 15 per cent of all advice, especially from friends, relatives and parents.

Overall, the best advice given was for respiratory complaints, the worst for psychiatric illness. One example of the patient sample was a village shopkeeper with a persistent cough. She received advice from her husband, an ex-hospital matron, a doctor's receptionist and five customers, three of whom recommended a patent remedy 'Golden Syrup', one a boiled onion gruel, and one the application of a hot brick to the chest. One middle-aged widower had come to see the doctor complaining of backache. He had consulted no one because he 'had no friends and anyway if I got some ointment there's no one to rub it in'.

Elliott-Binns (1986) repeated this study 15 years later, on 500 patients in the same practice in Northampton. Surprisingly, the pattern of self-care and lay health advice had remained largely unchanged; 55.4 per cent of patients treated themselves before going to the doctor, compared to 52.0 per cent in 1970. The only significant changes were an increase in impersonal sources of advice on health, such as home doctor books and television, and a decline in the use of traditional home remedies (although they still accounted for 11.2 per cent of health advice). In addition, the use of advice from pharmacists increased from 10.8 per cent in 1970 to 16.4 per cent in 1985. Overall the study suggests that, in Britain, self-care still remains the chief source of health care for the average patient.

REFERENCES

Anonymous (1982). Self-help groups for your patients. *Pulse*, 29 May, 51–2.

Anon (1989). What is the British Holistic Medical Association? *Holistic Health*, 22, 36.

Blaxter, M. and Paterson, E. (1980). *Attitudes to health and use of health services in two generations of women in social classes 4 and 5*. Report to DHSS/SSRC Joint Working Party on Transmitted Deprivation (unpublished).

British Astrological and Psychic Society (1998). *British Astrological and Psychic Society: Society Information: New Edition – May 1998* (pamphlet). Nutfield.

British Medical Association (1993). *Complementary Medicine: New Approaches to Good Practice*, pp. 28–30. British Medical Association.

British Medical Association (1993). *Complementary Medicine: New Approaches to Good Practice*, p. 67. British Medical Association.

Cant, S. L. and Sharma, U. (1996). Professionalization of complementary medicine in the United Kingdom. *Compl. Ther. Med.*, 4, 157–62.

Department of Health and Social Security (1982). Personal communication, 24 November.

Dunnell, K. and Cartwright, A. (1972). *Medicine Takers, Prescribers and Hoarders*. Routledge and Kegan Paul.

Elliott-Binns, C. P. (1973). An analysis of lay medicine. *J. R. Coll. Gen. Pract.*, 23, 255–64.

Elliott-Binns, C. P. (1986). An analysis of lay medicine: fifteen years later. *J. R. Coll. Gen. Pract.*, 36, 542–4.

Hindmarch, I. (1981). Too many pills in the cupboard. *New Society*, 55, 142–3.

Horoscope (1981). Advertisement 29, p. 36.

Hyde, F. F. (1978). The origin and practice of herbal medicine. *MIMS Magazine*, 1 February, 127–36.

Institute for Complementary Medicine (1989). Personal communication, 17 July.

Jefferys, M., Brotherston, J. F. and Cartwright, A. (1960). Consumption of medicines on a working-class housing estate. *Br. J. Prev. Soc. Med.*, 14, 64–76.

Levitt, R. (1976). *The Reorganized National Health Service*. Croom Helm.

Levy, L. (1982). Mutual support groups in Great Britain. *Soc. Sci. Med.*, 16, 1265–75.

Merry, P. (ed.) (1993). *NHS Handbook*, 8th edn, p. 10. JMH Publishing.

National Federation of Spiritual Healers (undated pamphlet). *About the National Federation of Spiritual Healers*. NFSH.

Office of Health Economics (1981). *OHE Compendium of Health Statistics, 1981*, 4th edn. OHE.

Pattison, C. J., Drinkwater, C. K. and Downham, M. A. P. S. (1982). Mothers' appreciation of their children's symptoms. *J. R. Coll. Gen. Pract.*, 32, 149–62.

Qureshi, B. (1990). British Asians and alternative medicine. In: *Health Care for Asians* (B. R. McAvoy and L. J. Donaldson, eds), pp. 93–116. Oxford University Press.

Robinson, D. and Henry, S. (1977). *Self-help and Health: Mutual Aid for Modern Problems*. Martin Robertson.

Sharpe, D. (1979). The pattern of over-the-counter 'prescribing'. *MIMS Magazine*, 15 September, 39–45.

Stacey, M. (ed.) (1976). *The Sociology of the National Health Service*. Croom Helm.

Stimson, G.V. (1974). Obeying doctor's orders: a view from the other side. *Soc Sci Med.*, 8, 97–104.

Thomas, K. J., Carr, J., Westlake, L. and Williams, B. T. (1991). Use of non-orthodox and conventional health care in Great Britain. *Br. Med. J.*, 303, 207–10.

Wadsworth, M. F. J., Buttertield, W. J. H. and Blaney, R. (1971). *Health and Sickness: the Choice of Treatment*. Tavistock.

Warburton, D. M. (1978). Poisoned people: internal pollution. *J. Biosoc. Sci.*, 10, 309–19.

CHAPTER 11

WHAT IS DISTINCTIVE ABOUT COMPLEMENTARY MEDICINE?

Annie Mitchell and Maggie Cormack

An emphasis on self-healing gives rise to several distinctive features of complementary treatment which have been summarized by Fulder (1996) and which we will consider here in turn for their implications for the therapeutic relationship.

Distinguishing features of complementary medicine

- Symptoms may only be assessed in relation to a particular person.
- Mental, physical and spiritual aspects of the person may be seen as interdependent.
- A broad definition of health is used.
- There is an emphasis on treating chronic disorders.
- There is a relatively low risk of side-effects.
- The patient is expected to do what he can to help himself.
- There is an emphasis on the patient's perspective.

SYMPTOMS MAY ONLY BE ASSESSED IN RELATION TO A PARTICULAR PERSON

The complementary practitioner aspires to treat the person rather than the disease. The person's difficulties are considered to be only understandable

Edited from Mitchell A, Cormack M. pp 9–15 *The Therapeutic Relationship in Complementary Health Care*. Edinburgh: Churchill Livingstone, 2003.

in the context of his constitutional background, life history and current circumstances. Treatment seeks to restore the person to his developmental potential through realigning and restoring imbalances, defects and destructive patterns. Therefore, it is believed to be important to assess both how the impediments to development arose in the first place and what is maintaining the difficulties now. This requires taking a detailed history of the person's past and current experiences. Doing so has significant implications for the therapeutic relationship: telling one's story to someone who is genuinely concerned and interested, who listens, who appreciates its relevance to the person's difficulties can be a profoundly therapeutic experience in itself. Many patients feel that, at last, they and their suffering have been taken seriously.

MENTAL, PHYSICAL AND SPIRITUAL ASPECTS OF THE PERSON MAY BE SEEN AS INTERDEPENDENT

In complementary therapy, the patient is treated as a whole person, with no barriers between mind, body and spirit. This approach gives him the opportunity to make links between his psychological and physical symptoms, his past and current lifestyle and the issues and events which have been important to him.

Certainly, it is now accepted that physical and psychological distress occur together more frequently than chance alone would allow, and the developing field of psychoneuroimmunology is providing insights into the mechanisms underlying the relationship between the mind and the body (Martin, 1997). It is already well established that people with more diversified social networks live longer than their counterparts with fewer types of relationships (House et al, 1988) and have less anxiety, depression and non-specific psychological distress (Cohen and Wills, 1985). Participation in a more diverse social network may influence motivation to care for oneself by promoting feelings of self-worth, responsibility, control and meaning in life and it seems that the impact of these processes on health and illness may be mediated via the immune system. In terms of both causation and maintenance of disorder, as well as in recovery, the traditional distinctions in orthodox medicine between psychiatric disorders, physical disorders in which a psychological component can be identified (psychosomatic disorders) and physical disorders without psychological involvement are now outmoded. Rather, psychosocial factors as well as organic factors may influence the whole spectrum of health disorders (Steptoe, 1991).

A report on the psychological care of medical patients by the Royal College of Physicians and the Royal College of Psychiatrists (1995) concluded that modern medicine is orientated towards technological investigations which may divert attention away from psychological problems. The bodily expression of psychological distress can lead to costly but unrewarding searches for organic disease while patients may not be receiving the real help they need. It was reported that between a quarter and half of all new medical outpatients experience physical symptoms that could not be explained on the basis of organic disease alone and up to half of such patients had underlying anxiety and depression. Equally, patients who present to orthodox medicine as primarily psychologically distressed frequently do not receive medical recognition or care for their bodily disorders. Maguire and Granville-Grossman (1968) found one-third of consecutive psychiatric inpatients had significant physical illness which had not been treated and Hall et al (1980) discovered physical illness requiring medical treatment in 80% of patients in a US psychiatric assessment centre.

The difficulty for orthodox approaches is that the dualistic thinking which separates physical from psychological functioning leads to an assumption that illness or symptoms are either physical or mental, thus leading to the neglect of whatever is less salient in the person's initial presentation. The advantage of complementary approaches for the patient is that he can be seen as a whole person whose psychological and physical suffering and distress permeate his whole being. Treatment need not separate out his experiences arbitrarily but, rather, he can be treated in a way which validates his experience of himself as a coherent being.

A BROAD DEFINITION OF HEALTH IS USED

An emphasis on the positive aspects of health involves taking seriously, and treating, patients' poor vitality and low resistance. There is a recognition, too, of the significance of convalescence, of the patient gradually building up his reserves of strength and energy after a period of illness. The intention is to help the patient to reach, or regain, a position of optimum well-being so that he is less vulnerable to disease and illness or so that he is better able to cope with chronic conditions which cannot be cured. To do so requires enhancing morale as well as bodily well-being through the therapeutic relationship.

THERE IS AN EMPHASIS ON TREATING CHRONIC DISORDERS

Complementary approaches are most at home when dealing with chronic, psychogenic or organic disorders where the patient's own resilience plays a large part in his coping or recovery. This is the area of health care in which orthodox medicine has been less successful. By contrast, orthodox medicine has been strikingly successful in dealing with more acute diseases and injuries, where complementary approaches may have more of an adjunctive role to play. Again, as we will explore, the personal aspects of a positive therapeutic relationship have an essential part to play in promoting resilience.

THERE IS A RELATIVELY LOW RISK OF NEGATIVE SIDE-EFFECTS

The low incidence of side-effects is often considered to be one of the positive aspects of complementary health care. It is not necessarily always the case that complementary procedures, techniques or remedies are harmless even when practised or prescribed competently; indeed, anything which may have the power to heal may also have the power to harm. However, to the extent that treatment is aimed at self-righting the organism or promoting self-healing as opposed to directly challenging symptoms or diseases, then the risk of direct damage is considered small compared to the risks of more powerfully interventionist treatment.

Nevertheless, Coward (1989) has rightly warned against an assumption that complementary approaches are in some sense 'natural' or, indeed, that naturalness can be equated with harmlessness. It is important to recognize that patients' vulnerability inevitably exposes them to risk of damage as well as the possibility of beneficial change in relation to the practitioner's power, whether that power is personal or technical. For now, it is enough to recognize that the dangers of the abuse of the practitioner's power will be minimized if the patient's own central role in treatment and healing is recognized and strengthened. At the same time, practitioners of all disciplines need to retain an awareness of the limits of their own skills, abilities and knowledge (as well as the limits of the therapies they practise) so that patients are not denied treatment which may be more relevant, appropriate or effective for their needs.

THE PATIENT IS EXPECTED TO DO WHAT HE CAN TO HELP HIMSELF

In most complementary therapies, the patient is seen as an active participant rather than a passive recipient of treatment. This is really quite different from some orthodox health care where patients may be expected to 'comply' with medical treatment but not necessarily to take steps to promote their well-being through changes in lifestyle. Doctors and nurses in orthodox settings often express exasperation that many of their patients, especially those with chronic disorders, do not do enough to help themselves. Indeed, some orthodox practitioners in workshops have expressed envy of complementary practitioners whose patients, almost by definition, are those who have decided to do things differently, take matters into their own hands and who are therefore more likely to be receptive to ideas about taking responsibility for their own health.

In orthodox health care, any inclination the patient may have to take personal responsibility can sometimes be difficult to act on because of the long tradition of authority in medicine, where the doctor has greater technical knowledge and the patient's knowledge may not be viewed as relevant. Moreover, many orthodox doctors feel that the real time constraints in their consultations do not allow them the opportunity to explain and to share information which would motivate the patient to take responsibility for change. The approach in complementary health care makes it easier for practitioners to adopt a more collaborative style with their patients. The aim should be to help the patient to take responsibility for his health, but not to take the blame for his illness.

THERE IS AN EMPHASIS ON THE PATIENT'S PERSPECTIVE

We wish to encourage practitioners to continue, throughout their career, to recognize and respect the wisdom of their patients. We also encourage practitioners to heed the words of Oliver Sacks:

> There is only one cardinal rule: one must always listen to the patient and, by the same token, the cardinal sin is not listening, ignoring. Prior to any and all specific approaches, there must be this general approach, the establishment of a relation, a communication with the patient, so that patient and physician understand each other. A relationship, moreover, in which the patient is not entirely passive and compliant, believing and doing what he is told, and taking what is 'ordered'; a relationship which is, essentially, collaborative. (Sacks 1992: 252)

REFERENCES

Cohen S, Wills T A 1985 Stress, social support and the buffering hypothesis. *Psychological Bulletin* 98:310–357.

Coward R 1989 *The whole truth: the myth of alternative health*. Faber and Faber, London

Fulder S 1996 *The handbook of complementary medicine*. Oxford University Press, Oxford

Hall C W, Gardner E R, Stickney S L, LeCann A F, Popkin M K 1980 Physical illness manifesting as psychiatric disease. *Archives of General Psychiatry* 37:989–995

House J S, Landis K R, Umberson D 1988 Social relationships and health. *Science* 241:540-545

Maguire G P, Granville-Grossman K L 1968 Physical illness in psychiatric patients. *British Journal of Psychiatry* 114:1365–1369

Martin P 1997 *The sickening mind: brain, behaviour, immunity and disease*. HarperCollins, London

Royal College of Physicians and Royal College of Psychiatrists 1995 *The psychological care of medical patients. Recognition of need and service provision*. Royal College of Physicians and the Royal College of Psychiatrists, London

Sacks O 1992 *Migraine*. Picador, New York

Steptoe A 1991 The links between stress and illness. *Journal of Psychosomatic Research* 35(6):633–644

CHAPTER 12

THE THERAPEUTIC RELATIONSHIP UNDER FIRE

Merrijoy Kelner

We are witnessing a remarkable and widespread surge of interest in complementary & alternative medicine (CAM) and an increasing use of CAM practitioners (Eisenberg et al, 1993, 1998; McGregor and Peay, 1996; Lloyd et al, 1991; Thomas et al, 1991; Mills and Peacock, 1997; Lewith and Aldridge, 1993; CTV/Angus Reid Group, 1997). One of the reasons that has been cited for the current attraction to CAM practitioners is that they are more empathic and collaborative than physicians and take a greater interest in the individual psycho-social aspects of their patients' lives (Bakx, 1991; Oths, 1994). Patients are said to choose CAM practitioners because they seek a more satisfying therapeutic relationship (Brinkhaus et al, 1998). It has also been suggested that the high degree of rapport that exists between the alternative practitioner and his/her patient has a powerful placebo effect and may indeed be the key factor in the ability of these practitioners to help their patients (Ernst, 1995). However, the assumption that CAM patients have more positive and valuable relationships with their practitioners than do patients of family physicians has not yet been subjected to rigorous research (Mitchell and Cormack, 1998). It is a notion that requires serious examination rather than stereotypical thinking.

This paper will explore the nature of the therapeutic relationship between patients of family physicians and patients of selected alternative practitioners and compare the way these two sets of patients perceive and describe their practitioners. Based on the assumptions noted above, it can

Edited from Ch 4, pp 79–99 in Kelner M., Wellman, B., Pescasoliolo, B. and Sales, M., *Complementary and Alternative medicine: Challenge and Change,* Amsterdam: Harwood Academic Publishers, 2000.

be expected that patients of CAM practitioners will be more likely to describe their therapeutic relationships in a positive manner and to depict them as collaborative, empathic and personal.

MODELS

Models of the therapeutic relationship have been developed almost exclusively on the basis of the doctor-patient-relationship. The three most commonly mentioned models are: the paternalistic, the shared decision-making, and the consumerist. This paper looks not only at the doctor-patient-relationship, but also at patient relationships with a range of alternative practitioners, and examines the extent to which the existing models can be applied to them.

The Paternalistic model

Beginning in the 1950s, Parsons (1951) posited the relationship between physicians and their patients as the functional interplay between two social roles with inherent duties and responsibilities. The patient assumes a 'sick role' which exempts her/him from the normal obligations of life, but in turn, is obliged to comply with the physician's prescribed treatment and to strive to recover. While the patient always has the option to refuse treatment, s/he is not involved in the process of choosing among treatment options; the physician decides on the preferred option and then presents it to the patient. Parsons later revised his model to acknowledge the patient's participation in decision-making in the context of chronic illness (Parsons, 1975), but he still viewed the relationship as essentially a paternalistic one.

In this model of the therapeutic relationship, physician-patient interaction is said to be characterized by limited and didactic communication on the part of the physician, reluctance to give sufficient information to the patient about his/her condition, the use of medical jargon in discussions with the patient, and evasion of direct questions about diagnosis or treatment (Skipper, 1965).

The shared decision-making model

Szasz and Hollender (1956) have termed this the model of mutual participation. In this shared approach, the physician's expertise lies in his/her clinical knowledge, while the patient's expertise stems from knowledge of the contextual facts about his/her own personal situation. The role of the physician is to assist the patient (or the client) to make the treatment choice that is most appropriate through an understanding of how the medical information relates to his/her unique situation. This kind of encounter is particularly suited to the management of most chronic illnesses, where the patient's own experiences provide important clues for therapy. The patient accepts responsibility for carrying out changes in lifestyle recommended by the practitioner as part of the therapy. Such a model requires that there be ongoing dialogue between physician and patient (Katz, 1984).

The consumerist model

In striking contrast to the paternalistic approach and an extension of the shared decision-making pattern is the consumerist model. It places decision-making firmly in the hands of the patient/consumer (Emmanuel and Emmanuel, 1995). Physicians are viewed as service providers in the sense that while the doctor outlines the relevant clinical information to the patient, it is the patient who chooses the type of medical intervention that s/he wants. It is then up to the doctor to execute the chosen option.

The question examined here is which model of the therapeutic relationship best characterizes the needs and desires of health care providers and their patients in today's society. A second, but no less relevant question is what are the key elements of patient satisfaction driving the need to reexamine this relationship

PATIENT SATISFACTION

Analyses of modern medicine often point out that while medicine is at a technological high point in its development, patient satisfaction with medical care seems to be at an all time low (Balint et al, 1993). Research on patient satisfaction with medical care (Lewis, 1994; Greene et al, 1994; Lupton, 1996) makes it clear that patients today want to have more personal, less distant relationships with their physicians; more sharing of information; more time for consideration of their individual needs, including psycho-social issues, and greater opportunities to participate in decision making. In other words, patients are showing a preference for a model of care that most closely resembles the shared decision-making one. However, the current economic pressures on industrialized countries have made it difficult for physicians to give patients the amount of time and attention required to deliver care in this way.

It has been demonstrated that lack of satisfaction not only influences the extent of adherence to therapeutic advice (Linn et al, 1982; DiMatteo et al, 1985), but also that it frequently leads to 'doctor-shopping' (Kasteler et al, 1976; Haug and Lavin, 1983) and to changing doctors (Marquis et al, 1983; Ware and Ross-Davies, 1983).

COMPARING PATIENTS OF ALTERNATIVE PRACTITIONERS WITH PATIENTS OF FAMILY PHYSICIANS

At the outset of this comparison, the therapeutic relationships between CAM practitioners and their patients were expected to closely resemble the model of shared decision-making or the more extreme consumerist model. In comparison, the therapeutic relationships between physicians and their patients were still expected to adhere more closely to the model of paternalism. This supposition is examined by comparing the way patients of family physicians describe and evaluate their relationships with their doctors, with the way that alternative patients talk about their practitioners.

It was possible to make these comparisons on the basis of a research project designed to investigate the health beliefs and practices of a sample of 300 patients in the city of Toronto, Canada during 1994–95. At the time, these patients were consulting either family physicians (general practitioners) or one of four types of alterative practitioners: chiropractors, acupuncturists/traditional Chinese doctors, naturopaths or Reiki healers. These five types of practitioners were selected to represent a broad spectrum of the many types of health care currently available in Canadian society.[1]

COMPARING THE SAMPLE OF PATIENTS

Demographic characteristics – A comparison of the demographic characteristics of those who were consulting alternative practitioners with people who were seeing family physicians for their primary health problem, reveals that there are marked differences between the two groups of patients (see Kelner and Wellman, 1997a).

The patients consulting alternative practitioners are more likely to be female, young, married, highly educated, in higher level occupations, more likely to be employed full time and to have high incomes. Patients who consult alternative practitioners are also more likely to report their ethnic origin as Canadian, to have no formal religious affiliation but on the other hand, to consider spirituality an important factor in their lives.

Primary health problems – Patients of family physicians most frequently mentioned life threatening problems such as heart problems, high blood pressure and high cholesterol while none of the alternative patients reported cardiovascular conditions as their main reason for seeking care from their practitioners. Patients consulting alternative practitioners were seeing them for chronic conditions like musculoskeletal problems, headaches and for health maintenance.

COMPARING THE NATURE OF THE THERAPEUTIC RELATIONSHIP

Family physicians and their patients

A typical setting for the doctor patient relationship is formal and often institutional. The physician wears a white coat and practices in a professional office with a receptionist or nurse who sees the patients first. When patients are ushered into their physician's office, the doctor usually sits behind a desk and takes control of the interaction, posing a series of questions to the patient allowing little time for response. If a physical examination is required, patients move to another room, usually removing at least some of their clothing, and then return to the doctor's office to learn their diagnosis and hear the recommended treatment. This kind of setting contributes to social distance and establishes the physician's authority in the healing process.

The surprising finding here is that so many patients of family physicians reported that they had a good sense of rapport with them. In contrast to the studies cited above, where patients complained of a lack of interest and impersonal treatment, this was not the case for the family physicians' patients in this study.

How do these findings compare to the way the CAM patients describe their relationships with their practitioner?

CAM practitioners and their patients

CAM practitioners are not a homogeneous group; their practice patterns differ according to type of modality and also within each modality. Nevertheless, for purposes of analysis, the four types of CAM practitioners are mainly treated here as one group, although from time to time, the more striking differences between them are identified.

In comparison to the settings of the physician-patient encounter, CAM practitioners meet their patients in a less formal and structured environment. The practitioner may practice in an office or at home (chiropractors are more likely than homeopaths or Reiki healers to work in offices), but even in offices, the ambience is informal, with personal touches provided by signs and children's drawings on the walls. Most CAM practitioners eschew white coats and present themselves in a more informal manner. Some do not even use a desk, but prefer to sit close to their patients without any barriers between them. History taking, diagnosis and treatment often take place in the same room and the whole interaction seems more like a visit than a consultation.

Like the family physician patients, the CAM patients expressed high levels of satisfaction with their current practitioners.

Although both groups of patients expressed satisfaction with their current practitioners, they frequently had negative comments about the relationships they had with the health care providers they had seen in the past (mainly specialist physicians but also some CAM practitioners).

PAST EXPERIENCE

Reasons for dissatisfaction with past therapeutic relations related both to patients' expectations about receiving help and also to the way they were treated. They complained that their previous physicians or CAM practitioners were unable to give them relief from their health problems, or that the help they received was only short-lived. Other complaints, directed primarily at medical specialists, included inadequate or mistaken diagnoses, not being listened to or treated with respect, being rushed, lack of interest in their specific situation and too great a reliance on drugs and surgery instead of trying to get to the root of the problem.

The fact that the patients expressed considerable dissatisfaction with their previous health care providers is not surprising. If they had received the help they sought and had been able to develop a positive therapeutic relationship they would not have decided to look elsewhere. What we do not know is how the patients will feel in the future about their current physicians or CAM practitioners if they fail to meet their expectations. This research captures patients at only one point in their search for improved health and thus can not reveal the whole story.

DISCUSSION

Physicians and their patients relate to one another within the framework of the biomedical model, whereas CAM practitioners relate to their patients within a more holistic framework. Yet this study shows that in some ways, the relationships between CAM patients and their practitioners do not differ much from the relationships between family physician patients and their doctors. Both groups reported overall satisfaction with their health care providers and said they would recommend them to others. Both groups found care givers who will usually answer their questions, give them explanations, understand their perspective and to a lesser extent, involve them in decisions concerning their health care. It is important to remember that the respondents for this study were recruited in the offices of their health care providers and are thus likely to be satisfied consumers. Unfortunately, we do not know how those who have departed due to dissatisfaction would feel about their caregivers.

Where the two groups of respondents differed most was in the basis for their satisfaction. While only a small percentage of the physician patients were getting positive results from their current treatment, most of them nevertheless expressed trust in the skills and expertise of their doctors and some also mentioned rapport with them as an important element in the healing process. The CAM patients, on the other hand, placed most emphasis on positive results such as less pain and discomfort. Their relationships with their practitioners were largely pragmatic; if the practitioners could help them, they would continue to see them; if not, they would move on to try another practitioner or another kind of therapy.

The other major difference between the groups of patients was the role they saw for themselves in the healing relationship. While almost all respondents expected to have input into decisions about their care, there were differences in emphasis. Most family physician patients believed that their doctors should play the key role. CAM patients, on the other hand, typically believed each patient should have the main responsibility for their own health and decisions about which kind of treatment to pursue. Whereas physicians' patients favoured provider-control and placed their trust in their doctors, CAM patients more often favoured self-control and placed their confidence in themselves, or in themselves in partnership with their practitioners.

These findings indicate that the popularity of CAM practitioners can be attributed in large part to the search for relief from persisting chronic conditions. These patients want a practitioner who can help them cope with their ongoing problems. While physicians have had extraordinary successes with many acute illnesses such as polio, pneumonia and heart conditions, they have not been able to offer much assistance to their patients who suffer with chronic problems. Medicine continues to rely on its existing armamentarium of solutions such as drugs and surgery for conditions which require different and less drastic approaches. Physicians often discourage patients from presenting painful chronic conditions as their primary problems because there is little they can do to help.

The explanation presented at the beginning of this chapter that it is the more intimate and sympathetic style of interaction employed by CAM practitioners that explains their popularity was not upheld by the findings. Instead, they emphasize the continuing search for relief from chronic problems. This finding throws doubt on the claim that it is the response of CAM patients to their practitioners' holistic interest in them that is the chief reason for the ability of CAM to help chronic illness. While there is no question that patients' perceptions of the nature of the therapeutic relationship can have a significant influence on the outcome of their treatments, all kinds of interventions – medical and alternative, have a degree of placebo effect on the healing process (Lewith and Aldridge, 1993; Goldstein, 1999).

When we look at the continuum of care delineated by the three models of the doctor-patient-relationship: (1) paternalistic, (2) shared decision-making and (3) consumerist, we see that each model directs attention to different aspects of how the therapeutic relationship is structured. The paternalistic model was only minimally evident in the reports of the current experiences of all the patients, although one key element of the paternalistic model was still apparent in the relationship between most family physicians and their patients. It was the physicians who made the decisions about treatments and the patients who trusted in these decisions.

Paternalism was clearly evident, however, when it came to the stories that both groups of patients recounted about their past experiences with medical specialists. In many instances they reported evasion of their questions, limited communication, and complete physician control of decision-making. A distinction was thus apparent in the type of relationship the patients experienced with family physicians, as compared to the more authoritarian and remote medical specialists they had consulted.

It was the mid-point on the continuum, the shared decision-making model, that best reflected the relationships of most patients with their health care providers. Both groups reported that they typically shared clinical information with them, communicated well and proffered emotional support. The model fitted therapeutic relationships with CAM practitioners more closely, however, due to the partnership role they took with patients, particularly around psychosocial issues and recommended lifestyle changes.

At the far end of the continuum, the consumerist model was reflected in the desire of both kinds of patients to find a successful resolution to their chronic problems. This was particularly apparent when patients spoke of their past health care experiences. The pattern was that if the practitioner was found to be unable to help them, or failed to respect them and their opinions about treatment, most decided to act as 'smart consumers' and search for another physician or CAM practitioner who would listen more attentively and make more appropriate, individualized recommendations.

To reiterate, most of the relationships experienced by patients in this study fall somewhere in the middle of the continuum. Paternalism appears to be disappearing for family physicians, who are relating to their patients in more open ways. The authority of the physician over health care decisions is no longer as influential. They are not, however, assuming partnership roles with their patients to the same extent that characterizes therapeutic relationships with CAM practitioners and their patients. An interesting question for the future is whether patients of family physicians will come to expect the same kind of consultative and egalitarian relationship from their doctors that they have been experiencing with their CAM practitioners.

This study demonstrates that models of the practitioner-patient-relationship that were developed solely on the basis of doctors and their patients can be expanded to apply to relationships with patients and CAM practitioners as well. While the models do not fit the realties of health care perfectly, they do direct our attention to salient points concerning the ways in which both physicians and CAM practitioners relate to their patients, and they also enable us to see interesting differences between various types of CAM practitioners.

CONCLUSION

The key finding here is that while there are overarching differences in the nature of the therapeutic relationship that exists in medicine and in alternative care, both kinds of relationships are nevertheless positive and valuable, and not mutually exclusive. The physician relationship is based primarily on trust in expertise, while the CAM relationship is based principally on partnership in healing. The opportunity to take an active role may well be part of the attraction of CAM for patients. The research reported here, however, indicates that their primary motivation is the continuing search for relief from chronic problems. This motivation is not restricted to Canadians who use CAM, but also applies to patients in Britain, the United States and other countries where CAM is currently popular.

Further research on the nature and significance of the therapeutic relationship in CAM is needed to flesh out the picture portrayed here. Rather than rely on patients' accounts of past and present health care experiences, scholars can pursue this topic in depth through use of tape recorders and video cameras during the actual encounters, as Mishler and his colleagues have done for the doctor-patient-relationship (Mishler, 1984). Analysis of the content, the tone and the timing of the consultation between CAM practitioners and their patients can reveal the nuances of the dynamics involved in the healing encounter. Some questions that could be answered using these research methods include: (1) Do different types of CAM practitioners have different kinds of therapeutic relationships with their patients? (2) Do age, gender, and cultural differences generate different kinds of therapeutic relationships with a CAM practitioner? (3) At what point in the treatment process do CAM patients show an interest in the healing philosophy of their practitioners? (4) Do the characteristics of the therapeutic relationship vary according to different societal conditions and contexts? and (5) Will the increasing professionalization of CAM practitioners change the dynamics of the therapeutic encounter in the future? The nature of the relationship between patients and their CAM practitioners has yet to be fully identified.

REFERENCES

Bakx, K. 1991. 'The "Eclipse" of Folk Medicine in Western Society.' *Sociology of Health and Illness* 13:20–38.

Balant, E., M. Courtney, A. Elder, S. Hull, and P. Julian. 1993. *The Doctor, the Patient and the Group*. London: Routledge.

Brinkhaus, B., G. Schindler, M. Linder, A. Malterer, W. Mayer, R. Kohnen, and E.G. Hahn. 1998. 'User Profiles of Patients in Homeopathic and Conventional Medicine.' in *5th Annual Symposium on Complementary Health Care*. Exeter, UK.

DiMatteo, M.R., S.L. Linn, B.L. Chang, and D.W. Cope. 1985. 'Affect and Neutrality in Physician Behaviour: A Study of Patient's Values and Satisfaction.' *Journal of Behavioural Medicine* 8:397–409.

Eisenberg, David M., Ronald C. Kessler, Cindy Foster, Frances E. Norlock, David R. Calkins, and Thomas L. Delbanco. 1993. 'Unconventional Medicine in the United States: Prevalence, Costs and Patterns of Use.' *New England Journal of Medicine* 328:246–252.

Emmanuel, E.J., and L.L. Emmanuel. 1995. 'Four Models of the Physician-Patient Relationship.' Pp. 163–178 in *Health Care Ethics in Canada*, edited by F. et al. Baylis. Toronto: Harcourt Brace.

Ernst, Edzard. 1995. 'Placebos in Medicine.' *Lancet* 345:65.

Goldstein, Michael. 1999. *Alternative Health Care: Medicine, Miracle or Mirage?* Philadelphia: Temple Union Press.

Greene, M.G., R.D. Adelman, E. Friedmann, and R. Charon. 1994. 'Older Patient Satisfaction with Communication During an Initial Medical Encounter.' *Social Science and Medicine* 38:1279–1288.

Haug, Marie R. & Bebe Lavin. 1983. *Consumerism in Medicine: Challenging Physician Authority*. Beverly Hills: Sage.

Kasteler, J., R. Kane, D. Olsen, and C. Thetford. 1976. 'Issues Underlying Prevalence of "Doctor-Shopping" Behaviour.' *Journal of Health and Social Behaviour* 17:328–338.

Katz, Jay. 1984. *The Silent World of Doctor and Patient*. New York: The Free Press.

Kelner, Merrijoy, and Beverly Wellman. 1997a. 'Health Care and Consumer Choice: Medical and Alternative Therapies.' *Social Science and Medicine* 45:203–212.

Lewis, J. Rees. 1994. 'Patient Views on Quality Care in General Practice: Literature Review.' *Social Science and Medicine* 39:655–670.

Lewith, George T., and David Aldridge (Eds.). 1993. *Clinical Research Methodology for Complementary Therapies*. London: Hodder & Stoughton.

Linn, M.W., B.S. Linn, and S.R. Stein. 1982. 'Satisfaction with Ambulatory Care; and Compliance in Older Patients.' *Medical Care* 20:606–614.

Lloyd, P., D. Lupton, and C. Donaldson. 1991. 'Consumerism in the Health Care Setting: An Examploratory Study of Factors Underlying the Selection and Evaluation of Primary Medical Services.' *Australian Journal of Public Health* 15:194–201.

Lupton, Deborah (Ed.). 1996. *Your Life in their Hands: Trust in the Medical Encounter*. Cambridge: Blackwelt Publishers.

Marquis, M.S., A.R. Davis, and J.E. Ware. 1983. 'Patient Satisfaction and Change in Medical Care Provider: A Longitudinal Study.' *Medical Care* 21:821–829.

McGregor, Katherine J., and Edmund R. Peay. 1996. 'The Choice of Alternative Therapy for Health Care: Testing Some Propositions.' *Social Science and Medicine* 43:1317–132.

Mills, S., and W. Peacock. 1997. 'Professional Organization of Complementary and Alternative Medicine in the United Kingdom.'. Exeter: Centre for Complementary Health Studies, Department of Health, University of Exeter.

Mishler, E.G. 1984. *The Discourse of Medicine: Dialetics of Medical Interviews*. Norwood: Ablex Publishing Company.

Mitchell, Annie, and Maggie Cormack. 1998. *The Therapeutic Relationship in Complementary Health Care*. London: Churchill Livingstone.

Oths, K. 1994. 'Communication in a Chiropractic Clinic: How a D.C. Treats his Patients.' *Cultural Medical Psychiatry* 18(1):83–103.

Parsons, Talcott (Ed.). 1951. *The Social System*. Glencoe, IL: Free Press.

Parsons, Talcott. 1975. 'The Sick Role and the Role of the Physician Reconsidered.' *Millbank Memorial Fund Quarterly* 53:257–278.

Skipper, J. 1965. 'Communication and the Hospitalized Patient.' Pp. 61–82(21) in *Social Interaction and Patient Care*, edited by J. Skipper and R. Leonard. London: Pitman Medical.

Szasz, Thomas S., and Marc H. Hollender. 1956. 'A Contribution to the Philosophy of Medicine: The Basic Models of the Doctor-Patient Relationship.' American Medical Association: *Archives of Internal Medicine* 97:585–592.

Thomas, Kate J., Jane Carr, Linda Westlake, and Brain T. Williams. 1991. 'Use of Non-orthodox and Conventional Health Care in Great Britain.' *British Medical Journal* 302:207–210.

Ware, J.E., and A. Ross-Davies. 1983. 'Effects of the Doctor-Patient relationship on Subsequent Patient Behaviours.' in *American Public Health Association*. Dallas, TX.

ENDNOTE

1. In the Canadian national health insurance scheme, all medical services are covered by government insurance. Alternative care, on the other hand, is paid for by patients out of their own pockets, with the partial exception of chiropractic.

CHAPTER 13

I'M NOT ILL, IT'S JUST THIS BACK: OSTEOPATHIC TREATMENT, RESPONSIBILITY AND BACK PROBLEMS

Geraldine Lee-Treweek

In this article, osteopathic patients' accounts of treatment and attempts outwith the practice room to prevent further episodes are discussed. The article illustrates that the main strategy discussed by patients for controlling back pain recurrence was 'being careful'. The implications of these findings for osteopathic practice and the practitioner/patient relationship are outlined.

THE BODY AND ILLNESS

Academics from a number of disciplines and research perspectives have been interested in the problems raised by illness for the individual sufferer. Although their methods involve different procedures, their overall aim has been the same: to examine the complex experience of illness and to understand the social and individual meanings which the state of ill-health involves.

Prior to the onset of illness the individual is unreflective about their body, a consequence of which is that most people act in the world with little consideration of the body itself (Merleau Ponty, 1962). Therefore,

Edited from *Health* 5(1):31–49. Copyright © 2001. SAGE Publications, London, Thousand Oaks and New Delhi.

even though it is the vehicle of social life, the well body is almost invisible to the individual. As Williams notes: 'Bodies are a spontaneous unity or synthesis of powers ... we both feel and are embodied' (1996: 25). In the particular case of back problems the back is invisible to our everyday lives; it is used almost without thought, unless something has directly drawn our attention to its use, such as a back care training course, or if the onset of serious symptoms focuses our thoughts upon it. Illness makes the sufferers feel that they have a body, rather than simply being the body (Lupton, 1994: 79). As Williams (1996: 26) highlights, there is a sense of betrayal and alienation for sufferers of ill-health when the body fails to perform in the way it normally would. At the same time sufferers' attitudes towards the body become pragmatic as they begin to act towards it in an attempt to find relief and/or develop coping strategies (Williams, 1996: 26). In the case of long-term problems, life can be transformed into a continual evalution of one's symptoms which sufferers construct as an 'it'; something separate and different from themselves.

This separation between body and mind is shaped and confirmed in western society by allopathic medical discourse. The authoritative ascribing of health and illness labels has become the sole preserve of medical personnel (Taussig, 1992). The 'expert's' interpretation of the body is the dominant one and from health care interactions patients receive instruction on how to view illness. In effect the patient is reliant upon the medical profession to interpret the body, as Taussig notes: 'The sick person is a dependent and anxious person, malleable in the hands of the doctor and the health care system' (1992: 86).

However, although society has become reliant on a dependent relationship with medicine, allopathy remains unable to answer some of the central questions raised by the experience of illness. Specifically Taussig (1992: 85) notes that doctors are often able to pinpoint causes for disease and explain likely prognosis but the issues of 'why now?' and 'why me?' are not addressed. While these questions are generally peripheral to the interests of medical personnel they are of central concern to the sufferer. Patients are left to scrutinize their lives seeking within their biographies and personal behaviours reasons for illness. We could add to Taussig's unanswered questions, that of 'what next?'

The criticism of allopathy as encouraging a dependent relationship between patient and practitioner, can also be seen to be relevant to the practice of alternative and complementary health care work. The category of alternative/complementary medicine does, of course, embrace a wide range of practitioners, aetiologies and treatment styles (Sharma, 1992: 6). However, all provide patients with readings of the body and practitioner-led opinion on health. Alternative or complementary medicines, similar to allopathic practitioners, have power to define individuals as healthy or ill and guide patients towards particular understandings of the body (Coward, 1989). Through their interactions with practitioners, patients also learn to attend to the body in particular ways, so that the experience of the body and symptoms is mediated through the description, explanation and even language of the practitioner giving treatment (Csordas, 1993). In osteopathy responsibility for one's health state is individualized and the wider social factors which affect health and illness are generally ignored (Sharma, 1992: 181).

Although there has been great debate over the role of complementary therapies in society, as yet there is relatively little qualitative research on how patients themselves view the accounts they are presented with by this growing sector of health care. This article examines osteopathic patients' accounts of their use of osteopathy for back problems. In general they reported a rejection of medical and osteopathic accounts of the back and little understanding and concern with treatment practices. Although this could be interpreted as a rejection of professional notions of the back and as a manifestation of the agency of the patient, the article shows the subtle ways that patients did accept professional management and a particular view of their symptoms. The article also examines how patients attempted to attend to the back as a daily concern of management, even while admitting they had no way of controlling it. This raises interesting questions for osteopathy itself about how patients are taught to view their personal health responsibilities outside the practice room, and the dependency created by osteopathic discourse and treatment.

THE APPROACH OF THE STUDY

An osteopathic practice was selected within the Glasgow area. Sixteen patients, eight men and eight women who attended over one day in March 1997 with what they self-defined as 'back problems', were interviewed in-depth for about an hour about their experiences. The patients were aged between 17 and 72 with the majority in their forties and fifties.[1] All except two patients, had attended the osteopath for over six months, with many having done so on and off for some years. One of my core questions for the research was, how do people use osteopathy when experiencing back pain? Do they combine it with other treatments, lay remedies or over-the-counter medications? Second, I was interested in how they said they understood the back. Third, I focused upon the strategies developed to cope with having back problems and the consequences of such strategies.

OSTEOPATHIC KNOWLEDGE AND PATIENT PARTICIPATION

In this article, I am not concerned with discussing the efficacy of osteopathic practices, however, a brief introduction to osteopathic thinking is needed to provide context to patients' accounts of treatment. Osteopathy involves a broad set of practices and treatments but in general could be said to have a focus upon the wholeness of the body and the correct functioning of movement within and between structures (Sneddon and Coseschi, 1996:11). Therefore, the term osteopathy (literally, suffering of the bone) is slightly misleading as osteopaths are also concerned with creating good muscular skeletal functioning generally. Furthermore, it is a 'hands on' treatment which can involve massage and various physical treatments of the spine and other structures, in a one-to-one patient/practitioner relationship.

Unlike some other complementary therapies, osteopathy is not directly concerned with lifestyle change as a therapeutic issue. Sharma (1992: 181) argues that the dominant osteopathic view of the body is mechanistic and, although it is opposed to drug use and heroic intervention, the nature of treatment is often physical and individual. Osteopathy is, of course, a 'fairly broad church' (Sharma, 1992: 181) however, conventional practice still leans towards a mechanistic approach.[2] For most osteopaths, working for themselves or for more established osteopaths in private practice, such changes have had little effect on their work. Mr D worked in a private capacity with a patient group who self-referred. He used the phrase 'drugless practitioners' to describe the role of the osteopath in relation to allopathic practitioners. However, his attitude was not negative to orthodox practice and he argued that there was a need for diversity.

Mr D was interviewed at the beginning of the research and on a number of occasions as the research progressed. One might expect him to have a profound effect upon patients' conceptualizations of their health through treatment and advice. Indeed he provided patients with a free leaflet he had written himself, about the nature of osteopathic treatment. In this, an explanation was given of the spine's role in overall health and the broad application of osteopathy as a system of medicine was explained. However, Mr D felt that providing information was often problematic.

> I know the patients read into what they are told what they want to hear ... I know the things that I would never say to a patient but the patient you've seen will come back and see you a week later and tell you what you said and you know you haven't, because they take the words you say and in some way they transform them.

Mr D argued that patients arrived with ideas about back problems and selectively constructed an understanding of their bodies and the treatment. Furthermore, he also felt that this led to a problem in interpreting patients' accounts of other practitioners and his policy was to treat what he found without judgement about previous practitioners. He therefore maintained that he followed a policy of basic and simple explanation of patients' conditions without presenting in-depth accounts which he felt might confuse patients.

In terms of self-treatment and lifestyle issues raised by their back conditions Mr D felt that expecting patients to change their lifestyles was ineffectual.

> People come up through life with a certain set of values which stick to them. You can get them to do some things but I never ask anyone to change their way of life because I don't think you can do it and will it make them any better in the end?

One could say then that Mr D's reported approach did not actively engage with patients' beliefs or confront them. He did not see the point of correcting ideas which he felt tended to persist even after explanation, Mr D argued that his role was to treat what he found through assessment of the body. Mr D's practice of osteopathy was firmly practitioner-led. Patients' words were, even at best, secondary to his professional reading of the body.

ROUTINE SCEPTICISM AND PATIENTHOOD

All of the patients were prompted to seek help in the first instance by back pain with immobility and swelling also mentioned as important symptoms. A small minority also mentioned the wish to dispel their fears that the pain indicated something abnormal. Referral was through friends and relatives, or in two cases, via checking the *Yellow Pages* telephone directory, not through medical recommendation. All had attended their general practice with back problems and many had seen other forms of orthodox practitioner for their backs on other occasions. Initially patients turned to the general practitioner but three-quarters of the patients noted dissatisfaction with the advice they obtained.

The main source of dissatisfaction was that general practitioners were perceived as carrying out only very basic examinations and not taking an active stance on treatment. A common idea was that something needed to be done, that active management was required. Therefore, the general practice stock advice of rest and painkillers was not interventionist enough for patients' expectations. Despite the lack of faith in doctors' treatment of bad backs, there was a common assertion that doctors could not be expected to know about backs. So typical comments were:

> It's not an illness, it's just something you get... I don't know what they [doctors] could do really because they don't do backs. (Margaret)

> I suppose he did his best but they can't know everything they're general aren't they, general practitioners. (Cliff)

The back was considered by the patients to be outwith the normal medical framework. This was despite the severity of some of the symptoms:

> I'm not ill, it's just this back ... I just can't stand up straight sometimes or move about. (Jonathan)

In this case back problems caused considerable difficulties for the patient making it hard for him even to move around his home. However, attendance at the general practice was not seen as a viable option for gaining treatment for back problems, no matter how invasive the symptoms.

Patients had similar experiences with other practitioners in the orthodox services. The typical career of the back pain sufferers in this group was of moving through different forms of care referred on by the general practitioner, arriving at the osteopath through self-referral when other forms of treatment had not worked.

Orthodox medicine was perceived as having lost interest in their backs, this was reinforced by the lack of action or explanation during meetings with health care professionals. It was a clear patient expectation that some kind of active management should be applied. Therefore, it is perhaps unsurprising that these particular patients sought such management through other means, in this case osteopathy.

Patients reported osteopathy as an immediate and accessible source of relief from symptoms. Indeed all of the patients noted a very definite positive change in their back problems after their first treatments, and this experience, along with their general scepticism with orthodox medicine, might suggest that the patients would report more acceptance of osteopathic ideas about the back. Indeed, the majority of patients argued that Mr D did not explain what was wrong with them and that they were not concerned with having a named condition.

> Mr D doesn't really tell you what's wrong. He just knows and I let him get on with it. (Albert)
>
> Well I don't ask questions, that's always been my problem. He goes straight to the pain and relieves it, I don't know how. (Muriel)

However, there was a high level of patient scepticism about Mr D's general description of their symptoms.

> He says it's joints, I think that's what he said anyway. Personally though, I think it's muscles, it's something in the muscles. (Teresa)

Mr D treats the back but it's up the leg really. (Cliff)

The patients exhibited a passive acceptance of osteopathic treatment itself but did not always accept explanation or osteopathic interpretation. As mentioned earlier, Sharma (1992: 30) has noted that it is possible for patients to use a complementary therapy and retain quite conservative notions of cause and the body. But also within the orthodox system, patients are used to being passive recipients of medical intervention; the body often being the object of medical inquiries in which they are not actively involved. In osteopathic treatment, the patients, in keeping with orthodox patterns of respect for medical knowledge, did not engage in the debate over what their symptoms meant. The difference here between their experience of orthodox medicine and osteopathy was that the osteopath showed interest in treating them, agreed that there was a problem, and demonstrated through physical treatments a willingness to manage the back for the patient. The osteopath can also be seen here as fulfilling a legitimating function, often at the end of a line of practitioners who had been perceived as uninterested.

TAKING CARE – A STRATEGY FOR COPING OUTSIDE THE TREATMENT ROOM

As has been noted, patients reported a lack of interest with osteopathic accounts of the back. Interestingly, patients also noted that they were not given much information on the back but suggested that they did not want it. In this section we look at the ways they reported they tried to protect the back in everyday life. This manifested itself in the practice of being careful or taking care. Twelve patients noted that taking care was, to a greater or lesser extent, the main way they looked after their backs. An exploration of these strategies indicates that taking care was a contingent matter which involved the scrutiny of everyday activities. As will be illustrated this task became impossible due to the uncertain notion of what constituted risk to the back. Despite patients' claims that osteopathy allowed them to live a normal life, most of them had become very concerned about the threat of everyday activity. Overall, patients were anxious about the issue of 'what next?' or how do I manage my back? All noted that although osteopathic treatment helped them keep going and reduced symptoms, such as pain and immobility, they were not provided with any means of assessing how their back was coping outside of treatment. By implication then, osteopathic treatment was accepted as the way of judging how the back was doing and patients did not rely upon their own feelings or evaluations. Furthermore, the back outside of the treatment room was at risk from the most innocuous of activities.

> He (Mr D) just says it's not the weight of a thing that might bring it on but the way you twist or turn at the time. You can put your back out cleaning your teeth. (Cliff)

As can be seen from the quotation above, patients did get information from Mr D that injury was possible from all kinds of movements, thus underlining the everyday problem of prediction.

'Being careful' was the patients' response to the uncertain world outside of the practice room but carefulness appeared to be assessed in an ad hoc and often contradictory way. For instance, one interviewee argued that she felt hockey may have contributed to her back problems so she no longer took part, however, she believed taking part in badminton and aerobics to be all right. Scrutiny of daily life was presented as one way of controlling possible damage to the back and therefore symptoms. However, notions of risk and threat to the back were applied in a contingent manner by patients as 'carefulness' was impossible to apply in any consistent way.

Failure to be careful was identified by seven people (five women and two men) as something which regularly made their backs bad. Here their own personal responsibility for lack of care was emphasized.

> I foolishly went to the library for an hour, it was probably a stupid thing to do because you're picking up books and they're high and low and I pushed it. (Jonathan)

When retrospectively considering the cause of episodes of back pain these participants tended to blame themselves for 'stupidly' doing such things as shopping for the family, carrying bags, bending over to plug things in, wearing higher than normal heels, lifting small children, dancing at a disco or tidying the house. Given the everyday nature of these activities it seems unlikely they could be avoided. However, these patients firmly placed the blame for injury upon their own foolhardy judgements of risk in daily life.

> That back problem came from stupidity or something I could have avoided. I bent down to get a piece of paper and I wasn't careful. I had the treatment and was fine but again was silly and pulled out the plug from my computer, bending over. (Julie)

Another common attitude was that carelessness in protecting the back was something which, although partially in the individual's power, was generally controlled by others. In the accounts of three men and two women, a notion of mitigated carelessness was expounded, with all citing work as the key constraining factor.

> I know if I've overdone it and I should stop but sometimes you can't do that in a job, you have to carry on so you try and compensate a little. (Susan)

> You can feel it going but you carry on ... I know that nobody can turn to you and say you don't have backache but it's hard to prove the thing. (Douglas)

These accounts moved away from total self-blame to arguing that the sufferer's failure lay in not being able to convey the risk to their back from various activities to colleagues at work. Furthermore, they were at fault for not refusing to undertake certain 'risky' tasks, even where it was clear their employment would be at threat if they did not. This group did not have as broad a notion of risk as the first group but restricted it to things such as lifting and carrying heavy or awkward weights, being sat in one position for a long period of time and bending and moving in small or difficult spaces. For this group a central problem was balancing the protection of the back with the demands of employment and their personal responsibility lay in conveying the need for protecting the back to others in this setting.

A last group of four participants, three men and one woman, did not discuss personal responsibility and blame for episodes of back problems. Two of the men had only experienced their back problems for around four months and were both certain that their problems were transient. The other two people were long-term sufferers who argued that sporting activities caused their problems. Both undertook sport every week, took it very seriously and appeared to expect physical damage. In comparison with the other patients, these people did not view general life as the cause of recurrent back problems and they argued that using osteopathic treatment was a way of maintaining their higher than normal levels of physical activity.

Patients' attempts to protect themselves from threat can be seen as related to the pattern of interactions they had with Mr D and with other health care practitioners in the past. At the same time, the world outside of the treatment room, and especially social and lifestyle factors which may impinge upon back health, are not addressed fully. Moreover, the patients' understanding of the back as constantly at risk is not identified or discussed in the practice room and in patients' accounts we see the tying together of symptoms (such as pain), fear of damage to the back and normal activity. For most patients, their attempts to protect the back are highly contingent and uncertain and self-blame is invoked when patients perceive themselves to be unable to prevent the recurrence of their back problems.

DISCUSSION

It is clear that the osteopathic patients discussed here expected and sought professional management of their backs. Although a small-scale qualitative study cannot provide generalizations, there are some interesting points to be drawn from these patients' accounts of their experiences. For instance, they reported a resistance to medical and osteopathic ideas about the back. There was a good deal of patient scepticism about medical and osteopathic explanation, terminology and diagnosis, with a tendency to not ask or question health care workers. It is interesting to consider the production of such passive patienthood. There was the belief that modern medicine should be able to 'do something'; to actively manage their symptoms for them. In the patients' search for actively managed care, most had moved through various orthodox practitioners and finally ended up at the osteopath. At this point the osteopath was noted by all the patients to provide what they perceived to be a high level of symptom control as part of actively managed care. Moreover, it could be argued the osteopathic encounter provided a continuous point of contact for the patients in which someone appeared to be interested in the patients' symptoms. The importance of this should not be underestimated; continuity is important to people with long-term illness and is often absent from their experience of health care (Murphy and Fischer, 1983). However, the orthodox experience of patienthood was duplicated in the patient/osteopath relationship and format of treatment. Mr D, as noted earlier, did not believe in providing too much information. It seems the patient is happy to be treated and acted upon by the osteopath with little understanding of what is happening.

The similarities between the allopathic and osteopathic patienthood are not surprising. As Sharma (1992: 181) argues, allopathic medicine, chiropractic and osteopathy share a mechanical construction of the body. Within this construction the patient's participation is minimal; their understanding is not required for treatment to work and they are consigned to an inactive role. Meanwhile legitimate knowledge about the back and the authority to interpret and define back problems remain the preserve of 'experts'. From this standpoint, the osteopathic patient with recurrent symptoms can be seen as an individual channelled through different objectifying health systems, which actively disengage them from their own care and reinforce the dependent attitude to health encouraged by modern health care systems.

However, the notion of complementary therapy patients as active agents in their own health care is compelling. The patients here chose to try osteopathy, arrived via self-referral and reported actively resisting practitioner accounts and meanings. The dependent relationship with treatment is visible in their need for ongoing and actively managed treatment; while at the same time they sought to identify and control risks to protect what they perceive to be the fragile back. The osteopath became the antidote to everyday living. In addition, the osteopathic approach to illness tends to minimize the impact of social and environmental causes of ill-health. As seen above, some patients did recognize the social constraints of the work environment but individualized this into a personal communication problem about their own inability to convey their need to be careful in the workplace. While the patient struggles to identify and predict risk to the back in their everyday activities, there is a danger that the carefulness and self-blame of patients will be interpreted by others (family, friends, colleagues, doctors, etc.) as overly cautious, or perhaps, even neurotic behaviour.

These findings raise important issues for osteopathic practice and indeed for any health workers involved in rehabilitation or care of patients with long-term symptoms. There are pragmatic concerns for the developing profession of osteopathy. But perhaps the real question raised by the findings here, is how can such dependent osteopathic patient/practitioner relationships be modified to empower the patient given their wish to be managed? Patients sought out treatment providing active management and were happy to place the responsibility for interpretation and treatment of their backs with Mr D. It would, of course, go against osteopathic tradition to encourage patients to be more independent and rely more on their own evaluations of their back health. It is difficult for the osteopathic profession to question its relationship to the patient. However, there are pragmatic concerns for the profession around the patient/practitioner relationship and it is to these I now turn.

As Taussig (1992) argues, patients in general are often more concerned with the *why?* rather than the *how?* of disease. However, patients are also concerned with the *what now?* In other words, they are concerned with issues of daily management and control and they look to health care professionals to provide guidance on how to do this. This article suggests that there is a gap in osteopathic treatment and argues that pragmatic changes are needed to provide patients with more guidance on back care. Osteopathic practitioners need to work on clearly communicating the sorts of activities that individual patients should be avoiding. The issue of patient self-blame could also be addressed at a training level so that osteopaths might qualify with a greater understanding of the individualization of health problems. It seems that at many points in the career of the back-pain patient it may be possible to provide more feedback and reassurance to patients. Osteopathic education might also focus more upon the practicalities of preparing patients to leave treatment, or in the case of chronic sufferers, encouraging a full engagement with everyday life without applying personal blame. Similarly, the social science component of education could focus more upon social and environmental constraints on patients' health states and link this more clearly to the experience students gain when meeting the general public in practice clinics. Attention could also be given to the subject of victim-blaming ideology in health care provision. This would be a step forward in raising practitioner awareness of the phenomenon of patient self-blame and also the wider issue of 'victim-blaming' ideology in health care provision (Crawford, 1980).

It is important to note that Mr D is not unusual in his practice of osteopathy and appeared to be trying to provide what he believed to be the best care for his patients. However, as the health care environment changes, the profession needs to become more reflexive and more willing to scrutinize its own practices. Further research needs to look closely at this interior of patient care and the ways that treatment might actually be contributing to patient anxieties.

NOTES

1. All patients referred to in this article and the osteopath, have been given pseudonyms to protect anonymity.
2. Other approaches such as cranial work are often popular at osteopathy colleges but are more difficult to practice in private practise, not least because patients expect particular treatments from an osteopath.

REFERENCES

Coward, R. (1989). *The whole truth: The myth of alternative health*. London: Faber.

Crawford, R. (1980). Healthism and the medicalization of everyday life. *International Journal of Health Services*, 10, 365–88.

Csordas, T. (1993). Somatic modes of attention. *Cultural Anthropology*, 8(2), 135–56.

Hyden, L.C. (1997). Illness and narrative. *Sociology of Health and Illness*, 19(1), 48–9.

Lupton, D. (1994). *Medicine as culture*. London: Sage.

May, C., Doyal, H. and Graham, C. (1999). Medical knowledge and the intractable patient: The case of chronic low back pain. *Social Science and Medicine*, 48A, 523–34.

Merleau Ponty, M. (1962). *Phenomenology of perception*. Translated by C. Smith. London: Routledge & Kegan Paul.

Sharma, U. (1992). *Complementary medicine today, practitioners and patients*. London: Routledge.

Sneddon, P. and Coseschi, P. (1996). *Healing with osteopathy*. Dublin: Gill & Macmillan Ltd.

Strauss, A. and Corbin, J. (1990). *Basics of qualitative research: Grounded theory procedures and techniques*. London: Sage.

Taussig, M.T. (1992). *The nervous system*. New York: Routledge.

Williams, S.J. (1996). The vicissitudes of embodiment across the chronic illness trajectory. *Body and Society*, 2(2), 23–47.

CHAPTER 14

WHOLENESS AND HEALTH

Fritjof Capra

Health care in Europe and North America is practiced by a large number of people and organizations, including physicians, nurses, psychotherapists, psychiatrists, public-health professionals, social workers, chiropractors, homeopaths, acupuncturists, and various 'holistic' practitioners. These individuals and groups use a great variety of approaches that are based on different concepts of health and illness. To integrate them into an effective system of health care, based on holistic and ecological views, it will be crucial to establish a common conceptual basis for talking about health, so that all these groups can communicate and coordinate their efforts.

It will also be necessary to define health at least approximately. Although everybody knows what it feels like to be healthy, it is impossible to give a precise definition; health is a subjective experience whose quality can be known intuitively but can never be exhaustively described or quantified. Nevertheless, we may begin our definition by saying that health is a state of well-being that arises when the organism functions in a certain way. The description of this way of functioning will depend on how we describe the organism and its interactions with its environment. Different models of living organisms will lead to different definitions of health. The concept of health, therefore, and the related concepts of illness, disease, and pathology, do not refer to well-defined entities but are integral parts of limited and approximate models that mirror a web of relationships among multiple aspects of the complex and fluid phenomenon of life.

Edited from Ch 10, pp 351–59 in Capra F, *The Turning Point; Science, Society and the Rising Culture*. London: Flamingo, 1983.

Once the relativity and subjective nature of the concept of health is perceived, it also becomes clear that the experience of health and illness is strongly influenced by the cultural context in which it occurs. What is healthy and sick, normal and abnormal, sane and insane, varies from culture to culture. Moreover, cultural context influences the specific ways people behave when they get sick. How we communicate our health problems, the manner in which we present our symptoms, when and to whom we go for care, the explanations and therapeutic measures offered by the doctor, therapist, or healer – all that is strongly affected by our society and culture (Kleinman, Eisenberg and Good, 1978). It would seem, therefore, that a new framework for health can be effective only if it is based on concepts and ideas rooted in our own culture and evolving according to the dynamics of our social and cultural evolution.

For the past three hundred years our culture has been dominated by the view of the human body as a machine, to be analyzed in terms of its parts. The mind is separated from the body, disease is seen as a malfunctioning of biological mechanisms, and health is defined as the absence of disease. This view is now slowly being eclipsed by a holistic and ecological conception of the world which sees the universe not as a machine but rather as a living system, a view that emphasizes the essential interrelatedness and interdependence of all phenomena and tries to understand nature not only in terms of fundamental structures but in terms of underlying dynamic processes. It would seem that the systems view of living organisms can provide the ideal basis for a new approach to health and health care that is fully consistent with the new paradigm and is rooted in our cultural heritage. The systems view of health is profoundly ecological and thus in harmony with the Hippocratic tradition which lies at the roots of Western medicine. It is a view based on scientific notions and expressed in terms of concepts and symbols which are part of our everyday language. At the same time the new framework naturally takes into account the spiritual dimensions of health and is thus in harmony with the views of many spiritual traditions.

Systems thinking is process thinking, and hence the systems view sees health in terms of an ongoing process. Whereas most definitions, including some proposed recently by holistic practitioners, picture health as a static state of perfect well-being, the systems concept of health implies continual activity and change, reflecting the organism's creative response to environmental challenges. Since a person's condition will always depend importantly on the natural and social environment, there can be no absolute level of health independent of this environment. The continual changes of one's organism in relation to the changing environment will naturally include temporary phases of ill health, and it will often be impossible to draw a sharp line between health and illness.

Health is really a multidimensional phenomenon involving interdependent physical, psychological, and social aspects. The common representation of health and illness as opposite ends of a one-dimensional continuum is quite misleading. Physical disease may be balanced by a positive mental attitude and social support, so that the overall state is one of well-being. On the other hand, emotional problems or social isolation can make a person feel sick in spite of physical fitness. These multiple dimensions of health will generally affect one another, and the strongest feeling of being healthy will occur when they are well balanced and integrated. The experience of illness, from the systems point of view, results from patterns of disorders that may become manifest at various levels of the organism, as well as in the various interactions between the organism and the larger systems in which it is embedded. An important characteristic of the systems approach is the notion of stratified order involving levels of differing complexities, both within individual organisms and in social and ecological systems. Accordingly, the systems view of health can be applied to different systems levels, with the corresponding levels of health mutually interconnected. In particular we can discern three interdependent levels of health – individual, social, and ecological. What is unhealthy for the individual is generally also unhealthy for the society and for the embedding ecosystem.

The systems view of health is based on the systems view of life. Living organisms, as we have seen, are self-organizing systems that display a high degree of stability. This stability is utterly dynamic and is characterized by continual, multiple, and interdependent fluctuations. To be healthy such a system needs to be flexible, to have a large number of options for interacting with its environment. The flexibility of a system depends on how many of its variables are kept fluctuating within their tolerance limits: the more dynamic the state of the organism, the greater its flexibility. Whatever the nature of the flexibility – physical, mental, social, technological, or economic – it is essential to the system's ability to adapt to environmental changes. Loss of flexibility means loss of health.

This notion of dynamic balance is a useful concept for defining health. 'Dynamic' is of crucial importance here, indicating that the necessary balance is not a static equilibrium but rather a flexible pattern of fluctuations of the kind described above. Health, then, is an experience of well-being resulting from a dynamic balance that involves the physical and psychological aspects of the organism; as well as its interactions with its natural and social environment.

The concept of health as dynamic balance is consistent both with the systems view of life and with many traditional models of health and healing, among them the Hippocratic tradition and the tradition of East Asian medicine. As in these traditional models, 'dynamic balance' acknowledges the healing forces inherent in every living organism, the organism's innate tendency to reestablish itself in a balanced state when it has been disturbed. It may do so by returning, more or less, to the original state through various processes of self-maintenance, including homeostasis, adaptation, regeneration, and self-renewal. Examples of this phenomenon would be the minor illnesses which are part of our everyday life and usually cure themselves. On the other hand, the organism may also undergo a process of self-transformation and self-transcendence, involving stages of crisis and transition and resulting in an entirely new state of balance. Major changes in a person's life style, induced by a severe illness, are examples of such creative responses that often leave the person at a higher level of health than the one enjoyed before the challenge. This suggests that periods of ill health are natural stages in the ongoing interaction between the individual and the environment. To be in dynamic balance means to go through temporary phases of illness that can be used to learn and to grow.

The natural balance of living organisms includes a balance between their self-assertive and integrative tendencies. To be healthy an organism has to preserve its individual autonomy, but at the same time it has to be able to integrate itself harmoniously into larger systems. This capacity for integration is closely related to the organism's flexibility and to the concept of dynamic balance. Integration at one systems level will manifest itself as balance at a larger level, as the harmonious integration of individual components into larger systems results in the balance of those systems. Illness, then, is a consequence of imbalance and disharmony, and may very often be seen as stemming from a lack of integration. This is particularly true for mental illness, which often arises from a failure to evaluate and integrate sensory experience.

The notion of illness as originating in a lack of integration seems to be especially relevant to approaches that try to understand living organisms in terms of rhythmic patterns. From this perspective synchrony becomes an important measure of health. Individual organisms interact and communicate with one another by synchronizing their rhythms and thus integrating themselves into the larger rhythms of their environment. To be healthy, then, means to be in synchrony with oneself – physically and mentally – and also with the surrounding world. When a person is out of synchrony, illness is likely to occur. Many esoteric traditions associate health with the synchrony of rhythms and healing with a certain resonance between healer and patient.

To describe an organism's imbalance the concept of stress seems to be extremely useful. Although it is relatively new in medical research (Selye, 1974), it has taken a firm hold in the collective consciousness and language of our culture. The stress concept is also completely consistent with the systems view of life and can be fully grasped only when the subtle interplay between mind and body is perceived.

Stress is an imbalance of the organism in response to environmental influences. Temporary stress is an essential aspect of life, since the ongoing interaction between organism and environment often involves temporary losses of flexibility. These will occur when the individual perceives a sudden threat, or when it has to adapt to sudden changes in the environment or is being strongly stimulated in some other way. These transitory phases of imbalance are an integral part of the way healthy organisms cope with their environment, but prolonged or chronic stress can be harmful and plays a significant role in the development of many illnesses (Pelletier, 1977).

From the systems point of view, the phenomenon of stress occurs when one or several variables of an organism are pushed to their extreme values, which induces increased rigidity throughout the system. In a healthy organism the other variables will conspire to bring the whole system back into balance and restore its flexibility. The remarkable thing about this response is that it is fairly stereotyped. The physiological stress symptoms – tight throat, tense neck, shallow respiration, accelerated heart rates, and so on – are virtually identical in animals and humans and are quite independent of the source of stress. Because they constitute the organism's preparation to cope with the challenge by either fighting or fleeing, the whole phenomenon is known as the fight-or-flight response. Once the individual has taken action by fighting or fleeing, it will rebound into a state of relaxation and ultimately will return to homeostasis. The well-known 'sigh of relief' is an example of such a relaxation rebound.

When the fight-or-flight response is prolonged, however, and when an individual cannot take action by fighting or fleeing to release the organism from the stressful state, the consequences are likely to be detrimental to health. The continual imbalance created by prolonged unabated stress can generate physical and psychological symptoms – muscle tension, anxiety, indigestion, insomnia – which will eventually lead to illness. The prolongation of stress often results from our failure to integrate the responses of our bodies with our cultural habits and social rules of behavior. Like most animals we react to any kind of challenge by arousing our organism in preparation for either physical fight or physical escape, but in most cases these reactions are no longer useful. In an intense business meeting we cannot win an argument by physically assaulting our opponent, nor can we run away from the situation. Being civilized, we try to deal with the challenge in socially acceptable ways, but 'old' parts of our brain often continue mobilizing the organism for inappropriate physical responses. If this happens repeatedly we are likely to get sick; we may develop a peptic ulcer or have a heart attack.

A key element in the link between stress and illness, which is not yet known in all its details but has been verified by numerous studies, is the fact that prolonged stress suppresses the body's immune system, its natural defenses against infections and other diseases. Full recognition of this fact will bring about a major shift in medical research from the preoccupation with microorganisms to a careful study of the host organism and its environment. Such a shift is now urgently needed, since the chronic and degenerative diseases that are characteristic of our time and constitute the major causes of death and disability are closely connected with excessive stress.

The sources of this overload of stress are manifold. They may originate within an individual, may be generated collectively by our society and culture, or may be present in the physical environment. Stressful situations arise not only from personal emotional traumas, anxieties, and frustrations, but also from the hazardous environment created by our social and economic system. Stress, however, comes not only from negative experiences. All events – positive or negative, joyous or sad – that require a person to adapt to profound or rapid changes will be highly stressful. It is very unfortunate for our health that our culture has produced an accelerating rate of change in all areas, together with numerous physical health hazards, but has failed to teach us how to cope with the increasing amount of stress we encounter.

Recognition of the role of stress in the development of illness leads to the important idea of illness as a 'problem solver.' Because of social and cultural conditioning people often find it impossible to release their stresses in healthy ways and therefore choose – consciously or unconsciously – to get sick as a way out. Their illness may be physical or mental, or it may manifest itself as violent and reckless behavior, including crime, drug abuse, accidents, and suicides, which may appropriately be called social illnesses. All these 'escape routes' are forms of ill health, physical disease being only one of several unhealthy ways of dealing with stressful life situations. Hence curing the disease will not necessarily make the patient healthy. If the escape into a particular disease is blocked effectively by medical intervention while the stressful situation persists, this may merely shift the person's response to a different mode, such as mental illness or antisocial behavior, which will be just as unhealthy. A holistic approach will have to look at health from this broad perspective, distinguishing clearly between the origins of illness and its manifestation. Otherwise it will not mean much to talk about successful therapies. As a doctor friend of mine put it forcefully, 'If you are able to reduce physical illness, but at the same time increase mental illness or crime, what the hell have you done?'.

The idea of illness as a way to cope with stressful life situations naturally leads to the notion of the meaning of illness, or of the 'message' transmitted by a particular disease. To understand this message ill health should be taken as an opportunity for introspection, so that the original problem and the reasons for choosing a particular escape route can be brought to a conscious level where the problem can be resolved. This is where psychological counseling and psychotherapy can play an important role, even in the treatment of physical illness. To integrate physical and psychological therapies will amount to a major revolution in health care, since it will require full recognition of the interdependence of mind and body in health and illness.

REFERENCES

Kleinman A, Eisenberg L, Good B (1978). Culture, illness, and care. *Annals of Internal Medicine*, February.

Pelletier KR (1977). *Mind as Healer, Mind as Slayer*. New York: Delta (London: Allen & Unwin, 1979).

Selye H (1974). *Stress Without Distress*. New York: Lippincott (London: Hodder & Stoughton, 1975).

CHAPTER 15

THE FANTASY OF THE WHOLE PERSON AND THE QUESTION OF PERSONAL BLAME

Rosalind Coward

Virtually all alternative therapies claim to be 'holistic', that is treating 'the whole system rather than the parts' (Pietroni, 1986). The claim is that, unlike conventional medicine, holistic approaches see health as the well-being of the whole person, and therefore involve not just a fit body, but a well mind or spirit. Holism has wondrous associations. It conjures up visions of a medicine which is preventive, gentle, and natural. This is an approach to the body that will not assault, attack or maim. It offers to integrate bits of our life, and bits of our bodies. Unlike conventional medicine, it will not increase our sense of fragmentation by treating bits of our bodies or different symptoms as if they were entirely separate from each other. Instead, holism suggests the possibility of integration, of feeling that all parts of ourselves belong to the same essential person and have meaning in relation to one another. Holism has almost religious connotations, suggesting that the whole person can be found and that when it is, the individual will be healed. 'To heal is to make whole. And what is whole can have no missing parts that have been kept outside.'[1]

'Holism' is the great strength of the alternative health movement. A holistic approach to treatment tends to mean a quality of personal attention and care which is total anathema to orthodox medicine. What is more, this holistic approach also appears to give an individual an unparalleled sense of participating in, perhaps even controlling, his or her own well-being. Yet this profound conviction that lying within each and every

Edited from Ch 3, pp 68–74 in Coward R, *The Whole Truth The Myth of Alternative*. London: Faber and Faber, 1990.

one of us is the kernel of a whole person is not without its own problems. Quite apart from the fact that the idea of a whole person might be a fantasy, there's a way in which the attempt at integrating all parts of a person to one central core has eased the way for a potentially highly moralistic approach to health. By relating the state of the body, the level of stress and so on to a deep meaning expressed by this kernel of the whole person, everything is made comprehensible by reference to this inner core. In the idea of the whole person, the possibility that an individual has control over health and the possibility that an individual is to be blamed for disease often shade into one another. And there are numerous ways in which a holistic approach to health gets tipped towards this more guilt-provoking idea of illness.

HOLISTIC TREATMENT: EMOTIONS AND MEDICINE

The precise definition of what is a holistic approach to health seems to vary a great deal between practitioners. Some talked of holism as simply the ability of an individual to integrate different treatments for different needs, such as using herbal medicine for a specific ailment, Alexander technique for working on body and posture, and psychotherapy for emotional distress. A small minority emphasized the social implications for the term holism; they stressed that holism implied the links between individual and environment and suggested treatments which would not only balance the internal parts of an individual but would also balance the relationship between the individual and her or his environment. More generally, however, practitioners and consumers alike defined holism as the treatment of the 'whole person', an approach which refuses to separate body, mind and spirit. Virtually all spoke of the tremendous difference which this approach actually made to *treatment* where a high premium was put on individuality and on exploring a whole range of aspects of an individual's life which conventional medicine would usually ignore.

There can be little doubt that this emphasis on the 'whole person' has produced techniques of treatment which diverge radically from most people's experience of routine consultations with conventional doctors. Almost all of the alternative therapies, apart perhaps from those which involve 'healing techniques at a distance' (e.g., radionics or diagnosis by hair), ask extremely 'intimate' questions about the individual involved. Consultations with many practitioners of alternative therapies involve detailed questioning about individual background, family history, history of illnesses, tastes and preferences, and current life situation. This individuality is frequently taken into account in the treatment. No two individuals should necessarily be given the same treatment. The healer or therapist must determine the individual's general state of physical, emotional and spiritual well-being before offering treatment.

The attention to the individual has been held by both supporters and critics of alternative therapies alike as one of its major strengths. Unlike conventional medicine, often overstretched in resources, and driven by professional divisions and hierarchies, these holistic therapies appear to offer a highly personalized approach to health problems. The founders of the Holistic Consciousness Foundation included amongst the reasons for the growth of popularity of alternative approaches to health those who turned to it 'seeking a re-assertion of individuality'. These are the patients who refused to be categorized as an NHS number and wanted to be treated as an individual.[2] More cynically, one interviewee described his sessions with an alternative therapist (acupuncturist and masseur) as just plain good value. For £15 he was given a solid hour's hard work on himself; he felt known and recognized as an individual.

But what exactly are these forms of attention to the individual which make alternative therapies so attractive, and how do they relate to the overall philosophies of health, well-being and disease? Time has always been cited as one of the main ways in which alternative therapies truly attend to the individual; whereas conventional doctors might see a patient for five to ten minutes, alternative therapists regularly see their patients for an hour or an hour and a half. They ask questions about changes in emotional state, and seek to find out about the apparently most minor physical symptoms. They want to know what we've been eating, how much exercise we have been doing, how much energy we have and how we are feeling. But it is more than just a question of time. Other factors include physical contact. Clients for Alexander technique, Shiatsu, or even a simple massage, all describe the experience of 'knowledgeable' hands holding, exploring, guiding and shaping the body, providing a wonderful sense that something is being done to help your body and overall well-being in a most tender and comforting way.

But perhaps most significant in the claims made for a whole person approach is the way in which emotions are integrated into treatment. This is particularly obvious in therapies based on some kind of medicine, as opposed to, say, manipulative therapies. In many cases this integration of the emotions is quite subtle and submerged, glimpsed in questions about patterns of mood, sleep and energy. But there are some practices for whom the emotions are absolutely central, like Bach flower remedies and aromatherapy. It is these therapies which most forcibly underline the distance between alternative and conventional medicine. In these practices it is far more common to find remedies offered according to a specific set of emotions or a personality type than it is to find the treatment of a specific illness. Bach flower remedies, for instance, offer thirty-eight remedies divided into seven groups to cover 'all the known negative states of mind'. The groups are fear, uncertainty, lack of interest in the present, despondency and despair, over-concern for the welfare of others, loneliness and oversensitivity. Thus a practitioner is likely to prescribe clematis for 'daydreaming and indifference, inattention and escapism' or chicory for 'possessiveness, self-pity, craving attention' (Inglis and West, 1983).

More than anything else it is this attention to moods, emotional states and predispositions of the personality which inform the idea of 'whole person' treatment. Examples could be endlessly duplicated but the following description of a homoeopathic approach to diagnosis could speak for a movement, 'all humans consist of the mind, body and spirit and all should be examined by any treatment. All patients should be treated as individuals, so diagnosis cannot be standardized. A diagnosis should be arrived at by examining all facets of a person's life; background, physical type, emotional state, body language, clothing etc. This creates an overall picture, that of the "whole person".'[3] Here then are all the aspects of a person which conventional medicine has regarded as irrelevant. Previously consigned either to psychotherapy or to astrology, and definitely considered irrelevant to the state of the body, they have now moved into the centre of the picture.

No one could deny the way in which conventional medicine overlooks personal and emotional factors which are likely to produce or foster illness – distress about poor social conditions, personal problems, and so on. Yet this new attention to previously neglected areas of the individual goes much further than simply including concern with all the factors in an individual's life as they are mediated through the emotions. The notion of the whole person very often merges indistinguishably with the concept of personality, or personality type. Homoeopathy is occasionally quite explicit about this. Its remedies are directed towards certain types of person with characteristic emotional states and often characteristic physical ailments: 'If you know your medicines very well and their mental and physical aspects and you know the mental make-up of the patient you can predict what his physical disease is going to be like and the other way around. If you know the physical make-up of the patient you can know what his temperamental nature must be.'

There is the very clear suggestion that medicine itself has definite emotional profiles, as if there were certain negative and positive emotions in nature which express themselves in persons and plants. This article from *Homoeopathy Today* goes on to give examples. The medicine, Arsenic album, for instance, is 'by nature very fussy, very meticulous'. The typical patient for Arsenic album 'is called the gold-headed cane patient – very trim and proper and the top of his cane must be well-polished.' At one level homoeopathy deals in personality types, offering constitutional medicine which is matched to the patient by the symptoms it produces. The Ignatia patient, for example, 'is a victim of modern society. Excessive social excitement and involvement exhausts them. Unlike the Sepia patient who is dull and stupid, the Ignatia personality is clever, highly refined, gentle and educated.'[4]

Much of this cannot fail to stir memories of the humoural medicine of the Middle Ages, which at its simplest classified people according to four distinct personality types and treated all ailments according to these dominant personality types rather than the characteristics of the disease. Obviously it is harsh to draw these links with homoeopathy which is based on longstanding research into the effects on the body of various substances and which combines elements – characteristics and symptoms of the illness with the personality type of the patient – in arriving at treatment. But nevertheless it is important to recognize the forceful return of beliefs in 'constitutional' medicine, and of course, by implication, beliefs in the existence of definite constitutions or personalities as crucial factors in any diagnosis.

This reintegration of constitutions or personality types into medicine is not without some obvious problems. The very idea of a personality type tends to disregard social and cultural reasons for the differences between individuals and their reactions. Instead people are seen as having been born with fixed constitutions, certain predispositions and tastes which make up their essential being. This view of the individual lends itself all too readily to certain kinds of mysticism and it is no coincidence that, side by side with the 'respectable' medicines like homoeopathy and acupuncture, flourish the more arcane pursuits like astrological medicine. Indeed astrology in general is enjoying a second wind, under the protection of some alternative therapies. This is a practice which is founded on the idea of a limited number of personality types. And, unlike constitutional medicine, astrology has no hesitation in explaining the origins of these different personality types: it is all down to the arrangement of the stars at the moment of our birth. But if most of the therapies which use constitutional medicine would turn away from the idea of heavenly conditioning, nevertheless the prevalence of beliefs in personality types has left a space for the more mystical explanations of personality to flourish.

There appears to be something of a contradiction in the understanding of personality in these approaches to health. For a 'whole person' approach to medicine stresses the degree of control an individual can exercise through her or his ability to change. Yet beliefs in personality types tend towards fatalism. If you accept the idea that we are born with an essential constitution it is difficult to see how far individual actions are going to be able to change this basic inheritance. Most of the therapies do not *appear* fatalistic, that is they do not seem to say that you are born as you are and can do nothing to change it either because of inherent, inherited, or astrologically conditioned characteristics. On the contrary they appear to be offering remedies for change, arguing that personality type is merely one predisposing factor. Yet, as we shall see, the idea of personality type is actually extremely important in these new approaches to health *and* it sometimes carries with it associations of a static and limited model of a world of fixed emotions and personalities into which human behaviour, characteristics and illness can be fitted. In fact, the unresolved tension between calls for change and beliefs in fixed personality types has tended to be the way in which guilt-provoking and moralistic notions of illness have been able to grow.

NOTES

1 *A Course in Miracles*.
2 Interview with Douglas and Nina Ashby of the Holistic Consciousness Foundation.
3 Interview conducted at the British Holistic Medical Association.
4 *Homoeopathy Today*, Summer, 1986.

BIBLIOGRAPHY

Inglis, Brian and Ruth West, *The Alternative Health Guide*, London, Michael Joseph, 1983
Pietroni, Patrick, *Holistic Living: A Guide to Self Care*, London, J. M. Dent, 1986

SECTION 3

CAM IN DIFFERENT SETTINGS

INTRODUCTION

Tom Heller

In this section the selected readings analyse various aspects of the way that complementary and alternative medical approaches are used in a wide range of settings. Immediately the focus on place and setting raises questions about the nature of the therapies themselves as well as throwing light on the people who practice these therapies, either as therapists or 'users'. How much does the setting matter? Are the basic principles of the various therapies transferable across a range of settings? Does a change of setting or context make practitioners, or users, behave differently? ... and what about the exchange of money for the services of a CAM practitioner? Does this help or hinder the therapeutic process? These are some of the issues that the authors of the selected readings have boldly chosen to explore.

Gavin Andrews and his colleagues have contributed two readings in this section based on research funded by the Nuffield Foundation. His first contribution, 'Receiving money for medicine: some tensions and resolutions for community based private complementary therapists', reports the results of a study of 426 community-based private complementary therapists in the UK. The reading highlights some of the tensions, and indeed the resolutions, for these CAM therapists between the 'business' of caring and the 'business' of making money from the provision of services. The second reading he has contributed, 'Small business complementary medicine: a profile of therapists and their pathways to practice', looks more specifically at the journeys that people have made to become CAM practitioners. The diversity of their backgrounds and motivations is explored. It is reported that his sample of practitioners have entered the 'market' equally from non-traditional careers and from professional backgrounds; *'These are a diverse set of people, with a diverse set of motivations, providing a diverse range of health care.'*

More evidence of the diversity of CAM provision, even within statutory services, is provided by Donna Luff and Kate Thomas in their reading, 'Complementary therapy provision in primary care – policy considerations based on case studies in practice'. Their research highlights a number of distinctly different approaches to the provision of a range of complementary therapy services even within the British NHS and its potentially standardized primary care services. The previously apparent innovation and flexibility within the primary care system that has allowed so many different models of CAM provision to survive is highlighted with the conclusion that; *'These services will survive in their present form only if a margin of flexibility and innovation is retained at practice level.'*

Marion Bowman, in contrast, has provided a reading, 'Healing in the spiritual marketplace', that looks at the 'spiritual service industry' particularly those related to New Age phenomena, and the healing practices that increasingly have become an integral part of it. *'The idea that profit and spirituality cannot converge'* is critically examined.

An international dimension is added to this section through the work of Melinda Goldner, 'Expanding political opportunities and changing collective identities in the complementary and alternative medicine movement'. This reading reports her research into the CAM movement in one area of San Francisco. In this geographical area various groups of CAM practitioners have taken very different political and strategic directions during the time when the growth and development of various modalities has continued. It is not clear from her work whether the future of CAM development lies with those who would wish to remain 'alternative', or with those who strive to be 'integrative' and associate increasingly with orthodox medical care systems.

'Lessons on integration from the developing world's experience' are given by Gerard Bodeker.

The final reading is this section by Phil Nicholls, 'Homoeopathy, hospitals and high society', explores the relationship between homoeopathy and 'high society', particularly members of the Royal Family. Although this is a fascinating historical view on the subject, it is of course entirely relevant to our understanding of the contemporary growth of interest in CAM and the advocacy of integrative medicine by HRH Prince Charles.

CHAPTER 16

RECEIVING MONEY FOR MEDICINE: SOME TENSIONS AND RESOLUTIONS FOR COMMUNITY BASED PRIVATE COMPLEMENTARY THERAPISTS

Gavin J Andrews, Elizabeth Peter and Robin Hammond

Charging direct, out-of-pocket payments for healthcare and medicines is not an uncommon practice. Indeed, wherever state finance, private insurance and voluntary sector coverage is incomplete or absent, direct payment remains a common form of financial cost recovery.

The focus of discussions around direct payment is clearly centred on professional orthodox medicine (OM). However, consideration of the practice of paying directly for private complementary medicine (CM) is less common in health research. Nevertheless, this is a potentially important issue since, within many countries, CM is a very common example of healthcare providers charging directly at the point of their healthcare delivery. Professionalism and healthcare are intrinsically linked. However, unlike OM, the degree of professionalism in CM is debatable, and rather depends on the particular form or modality that it takes. Indeed, certain types of therapists may be regarded from outside the sector, or regard themselves, as professionals, whilst others may be regarded or regard themselves as aspiring to professional status. In the wider workforce and business-related literature, professionalism is widely thought to entail a common core of characteristics and professional status is conferred upon

Edited from *Health and Social Care in the Community* © 2003 Blackwell Publishing Ltd 11(2):155-67.

groups when they require a lengthy and significant education to gain membership, possess a unique body of knowledge, are autonomous in practice, are guided by a code of ethics and provide an altruistic service to society (Friedson, 1983; Lundberg, 1997). To some extent, all these characteristics are evident in the private practice of CM, perhaps with the exception of a dedicated and comprehensive education which very much depends on the particular modality of therapy practised and in what particular country (Sharma, 1995). Still, whatever the degree of professionalism in CM, it is the final characteristic that can pose particular ethical tensions for therapists, who, like many professionals, work most often on a fee-for-service basis. The available medically related literature describing this tension, although generally focused on orthodox physicians, has direct relevance to private complementary therapists. For example, Rodwin (1993, p. 1) stated that, 'medicine almost inevitably involves a tension between the physicians' commitment to healing others and their economic self-interest'. Nevertheless, professionals have often been regarded as fiduciaries who are trusted to not allow their material self-interests to override the best interests of their clients and the public (Lo, 1999; Sullivan, 1999).

Of course, money is an economic necessity in most societies and cultures, except those which still use the traditional and ancient exchange system of barter.

Indeed, May (1997) explained that financial compensation provides some stability between the professional and the client. The argument is developed that, if services depended solely on altruism or love, the inclination to provide them could easily wax and wane. Furthermore, in the absence of full state planning and provision, other than open market systems, few other economic systems are likely either to produce an appropriate distribution of services, or encourage technological advancement and economic growth. In whatever guise, the market delivery system's reliance on providers as profit maximisers and purchasers as utility maximisers, each working in their own self interest, undoubtedly has its flaws and few markets actually reach an equilibrium like the stylised markets of economic theory. However, despite potential allocative failures, the market mechanism is regarded as an extremely efficient distributor of scarce resources. On a related and more humanistic note, May (1997) also described how money and the payment for goods and services connects strangers. For example, the professional's skills and services are not just available to family and friends, they are also available to many, distributed and regulated through the market mechanism. Finally, for professionals, or at least aspiring professionals, money often signifies a personal worth, particularly when one is selling one's skills (May, 1997).

Therefore, it would seem that, if society is willing to pay for a service, the payment confers a type of merit that freely given services do not. However, money cannot only facilitate caring and healing, it also has the potential to distract attention away from the focus on altruistic service. For complementary therapists, the resulting conflict of interest may express itself in several ways. First, a danger exists that therapists could encourage unnecessary, or even harmful, treatment for their own personal financial gain. This potential conflict of interest could be made more ethically problematic because therapists are recommending products that they are selling themselves (Rodwin, 1993). Indeed, as a result, professionals including therapists are required to be sufficiently distanced from their own interests to fully serve their clients' interests (May, 1997). Secondly, May (1997) described how a professional must sometimes go beyond responding to a client's self-perceived wants and address her or his deeper needs. In the case of CM, this process could entail, for instance, ending treatment even when a client insists on continuing. Alternatively, the potential for financial loss could lessen the likelihood of a therapist taking this sort of approach. Thirdly, therapists could also fail to refer a client when clinically necessary to another health professional, such as a family physician, in order to retain the person as a paying customer. The need to refer to others also requires therapists to acknowledge the limits of their expertise, and to appreciate the knowledge and skill of other providers. Fourthly, as May contended, money can also exclude. For example, those who cannot pay for a service cannot benefit from it. Alternatively, in related circumstances, there may be clients who initially have the means to pay for treatment, but who later can no longer afford to continue. In the case of CM, the question arises as to what therapists do in such situations. How can both the best interests of the client and the financial self-interests of the therapist be met? As Andrews and Phillips (2000, 2002) aptly demonstrated in the case of private residential care for older people, ultimately, the combination of profit making and professional altruism can potentially create morally complex conflicts of interests which are not easily resolved. For the first time, the present paper poses some of these questions to CM therapists, both hypothetically and relating to their actual courses of action in practice.

RESEARCH RESULTS

This paper reports on research on 426 community-based private complementary therapists in the UK. Using a combined questionnaire ($n = 426$) and interview survey ($n = 49$), the present paper considers the potential tensions and dilemmas which therapists face and the resolutions which they come to in being carers, but in market terms, also profit makers. The survey responses elicited 23 modalities which, given definitions of CM in the descriptive literature, were thought to be distinct enough to warrant their independent categorisation.

Out of the 426 respondents, 155 (36.4%) were male and 269 (63.1%) were female (0.5% non-response). The youngest of the respondents was 25 years old and the oldest 76 years, the mean age being 46.9 (SD = 10.0 years). Therefore, what is immediately striking is the female domination of CM private sector provision and a middle-aged age profile. Regarding the structure of their private businesses, 45.3% of therapists claimed to be practising CM part-time, 48.6% claimed to be practising full-time, whilst 2.3% just claimed that they worked 'as much as possible' (3.8% non-response). Reflecting the part-time nature of much private practice, 34.9% claimed to supplement their income with other forms of work and 27.6% by working in the same types of work which they were involved in prior to their involvement in a CM business. Respondents had been practising therapists for between 3 months and 43 years, the mean length of practice being 10.5 years (SD = 7.9 years). Indeed, many businesses were relatively new, reflecting the considerable growth in the private CM sector in the UK during the previous 15 years. Most therapists practised more than one therapy, the mean number being 1.9. Therapists' self-perceptions of their jobs were considered important, and in particular, issues surrounding business and care formed explicit and dedicated lines of inquiry in both the interviews and questionnaires. When questioned directly about their feelings about being both carers and business owners, 37.1% of respondents stated that they perceived themselves to be primarily a carer, 45.3% stated that they perceived themselves to be both carers and business people, whilst only 2.8% stated that they were primarily a business person (14.8% non- or other responses). Indeed, it is not unreasonable to suggest that, for many therapists, business ownership was simply a necessary by-product of practising CM that was endured, although not necessarily disliked. In this context, a therapist suggested:

> Business and caring? I do both, but my reason for practising is to care for people in the way that I want to. The business side can sometimes be a worry and sometimes it can be interesting, but it's not my main motivation.

Furthermore, 57.7% of respondents commented that some form of tension existed for them between the caring and business features of their jobs, whilst 38.3% claimed that such tensions did not exist for them (4% nonresponses). As the frequency of comment clusters in Table 16.1 identify, the most common cited tension between the caring and business features of private CM practice was that it was perceived by some that, in order to be a 'good' and accessible therapist, certain financial sacrifices have to be made at times. Indeed, these types of responses accounted for more than one-quarter of all comments. In particular, two respondents stated:

Table 16.1 Types of tensions between caring and business ownership

Tension	*Frequency of comment*	*Percentage of comments*	*Percentage of respondents*
Sacrificing income because of care needs	87	25.8	20.4
Regulating access to care	77	22.8	18.1
Direct conflicts of interest in practice	50	14.8	11.7
Perceived 'value' of the work	49	14.5	11.5
Charging for care (philosophical opposition)	35	10.4	8.2
Other tensions	39	11.6	9.2
Total	337	100.0	79.1

> I hate having to ask for money as I was used to being in the NHS and working for free. Often I do not ask. I saw a grieving woman last week, she left after 2 hours and I didn't ask for payment.

> I moderate fees to give the very sick access to treatment whilst I'm desperate for income myself.

On a related note, many therapists (18%) were concerned that they were unable to provide care for those who could not afford it. One commented:

> I feel really bad when people who are really sick can't come because they have no money.

Just under one in 10 therapists (8.2%) highlighted an almost diametrical philosophical opposition between caring and profit making, and certain therapists talked of charging being an unfortunate but necessary side effect of their private practice. One commented:

> I'd prefer to be paid by the Government instead of by the clients. I started reflexology because I wanted to make people feel better, not for any other reason ... Charging is a necessity, but part of my job that I don't really enjoy. Charging and caring don't always go well together, and it can feel a little awkward.

Other therapists (11.5%) were more comfortable with charging their clients for their services and their perceived tension did not regard the appropriateness of charging, but in contrast, concerned the perceived financial undervaluing of their work. Two respondents stated:

I would like my service to be available to everyone, yet I have to charge what is perceived to be a high fee and still won't cover my costs. Carers of all sorts, including mothers, are still not valued, and are still expected to give their service freely and willingly.

We have to pay the bills and live like everyone else. It sometimes seems wrong to charge when a client seems not to be able to afford it, but they would gladly pay for a TV or washer to be repaired. Why not their health?

Table 16.2 Reasons why tensions do not exist between caring and business

Reason	*Frequency of comment*	*Percentage of comments*	*Percentage of respondents*
Worth what we are paid	35	32.7	8.2
External mitigating factors	25	23.4	5.8
Donate some time	7	6.5	1.6
All businesses charge for services	6	5.6	1.4
Other	34	31.8	8.0
Total	107	100.0	25.0

As Table 16.2 indicates, certain therapists did not perceive there to be tensions between the business and caring aspects of their jobs. Thirty-five (8.2%) explicitly stated that their services were worth what they charged, and very evident in the tone of similar comments made during interviews was a firm belief in the market delivery system and the exchange of their services for financial compensation. Twenty-five (5.8%) suggested that they did not feel tensions because of external mitigating factors. These were diverse in nature, and included having another job as their main source of income, or being independently wealthy and thus financial compensation for their services not being a great concern to them. Meanwhile, a small number (1.6%) felt less concerned about charging because they donated a proportion of their sessions for free, or at a reduced rate, to those potential clients for whom payment was a problem. Therapists were asked explicitly under what circumstances they would either refuse or withdraw their services, and most (89%) claimed that they have had to do this on more than one occasion. Forty-one per cent of therapists stated that they would or have refused to treat a person because of their modality or expertise not being suited to the condition/illness (Table 16.3). One commented:

If I felt that I couldn't handle their problems effectively and creatively and if they had a condition that I did not feel qualified to treat.

Table 16.3 Reasons for the refusal or withdrawal of treatment

Reason	*Frequency of comment*	*Percentage of comments*	*Percentage of respondents*
Condition is outside the therapist's or their modalities' area	175	24.0	41.0
Potentially deleterious effect on the client's health	93	12.7	21.8
Concern for own personal safety	67	9.2	15.7
Client displays uncooperative behaviour	45	6.2	10.6
Client displays rude, abusive or obnoxious behaviour	42	5.8	9.9
Serious mental health problem obstructing awareness or reason	42	5.8	9.9
Suspicion of a sexual motivation or actual sexual comments	40	5.5	9.4
Client intoxicated with alcohol or illegal drugs	33	4.5	7.7
Client can not pay or has a poor record of payment	30	4.1	7.0
Personal conflict or unresolved disagreement	24	3.3	5.6
Client displays inconsistent or uncommitted behaviour	23	3.2	5.4
Treatment would conflict with another treatment	20	2.7	4.7
Client has very unrealistic expectations of treatment outcomes	18	2.5	4.2
Danger of personal infection	12	1.6	2.8
Client will not act on their doctor's advice	9	1.2	2.1
Client has very poor personal hygiene	7	1.0	1.6
Client displays deceptive behaviour	7	1.0	1.6
Unclear diagnosis	5	0.7	1.2
Client is a relative or a friend	4	0.6	0.9
Others	34	4.7	8.0
Total	730	100.0	–

As may be expected, many respondents (21.8%) stated that they do not or would not perform procedures which would be potentially harmful. One suggested:

> If I think that homeopathic treatment would delay normal medically urgent treatment, if I think that other urgent medical attention is needed and if the patient wants to cut all allopathic medicine completely against my advice.

Certain female therapists (15.7% of all respondents) stated that they do or would refuse or withdraw treatment if they feared for their own personal safety. Indeed, the issue of being alone and sometimes isolated with strangers was an everyday concern, and something to be constantly aware of. Two commented:

> I'd refuse if they sounded dangerous or perverted. I would first tactfully say that I don't think that I have the experience to help them or say that I have a long waiting list.
>
> I say no if I would be putting myself in danger. If I get bad vibes about their intentions. There are a lot of creeps out there.

A number of therapists stated that they had refused or would refuse a client: who was intoxicated by alcohol or illegal drugs (7.7%); who had a poor prior record of payment (7.0%); if there had been a personal conflict or unresolved disagreement with the client which may compromise either neutrality or objectivity (5.6%); if the client had previously wasted their time by not following their advice or by missing appointments (5.4%); or through fear of personal infection (2.8%). Therapists were asked what they would do if a client could no longer afford to pay for the continuation of their treatment but still wanted to continue. Indeed, this was also a reasonably common occurrence and 77% had encountered this scenario on more than one occasion. The majority of therapists (66.9%) claimed that they would negotiate, or at least attempt to negotiate, an affordable price on an individual basis, and would or do attempt to meet the client halfway (Table 16.4). This took a variety of forms. Two suggested:

> I reduce some fees to encourage the patient to continue until they are getting better.
>
> I organise a system of letting them pay later. So much a week until it is fully paid off. With no interest included.

Within this group, the informal exchange of goods (barter) was often a solution to financial dilemmas. Two suggested:

> Some times I do it anyway, but I like to try and barter.
>
> I may accept other things in exchange. A person may make some food or do something practical for me. It rather depends on who they are and what they do. It has to be friendly though and they have to suggest it first.

Some therapists (15.5%) stated that they would or do continue to treat the client for free regardless of their ability to pay at a later date. One suggested:

> I do offer free consultations and treatments, but I need to be very sure of their proclaimed poverty and the realistic chances of success.

Table 16.4 What therapists do/would do if a client could no longer afford to be treated

Course of action	*Frequency of comment*	*Percentage of comments*	*Percentage of respondents*
Negotiate a solution (meet halfway)	285	59.6	66.9
Treat the client for free	66	13.8	15.5
Very dependent on the individual	33	6.9	7.7
Refer to someone cheaper	22	4.6	5.2
Stop treatment	18	3.8	4.2
Provide self-healing/administered treatments for home	10	2.1	2.3
Other	44	9.2	10.3
Total	478	100.0	–

A very small minority (4.2%) suggested that they do or would simply stop providing their service, whilst 10 suggested that they would or do direct the client to undertake related self-administered care at home.

Table 16.5 What therapists do/would do if a treatment was not helping but a client insisted on continuing with it

Course of action	*Frequency of comment*	*Percentage of comments*	*Percentage of respondents*
Let them continue (qualified)	152	30.8	35.7
Refer them on (either to CM or OM practitioners)	132	26.8	30.1
Attempt to reach a resolution through discussion	95	19.3	22.3
Discontinue the treatment	72	14.6	16.9
Change the treatment type	27	5.5	6.3
Reduce the number of treatments	10	2.0	2.3
Do not know	4	0.8	0.9
Give a placebo	1	0.2	0.2
Total	493	100.0	–

Therapists were asked what they do or would do if a client insisted on continuing with an ineffective treatment. This scenario was rarely encountered and less than one-third (29%) were basing their responses on actual experiences. Over one-third of respondents (35.7%) suggested that they would or do continue the treatment (Table 16.5). However, this was almost always a qualified statement and often depended on the particular modality of CM that they practised. For example, two stated:

> What I do is beneficial to well-being and not harmful even if it doesn't cure a particular illness. If they know the limitations and are happy to continue, then so am I.

> I treat as long as the patient was not harmed, they fully realised my position and opinion, and still felt a benefit themselves. Also, there has to be no missed diagnosis to explain the lack of progress.

Some therapists also highlighted the potential differences in patients and their conceptions of the 'effectiveness' of treatments. Two commented:

> If they think that it is helping, then who am I to judge? Unless I thought that I was doing physical damage, I'd continue, and that's unlikely anyway.

> If they insisted on continuing, it would be because they are getting something from it. Perhaps not what I wanted, but I would have to look at my own arrogance and why in that case I thought that I knew best.

Just under one-third of therapists (30.1%) suggested that they would or do refer clients on to either an orthodox or complementary practitioner who may be more able to help them. Two suggested:

> This is unusual, but I would probably refer them on to another therapist.

> I would and do advise them to seek a different treatment, and would suggest alternative therapies that I think would help them.

A significant proportion (22.3%) suggested that they would or do attempt to find a resolution through discussion. Many of these respondents regarded an unnecessary dependence on therapies to be an illness issue in itself. Two suggested:

> I would ask them why and try to work with whatever the real problem was.

> I would not continue to treat them for the former problem, but I would work with them to deal with this dependency issue.

Other responses included: discontinuing treatment against the client's wishes, but for their own good (made by 16.9% of respondents); changing the types of treatment provided (made by 6.3% of respondents); and rather worryingly, in one isolated case, administering a placebo.

DISCUSSION

In the absence of previous dedicated research investigation, the present paper highlights some potential tensions and resolutions for complementary therapists as both carers and business owners. Regarding self-perceptions of their jobs, almost all respondents identified with either being primarily carers, or being equally both carers and business owners. Indeed, very few stated that they were primarily business owners. Although, in all cases, they actually undertake both roles, the data provide some interesting impressionistic evidence on how the providers of CM perceive their jobs. Over half of the therapists claimed that some form of tension exists for them between the caring and business aspects of their jobs, although the form of these tensions varied substantially, ranging from having to sacrifice income to be a good carer to the perceived societal undervaluing of their work. Those who did not perceive there to be tensions between caring and business ownership were quick to cite the undervaluing of their work, and a variety of external factors which made them feel better about charging their clients, such as donating a proportion of their sessions free of charge. Therapists were then given a number of scenarios which could either be hypothetical or real, depending on the individual and their experiences in practice. Most therapists had refused or withdrawn treatments at one time or another, and by far the most common reason was because the health problem was outside their area of expertise. Other common responses included a fear for their or their client's personal safety. Most therapists had also encountered a situation where a client was unable to afford to continue their treatment. Under these circumstances, most chose to negotiate a financial solution or, in some cases, forgo income in order to continue the treatment. Indeed, it is not unreasonable to suggest that few other types of small businesses would be prepared to give their customers such flexibility, albeit that these business owners are also healthcare providers, often with associated ethical codes of practice.

Far fewer therapists had encountered clients who insisted on continuing their treatment against their advice. Regarding this mostly hypothetical scenario, the majority claimed that they would continue treatment, but heavily qualified the responses with prerequisites concerning openness, the sharing of information and continued safety.

In some ways, the present paper poses more questions than it immediately answers. However, it does provide some food for thought and highlights some important areas for future research. In particular, the current research investigated actual or potential actions in different caring and business scenarios. However, questions are raised by the present investigations regarding how therapists feel about these scenarios, conflicts and tensions, and their potential resolutions, and also how much their businesses rely on these types of negotiations for their continued prosperity and survival.

REFERENCES

Andrews GJ, Phillips DR. Moral dilemmas and the management of private residential homes: the impact of care in the community reforms in the UK. *Ageing and Society* 2000;20(5):599–623.

Astin J. Why patients use alternative medicine: results of a national study. *Journal of the American Medical Association* 1998;279(19):1548–53.

Friedson E. The theory of professions: state of the art. In: R Dingwall and P Lewis (Eds) *The Sociology of the Professions*, pp. 19–37. Macmillan, London, 1983.

Greene J. Melatonin for the masses. Antiaging entrepreneurs peddle therapies that promise to cheat the clock. *Hospital Health Network* 1998;72(22):32–4.

Lo B. The patient-provider relationship: opportunities as well as problems. *Journal of General Internal Medicine* 1999;14(Suppl. 1):S41–4.

Lundberg G. The business and professionalism of medicine: a pendulum swings and a rocking horse rocks. *Journal of the American Medical Association* 1997;278(20):1704–5.

May WF. Money and the medical profession. *Kennedy Institute of Ethics Journal* 1997;7(1):1–13.

Sharma U. Complementary practitioners in a Midlands locality. *Complementary Medical Research* 1991;5:12–16.

Sharma U. *Complementary Medicine Today: Practitioners and Patients*. Routledge, London, 1995.

CHAPTER 17

SMALL BUSINESS COMPLEMENTARY MEDICINE: A PROFILE OF THERAPISTS AND THEIR PATHWAYS TO PRACTICE

Gavin J Andrews and Robin Hammond

SMALL BUSINESS COMPLEMENTARY MEDICINE

The provision and use of CM sector has grown rapidly in recent years. Indeed, Vickers (1994) suggests that between 7% and 11% of people visit complementary therapists every year, and Thomas et al (1995) estimates that 33% of the population have used some form of CM at least once in their lives. Meanwhile, the House of Lords Select Committee on Science and Technology (2000), estimates there to be 15 million users of CM nationwide. In the UK, a small but increasing number of therapists are funded directly by public finance, and work for the National Health Service (NHS) in hospital and community settings. However, the majority of therapists earn a living from direct out-of-pocket payments made by privately paying clients (Sharma, 1991, 1995; Zollman and Vickers, 1999). In financial terms, this represents a considerable expenditure. For example, White (1996) estimates the total out-of-pocket spending on private consultations to be between £500 million and £1000 million each year, which represents a figure equivalent to between 1.5% and 3% of the annual NHS budget. Most private therapists operate independently, either practicing alone or in shared facilities, whilst a smaller number are based in GP surgeries and in health centres. Nationally, the CM sector

Edited from *Primary Health Care Research and Development* 2003;5(1):40–51.

may enjoy a considerable financial turnover, but the organisational nature of the sector remains one of small private business, essentially a cottage industry (Fulder, 1996; Sharma 1995). The exact number of complementary therapists in the UK remains disputed because not all CM disciplines are regulated and therapists registered. Nevertheless, Zollman and Vickers (1999) estimate the numbers of therapists to have more than trebled from 13 500 in 1981 to 40 000 in 1997. Both Fulder (1996), and the House of Lords Select Committee on Science and Technology (2000), estimate there to be approximately 50 000 therapists in the UK. In contrast, there are approximately 32 000 GPs in the UK and arguably complementary therapists can sometimes compete, in market terms, with them to provide certain forms of primary health care (Fulder, 1996).

The current research provides evidence of the industries and professions that therapists came from and why they ended up in practice. Second, it provides a profile of their age, gender, and stage in the life course. Arguably, these are issues fundamental to any other consideration of therapists but are yet issues that are relatively under-researched. Therefore, this is a baseline study which contextualizes past and future research on therapists' practice decisions following their market entry.

FINDINGS

Of the 426 respondents, 155 (36.4%) were male, and 269 (63.1%) were female (0.5% non-response). The youngest of the respondents was 25 years old, and the oldest 76 years, the mean age being 46.9 and the standard deviation 10.0. What is therefore immediately striking is the female domination of CM private sector provision and a middle-aged, age profile. Indeed, these findings are supported by Sharma (1991, 1995) which found therapists to have a mean age of 42 years and most to be female. Regarding the structure of their private businesses, 45.3% of therapists claimed to be practicing CM part-time, 48.6% claimed to be practicing full-time, whilst 2.3% just claimed that they worked 'as much as possible' (3.8% non-response). Reflecting the part-time nature of much private practice, 34.9% claimed to supplement their income with other forms of work and 27.6% by working in the same types of work that they were involved in prior to their involvement in a CM businesses. However, a common aim of therapists was to develop their businesses and to eventually work full time. This is reflected in the infancy of many businesses. Indeed, the respondents had been practicing for between 3 months and 43 years, the mean length of practice being 10.5 years and the standard deviation 7.9 years. That many businesses were relatively new, reflected the considerable growth in the private sector in the UK during the previous 15 years.

Table 17.1 Types of therapies offered

Modality	*Frequency*	*Percentage of modalities*	*Percentage of therapists*
Massage	75	9.4	17.6
Homeopathy	75	9.4	17.6
Reflexology	66	8.2	15.5
Psychotherapy	65	8.1	15.3
Osteopathy	64	8.0	15.0
Hypnotherapy	55	6.9	12.9
Aromatherapy	52	6.5	12.2
Acupuncture	45	5.6	10.6
Herbal therapy	36	4.5	8.5
Chiropractic	34	4.2	8.0
Reiki	34	4.2	8.0
Counseling	30	3.7	7.0
Shiatsu	20	2.5	4.7
Alexander Technique	19	2.4	4.5
Nutritional advice	17	2.1	4.0
Naturopathy	13	1.6	3.1
Natural healing	13	1.6	3.1
Allergy advice	9	1.1	2.1
Stress management	7	0.9	1.6
Yoga	5	0.6	1.2
Kinesiology	4	0.5	0.9
Acupressure	3	0.4	0.7
Life Coaching	3	0.4	0.7
Others	57	7.1	13.3
Total	801	100.0	–

The 426 respondents practiced a total of 801 therapies (Table 17.1). Although it was most common for therapists to practice one modality of CM (mode=1), this was evidently not always the case and many therapists specialised in more than one. For the respondents, the number of therapies practiced by individuals ranged between 1 and 8, the mean number being 1.9. These findings support Davies (1984) who found over 50% of therapists to practice more than two therapies and 25% more than three.

The volume of different therapies differs from the findings of previous surveys, which questioned consumers not providers. Zollman and Vickers (1999) report that Which (1986), Mori (1989) and Thomas et al (1993) all list acupuncture as the most common CM modality followed by chiropractic, herbal medicine, homeopathy and osteopathy. Meanwhile, Ernst and White (2000), found herbal medicine to be most the common form of CM, followed by aromatherapy, homeopathy, acupuncture, reflexology, massage, osteopathy and chiropractic. In contrast, and as Table 17.1 identifies, the current study found acupuncture to be 8th most common, chiropractic 10th, herbal medicine 9th, osteopathy 5th and aromatherapy 7th. Massage was most common (practiced by almost one-in-five therapists), a frequency equalled by homeopathy, then closely followed by reflexology (3rd), psychotherapy (4th) and osteopathy (5th). However, an important point to be considered is that the above user surveys calculate frequencies of use and not frequencies of provision as in the current study. Therefore, the data from user and provider surveys may not be either directly comparable or indeed contradictory. More generally, what was also striking was the extremely wide-range of therapies practiced, especially considering that certain categories could include many different variants and sub-varieties. The category 'Massage', for example, included at least 6 variations, some specific to particular parts of the body, some with specific technical procedures and some with origins in specific geographical regions or countries. Swedish massage, deep massage, and therapeutic massage being examples. Indeed, a particular and challenging task during the analysis was identifying and categorizing sub-varieties of CM such was the diversity, specificity and obscurity of many responses.

As Table 17.2 identifies, previous forms of employment are varied. Furthermore a total of 485 responses indicates that respondents could have been employed in more than one job directly prior to their practicing CM. The most common category is 'skilled professional' (78) although this is perhaps slightly deceptive as a discrete category because it contains

Table 17.2 Therapists' previous employment types

Previous employment type	*Frequency*	*Percentage*
Skilled professionals (private sector)	78	16.0
Nursing	63	13.0
Education/teaching	57	11.8
None (student of CM)	52	10.8
Secretarial/clerical	39	8.0
Service sector	34	7.0
Arts-related	33	6.8
Social Care	27	5.6
Social Work	18	3.7
Local Government/civil service	11	2.3
Other NHS	10	2.0
Unskilled manual	10	2.0
Housewife	9	1.9
Private business	9	1.9
Skilled manual	7	1.4
Military	2	0.4
Unemployed	2	0.4
Retired	1	0.2
Missing (non-responses)	23	4.7
Total	485	100.0

a wide-range of former job types including for example, executives, chief engineers, architects, designers, bankers, and public relations managers. These types of jobs, along with some other categories, do though suggest a slightly middle-class, or at least affluent, profile for therapists and in many cases a radical change in job types.

The largest 'single job' category was nursing (63). For this group, a very specific set of 'push' factors from the NHS can be identified which are largely associated with wider structural and experiential issues in the NHS such as the long hours worked, the job pressures created by constant policy and management changes, changes in job roles and frustrations that CM was not adequately integrated into their former jobs. Related 'pull factors' may also be identified. Some are caring related, such as preferences for the way CM deals with patients and their welfare; the closer interpersonal relationships between patients and therapists and being able to help patients to a greater degree. This specific group of nurse-therapists is considered in a dedicated paper in relation to current nursing recruitment and retention debates (Andrews, 2003).

The other caring-related professions of teaching, social care and social work together accounted for almost one-quarter (21%) of all previous professions. The former teachers and social workers were not so explicit about their push factors and dissatisfactions with their former jobs as the nurses. However, given that the questionnaire was generalized and designed to capture the opinions of all professions, and that the researchers had no previous indication that they would arise in substantial numbers, there may well be underlying dissatisfactions that were missed in the current study and thus these therapists, and the issues surrounding their changes in careers, may be worthy of dedicated research investigation. Indeed, given recruitment and retention problems also facing these particular professions, the movement of teachers and social workers into CM is highlighted as an important area for future research.

A relatively small amount of therapists (52, 10.8%) entered the sector straight from education as their first career. Often these therapists were younger and had undertaken either a full or part time course as part of their training directly after school and sometimes within higher and further education institutions. Of the 52 therapists who entered practice straight from their education, 31 were osteopaths. Indeed, these 31 represent almost one-half of all the 64 osteopaths in the questionnaire survey. The first destination career tendency of osteopaths reflects osteopathy's increasingly professional status and the longer periods of often full-time education required to qualify and practice. It may be speculated that, in future, as a wider range of CM modalities gradually become more professionalised, and their training standardized and expanded, the proportions of these first destination career therapists may increase. However, at present, they remain a relatively small minority. Interestingly, very few therapists (1.9%) had owned a business prior to CM practice, yet small

Table 17.3 Motivations and circumstances for entering CM

Motivation	*Frequency of comment*	*Percentage of comments*	*Percentage of therapists*
Witnessed/experienced the success of CM	158	17.5	37.1
Developed a personal interest in therapy	141	15.6	33.1
Wanted to help people	126	14.0	29.6
Unhappy with orthodox medicine	99	11.0	23.2
Unhappy with previous job	55	6.1	12.9
The independence and flexibility of self-employment	52	5.8	12.2
To seek greater job-satisfaction	36	4.0	8.5
Re-evaluation of goals in life (often after crisis)	33	3.7	7.7
A mentor/therapist encouraged them	30	3.3	7.0
Previous job ended/had to leave previous job	23	2.5	5.4
Interpersonal (wanted more contact with people)	20	2.2	4.7
A unique opportunity arose	17	1.9	4.0
For financial benefit	16	1.8	3.8
For spiritual reasons	15	1.7	3.5
To increase personal skills	13	1.4	3.1
Other	68	7.5	16.1
Total	902	100.0	–

business ownership is a necessary bi-product of CM practice, and indeed all of the respondents in the current study ran some form of small private business. Indeed, in-the-light-of this lack of experience, business decisions and attitudes are highlighted as important areas for future research investigation.

As Table 17.3 identifies, over one-third of all therapists (158) stated that they were originally motivated to enter practice after experiencing successful treatment either directly themselves or indirectly by their family and friends:

> 'I received hypnotherapy myself in 1995 coupled with divorce. It was such a wonderful experience which allowed me to deal with all the emotional problems at that time. It has had a profound effect on my life ever since'

Just under one-third of all therapists (141) stated that over time they gradually developed a personal interest in CM, how particular therapies worked, and that this interest eventually led on to their practice. Two suggested:

> 'I began to be interested in the way emotions and spirituality affect physical health'

> 'I was interested in self-healing and then in healing others. I had an intellectual interest in Chinese medicine, anatomy and physiology and how energy works'

Another popular motivation for practice was wanting to help people (126). Indeed, this was a common and very basic caring-related motivation and often something that therapists thought that their former occupations lacked. The final quotation below demonstrates the potential for this motivation to be very personal in nature, and how it can be directly related to family and friends:

> 'I had found that these systems of healing could result in tremendous alleviation of mental, emotional and physical systems so wanted others to receive these benefits'

> 'My father died of cancer. I knew he would get ill before he died, he lost the will to live. No one was treating that and what I do now does. It makes me sad to see people suffer and glad to help'

Others (99) stated an unhappiness with OM, either in its financing, organizational structure or efficacy. For some, this unhappiness originated from direct and first-hand negative experiences of OM, for others it came from more general observations of the formal medical system, and in particular the perceived market connections between OM and pharmaceutical companies. In either scenario, by entering the private sector for CM, therapists had chosen to do something about their unhappiness:

> 'After a period of ill-health, I thought that there had to be a better way. Politically I was scandalized by the lack of choice and the ignorance in orthodoxy. As a biologist, homeopathy made intuitive sense to me'

> 'A realization that orthodox medicine is dominated by pharmaceutical companies aiming to make enormous profits. They exert massive influence on doctors with hard-sell propaganda and hidden bribes ignoring more effective, side-effect free, but less profitable treatments'

As Table 17.3 identifies other reasons included dissatisfaction with a previous job (55) and seeking greater job-satisfaction (36). Together these two work-related push factors accounted for just over 10% of responses. Wanting to be self employed (52), a re-evaluation of life's goals (33) and being encouraged by a mentor (30), were also common, whilst relatively few (16) cited financial motivations. Given that over 900 reasons were

Table 17.4 Satisfactions and rewards gained from practice

Satisfaction/reward	*Frequency of comment*	*Percentage of comments*	*Percentage of therapists*
Greater everyday job satisfaction	243	31.2	57.0
Ability to help people	226	30.0	53.1
Interpersonal relationships formed	62	8.0	14.6
Independence/autonomy/flexibility	55	7.1	12.9
Personal development/skills development	49	6.3	11.5
Interest/stimulating	35	4.5	8.2
Financial	30	3.9	7.0
Challenging	20	2.6	4.7
Spiritual	10	1.3	2.3
Ethical/moral	8	1.0	1.9
Less stress	6	0.8	1.4
Other	36	4.6	8.5
Total	780	100.0	–

cited by the 426 therapists, and the mixed reasons highlighted even in the above quotations, many respondents evidently had multiple motivations for entering CM. Indeed, the interviews often revealed complex and very individualised stories about therapists' particular pathways to practice. What is undeniable however is that these changes in mid-career and life course were not only highly and complexly motivated, they were often radical and substantial changes. As a consequence, respondents' day-to-day experiences of work life have changed considerably.

The survey also investigated the positives that therapists gained from CM. As Table 17.4 identifies, well over one-half of all respondents (243) cited greater 'everyday' satisfaction with their jobs. One commented:

> 'Connecting with the mysteries of life and living. I'm fascinated with life's process and always think wow, amazing. Extraordinary things happen and they do frequently'

Related to the caring motivation cited earlier for entry into the CM sector, over one-half of therapists (226) cited being able to help people and make a difference to their health and well-being as positive features of their jobs. In this respect, it seems that, for many, their hopes and needs had been met. Two respondents commented:

> 'I get a great sense of achievement and also a profound sense of privilege at being allowed to be with people at crucial moments of change and revelation in their lives'

> 'The joy of seeing people get better and become happier. It is quite common for peoples lives to change dramatically for the better after treatment'

Importantly, the above gains of 'everyday satisfaction' and 'helping people' account for over 60% of all responses. Other responses accounted for much smaller proportions. Sixty-two respondents, for example, cited interpersonal factors and enjoying close contact with people:

> 'Joy in giving and receiving, connecting with people in a full way; emotionally, mentally, spiritually and physically and thus connection is kept alive on a personal level'

Others cited the independence and flexibility of their job (55). Indeed, this reflects that, for many, a CM practice was their first self-owned private business and this, in itself, was an attractive feature of their working lives. Two respondents commented:

> 'I can have an independent view, flexibility and more time with patients and I'm able to adjust my hours to suit myself'

> 'I've the freedom to work with my own ideas, make my own decisions without the constraints of the NHS'

Interestingly, as with motivations, very few respondents cited financial rewards as an important feature of practice (30). Evidently, as with reasons for market entry, income was not a prime motivating factor (at least admitted). This is understandable given the context of the large proportion of part-time practice and given the secure professional jobs that many therapists had given up. Interviews also highlighted that each therapist had a very personalised story to tell. Many provided an example of an individual patient case when elaborating. One suggested:

> 'She use to come in and she looked lost. I've seen her confidence gradually grow and she seems like a different person. Now, I know its my job but just imagine how good that makes me feel. When the evidence is right in front of you, you know that you're doing a good thing'

However, as the total amount of comments (780) and the following quotation both suggest, quite often, respondents had a combination of gains:

> 'It's a good way to work with people and help people improve their lives. Its fascinating work, and very rewarding, satisfying and challenging. I enjoy working with people and interacting at a deep and meaningful level'

CONCLUSION

In the context of a relative paucity of dedicated research investigation, this paper highlights some broad trends in therapists and their pathways to practice, together with providing some detailed attitudinal data on their motivations and general experiences. Although many males were therapists, the sector is female dominated. Therapists are a wide-range of ages but tend towards the middle aged. They work a mixture of full and part-time hours, but many work part-time hours and supplement their income with other forms of work. The majority of businesses are relatively new, reflecting growth in the sector during the past fifteen years. Manual therapies such as massage and reflexology are the most common modalities, but many therapists practiced more than one modality. Complementary medicine was often a second career for therapists who entered the sector from a variety of former occupations. The most common 'group' were skilled professionals, however, this group was extremely varied. Many therapists came from caring-related professions such as nursing, teaching and social work, and in general there was a middle-class dominated ownership profile. A small amount of therapists were practicing as a first career and came straight from their education. This group was dominated by osteopaths who generally required longer and full-time periods of training in order to practice. Therapists were motivated by a combination of push and pull factors to enter practice which often related to being unhappy in their previous job, witnessing the success of CM and wanting to care for people. Their gains from practice were equally varied, ranging from an everyday job satisfaction to being able to help people, the interpersonal relationships formed though practice and being able to be flexible. Notably, pure business and financial reasons were rarely cited for both original motivations and personal gains.

More generally, the research demonstrates that providers of a range of private non-traditional primary health care are entering the market from equally non-traditional career and professional backgrounds. These are a diverse set of people, with a diverse set of motivations, providing a diverse range of health care. However, in terms of volume, they are effectively providing the majority of primary health care in the United Kingdom and arguably in the developed world, more so than even general practitioners/family physicians. The argument and research agenda is clear, and our point is simple; that surely a range and depth of research should mirror this fact. Currently the literature on CM provision is growing but extremely slowly and from a very small base. Researching CM is undoubtedly a trans-disciplinary social science research endeavor and one that, given the first-contact and dispersed nature of much provision, those interested in primary health care could meaningfully contribute.

REFERENCES

Andrews GJ. Nurses who left the NHS to practice private complementary medicine: Why did they leave? Would they return? *Journal of Advanced Nursing* 2003;41:1–13.

Davies P. *Report on trends in complementary medicine*. London: ICM.

Ernst E, White A. The BBC survey of complementary medicine use in the UK. *Complementary Therapies in Medicine* 2000;8:32–6.

Fulder S. *The Handbook of Alternative and Complementary Medicine*, Oxford: Oxford University Press, 1996.

House of Lords Select Committee on Science and Technology. Complementary and Alternative Medicine. HL paper 123, November, 2000.

MORI (Market and Opinion Research International). *Research on Alternative Medicine*, 1989.

Sharma U. Complementary practitioners in a Midlands locality. *Complementary Medical Research* 1991;5:12–16.

Sharma U. *Complementary Medicine Today: Practitioners and Patients*. London: Routledge, 1995.

Thomas K, Fall M, Nicholl J, Williams B. *Methodological study to investigate the feasibility of conducting a population-based survey of the use of complementary health care*. London: RCCM, 1993.

Thomas K, Fall M, Parry G, Nicholl J. *National survey of access to complementary health care via general practice: report of Department of Health*. Sheffield: SCHARR, 1995.

Vickers, AJ. Use of complementary therapies (letter). *British Medical Journal* 1994;309:1161.

Which. *Magic or Medicine?* 1986;October issue:443–7.

White A. Do complementary therapists offer value for money? In: *Complementary Medicine: An Objective Appraisal* Ernst E (ed). Oxford: Butterworth Heinemann, 1996.

Zollman C, Vickers A. The ABC of complementary medicine: users and practitioners of complementary medicine. *British Medical Journal*, 1999;319:836–8

CHAPTER 18

COMPLEMENTARY THERAPY PROVISION IN PRIMARY CARE – POLICY CONSIDERATIONS BASED ON CASE STUDIES IN PRACTICE

Donna Luff and Kate Thomas

Findings from a 1995 survey of a random sample of GP practices in England indicated that 6% of practices had a complementary health care practitioner working on the premises, while 21% of practices reported having a member of the primary health care team who provided a complementary therapy to the practice patients, and 25% of practices reported making NHS referrals for complementary therapies (1st Access study). The present study addressed the need to increase our understanding of how these schemes operate in *practice* (e.g. how do the schemes work and what needs are they expected to meet), in order to inform policy making in a context of rapid change. The study was conducted in 10 purposively selected sites across England in 1998. The sample was designed to include the *range* of complementary therapy services currently available. The study generated in-depth case studies by employing multiple research methods including observational site visits and interviews with GPs, practitioners and patients.

The study was not an evaluation of individual services, rather it aimed:

- To give a full descriptive analysis of a purposively selected sample of ten schemes covering the range of provision currently provided, including the rationale for service development.

Edited from a report published by Medical Care Research Unit, School of Health and Related Research, University of Sheffield.

- To assess perceptions of the impact of the schemes on the organisation of each practice, on patient satisfaction, and on practice costs.
- To identify the potential problems and perceived benefits as they apply in general to the provision of complementary therapies in primary care, and as they are specific to particular modes of organising such a service.

THE FUTURE OF COMPLEMENTARY THERAPIES IN A PRIMARY HEALTH CARE LED NHS

The research findings presented here contribute to a growing literature and debate about the integration of complementary therapies in primary care. Here we consider the main issues highlighted by this research relating to the organisation and sustainability of the different services studied and situate them within the wider policy-related debates about the provision of complementary health care within primary care.

We characterised the services in the case studies presented according to their structural features, their primary funding source, and their philosophical approach (i.e. the dominant stated rationale behind the service offered). Each of these was shown to have an identifiable impact on the character and sustainability of the services offered.

IN-HOUSE OR OFF-SITE PROVISION?

Structural features include the physical location of the service, (in-house or off-site), the scope of the service (exclusive to the practice or offered to a wider population), administrative arrangements, and level of GP control (GP instigated and part of the practice or independent of the practice). Whilst structural features are useful for distinguishing between types of provision, in practice they are not always mutually exclusive. Thus it is possible to have a 'semi-detached' service, where the complementary medicine service operates in adjacent property to the practice, with a shared administrator, is GP instigated but offers a large degree of autonomy to the practitioners.

This study has shown that there are many perceived benefits of complementary practitioners working on-site within a GP surgery. For GPs and complementary practitioners alike it offers an opportunity for the structural integration of complementary therapies into the routine work of the primary care team. It also offers ease of access to facilities and greater opportunities for communication and education. In the on-site models ease of access to tests, patient notes and further referrals was seen as a notable advantage by complementary practitioners. From the GP perspective, the on-site model also allows a considerable degree of control over the shape and scope of the service, and the opportunity to tailor it to the perceived needs of the practice population. These characteristics of on-site services may serve to enhance the actual and potential benefits to patients and provide continuity of care. However, it is clear that these should be regarded as *potential* rather than *guaranteed* benefits of being on-site.

On-site services tend to offer a limited range of therapies and are usually restricted to providing care to patients registered with the practice. The exception to this is the service which cuts across the distinction between the inclusive/exclusive patient population provision by offering some access to the practice population as an NHS service, whilst at the same time operating as a private service for the wider community. The ability to do this stems from the structural separation of the service from the practice. This model of provision clearly also has the capacity to extend its services to NHS patients from other practices in the locality. At the time of the study, another practice which was part of the same multi-fund as the sampled practice, also made NHS referrals to the service.

Services located off-site, in a referral centre accessible to local GPs, create conditions for greater complementary practitioner control over the ethos and running of the centre. Inevitably, this means that GPs have less scope for shaping the service to suit their perception of particular patients needs, and the scope for communication and mutual education is restricted by the absence of any shared space. Problems relating to communication with primary care teams and ease of access to the services which are more readily available on-site are also important considerations which are confirmed in the existing literature (Reid, 1993; Richardson, 1995). On the benefits side, off-site referral centres can clearly offer services to many general practices within an area. In terms of the stated desire of policy makers to consider equity of access in complementary therapy provision (Smith and Wilton, 1998; Trevelyan, 1998), referral centres may therefore have advantages over on-site services. In practice, however, this capacity will be mediated by the willingness and financial ability of local primary care teams to make referrals to a complementary health care centre. In the absence of a common policy of how to use the referral centre and general commitment from the primary care teams in the area, differential access to services are likely to remain a feature of this model of provision.

FUNDING AND EQUITY

While structural features clearly have an important role in the way a service is delivered and its capacity to respond to external policy changes, other factors also impact on the service development and organisation, most notably the issue of funding. The funding of complementary therapies in primary care is perhaps the central issue which cuts across all the lessons that can be drawn from existing models. Whether and how to fund such provision, and which therapies should be routinely funded within the NHS are key policy questions.

The current picture with regard to the funding of existing services is one of innovation and seizing opportunities as they emerge, with a background perception that the long term future of the service is uncertain. Funding arrangements currently include various NHS sources (local Primary Care Trust development monies, and ancillary staff budgets), patient out of pocket expenditure, donations and charitable trust funding.

Many of the cases investigated have negotiated a variety of funding sources over time and there are important lessons to be drawn from this. As has been noted elsewhere complementary therapy provision remains a 'marginal' if widespread activity in the NHS (Thomas et al, 1995; Trevelyan, 1998) and as such practices have been forced to be creative in securing and maintaining funds for their services.

The cases that exhibit the highest levels of anxiety about funding are directly dependent on Health Authority or PCT decision-makers for monies. A perception of greater flexibility and stability is exhibited in the private, charitable and GP fundholding models. Whilst private models currently contribute much to primary care complementary therapy provision, there are important issues of equity of access which give cause for concern to many GPs and complementary practitioners alike. NHS-funded sites reported that a key benefit of complementary therapies as part of primary care was increased equality of access for those who otherwise would be unable to afford such services. In the one site where all provision was privately financed by patients, it was recognised that this avenue was only possible for the relatively affluent section of the patient population, and GPs and practitioners alike expressed a high degree of frustration about funding and concerns about widening the health divide.

Charitable funding, managed via a trust fund, can be seen as a 'halfway house' in addressing this issue, with greater possibilities for the routine reduction or wavering of direct charges to patients. However these schemes require high levels of personal commitment to the time consuming activities of continual fund-raising, and there may be issues about their viability and expansion, particularly in deprived locales, without some statutory support or 'national' profile. In terms of equity of access, the majority of respondents in this study would support the view that 'long term NHS funding' is essential for the secure maintenance of services free at the point of delivery to patients on any large scale (Hills and Welford, 1998).

In the current climate of change within primary care, consideration needs to be given at a policy level both to the continuity of successful schemes of complementary therapy provision already in existence, and to fostering a greater equity of such provision so that the current pattern of provision, favouring certain sections of the patient population, is not further replicated.

The fact that many of these services are maintained through the vision and commitment of key individuals underpins both the strength and the vulnerability of many of these services. The history of the services described in these case studies suggests that while they may be vulnerable to funding changes, they are clearly also characterised by their ability to respond and adapt to new contexts. Their longevity appears to be related to their ability to identify emerging funding sources, coupled with the determination and drive of the key instigators. The services described in this study are by definition experimental and innovative. They have developed in a context which is not generally supportive, and it is clear that the existence of a key advocate of the service is necessary for their continued existence. To a greater or lesser degree, this means that the services themselves reflect the priorities and beliefs of the instigators. This includes the range of services on offer and the mode of delivery, as well as the degree of integration between conventional and complementary medicine.

To date, the use of fundholding savings has provided the most accessible source of NHS finance for complementary therapy services in primary care. The flexibility afforded by GP fundholding has enabled many of the existing schemes to develop and has facilitated a growth in complementary provision within primary care overall. However, these developments have been ad hoc and depend critically on the beliefs and commitment of lead GPs. The need for research-based evidence to guide future developments, and to help them to distinguish between 'core' and 'fringe' therapies was expressed by a number of GP respondents.

A 'SUPERMARKET' OR 'DELI' SERVICE?

The non statutory nature of these services, and the consequent funding patterns have led to an idiosyncratic pattern of provision around the country, and an absence of any overarching vision of the role of such therapies in the future of a primary-care led NHS. As this study has shown, at one level each of the services has its own 'personality', and no two services were found that were similar in all respects. In practice, structural features are mediated by operational and cultural features which play a large role in defining the character of each service.

This guiding rationale for the complementary care service within the practice is related to the overall vision of the style of primary care offered by the practice. This has a clear and identifiable impact on all aspects of the way in which a service operates and develops. In particular it impacts on the ways in which the appropriate style of service delivery is viewed. Shopping metaphors may illustrate this point. Within existing services there are both 'supermarket' and 'deli'-style approaches to the provision of complementary health care. In a 'supermarket' the principle is to maximise choice with minimal control on decisions about which product (therapy) to choose. In contrast in a 'deli' the aim is to provide specialised services, pre-selected and evaluated in some way. The policy question would appear to be whether we are happy to accept a plural model where both styles of provision can exist depending on local needs, visions and circumstances or are we arguing that one style is preferable or more desirable than the other? A key issue here seems to be about the control that GPs and primary care organizations keep over the integration of complementary health care, that is the extent to which they remain gatekeepers for funded services, and this is an area that needs further debate and discussion.

'ADDITIVE' OR 'TRANSFORMATIVE'?

Another defining characteristic lies in the philosophical approach, or rationale, for the service. Two broad rationales were identified from the case study data – the perceived need to extend existing services to enhance the choice offered to patients ('additive'), and the perceived need to offer more appropriate services in the context of a desire to change the character of primary care ('transformative'). In any single case both these rationales could be in evidence, but in practice one of them tends to dominate, and provides the driving force for establishing and maintaining the survival of the service.

PROFESSIONAL INTEGRATION AND TEAM WORK

The dominant rationale for the service also has implications for the nature of the working relationships between the GPs and the complementary therapists. Concerns amongst complementary practitioners about their role and autonomy within NHS primary care are played out against a background of funding arrangements which place GPs firmly in the role of gatekeeper and arbiter of services. In this study we found mixed responses to incorporation within the NHS, but concerns were frequently expressed by practitioners about their status and autonomy. Interestingly, practitioners working in those practices where the 'additive' approach dominated were no more likely to express these concerns than those working in practices with a dominant 'transformative' philosophy. Considerable variation was observed in the way in which service rationale and leadership impacted on expectations regarding control, teamwork, communication and shared learning. The extent to which each of these services was successful, and worked well on its own terms, appeared to be dependent, in part, on the existence of a shared vision of the service, its aims and potential. Agreement about joint working methods and functional day-to-day relationships followed from this. In this respect as well, each service studied was slightly different and none offered an obvious solution to the problems inherent in the practice of integration.

THE NEED FOR MORE RESEARCH

The evidence base for complementary therapies in primary care is limited and, not surprisingly perhaps, plays a relatively small part in the way that services have been set up and operate. However, there is a clear, expressed need for more research in the area of complementary therapies and primary care. The types of research advocated by service providers covers clinical effectiveness, patient satisfaction, service evaluation and cost-effectiveness. The perceived need for further research by this group stems in part from the recognition that evidence is required to support the process of obtaining and securing reliable funding. With some notable exceptions, practices in our sample lacked the skills and resources to undertake extensive research, although a number of practices were undertaking some form of internal monitoring of the service they offered.

There was evidence of a widespread belief in the cost-effectiveness of complementary therapy provision within primary care, alongside a belief that this was difficult to prove within the models studied. In particular, the difficulties of conducting cost-effectiveness research in an established service were presented as a barrier. The perceived ability of complementary medicine to 'make in-roads into areas of care where conventional medicine has been singularly unsuccessful' (Smith and Wilton, 1998) may be of particular significance in evaluating the cost implications of such services. Work on cost-effectiveness would be welcomed as timely and helpful to inform debates about the direction and development of existing services. Whilst there would seem to be a particular need for cost-effectiveness studies, the logistics of doing this kind of research within primary care are complicated, as the feasibility study conducted in this research has illustrated.

Where it existed within the cases involved in this research, patient feedback was positive. The level of patient demand is also seen as a key indicator of the desirability and success by service providers and users. The patient interviews conducted specifically for this study would further support an overwhelmingly positive valuation of complementary therapy provision by patients. In particular the following aspects of complementary treatment seem to be prized: the caring nature of complementary practitioners; the holistic approach, in particular the explanations for ill-health and the control over/responsibility for health offered; clinical benefits and health outcomes, i.e. that it 'works', at 'best' producing complete cures, at 'worst' ameliorating chronic problems and improving quality of life. These results are comparable to those reported elsewhere that indicate that patients have a positive response to the complementary treatment approach, value gaining more insight and understanding of their problems, and report significant changes in their health status (Hills and Welford, 1998; Richardson, 1995).

Whilst the patient research from this study was limited in many aspects, the correlation of the findings here with other studies suggests that the qualitative methodology used was equally successful in drawing out the significant dimensions of patient satisfaction whilst also avoiding some of the noted pitfalls of questionnaires, for example their acceptability to disadvantaged patient groups (Hotchkiss, 1995). However, the highly positive levels of satisfaction found in this study did not appear to be related to the type of therapy provided or to the model of provision. Whilst high levels of reported patient satisfaction can be taken as indicative of the value and overall acceptability of such provision, outcome studies are still needed to assess longer term benefits and to identify the specific health gains for particular patient groups (Hills and Welford, 1998).

Overall, there are clear opportunities to learn from, and utilise, the experiences of existing services through appropriate research interventions. The sites involved in this study saw the generation of research and audit evidence from their experience as important, but most felt constrained in these activities by resources, time and expertise. The majority had conducted some form of audit and/or evaluation of the service but in many cases this was limited or sporadic. Interviewees at several of the sites studied expressed a keen interest in conducting research. In practice many services may be caught in a double bind; they perceive a need for research based evidence to develop future plans for the service or to secure future funding, but the ability to conduct such research rests critically on the existence of a stable service.

THE FUTURE OF COMPLEMENTARY THERAPIES IN A PRIMARY HEALTH CARE LED NHS

The purpose of this study was to inform policy making in a time of change, to draw lessons from the current situation which can be transferred into new and emerging contexts. In the event, NHS primary care policy has altered significantly with the publication of the NHS white paper (Secretary of State for Health, 1998). The ending of GP fundholding in 1999 and the introduction of locality commissioning through primary care trusts will set the context for the survival and the development of complementary health care services in primary care in the foreseeable future.

It seems possible that funding for commissioning complementary health care could be made available to primary care trusts in response to the charge of developing new services to meet local demands and needs. In terms of their practical characteristics and location within primary health care structures, each of the models described in this study has the potential to respond to locality commissioning strategies. In practice, it seems likely that any such development will happen most readily in areas with existing services and build on current practice. For this to happen, existing services will have to survive a period of change and uncertainty affecting all aspects of primary care. In-house services financed by fundholding savings will perceive themselves to be at risk with the end of fund-holding. These services will survive in their present form only if a margin of flexibility and innovation is retained at individual practice level. The potential for these in-house services to offer care to a wider population depends, in part, on their capacity for expansion, which in turn, will depend on practitioners' willingness to increase the number of sessions which they currently offer, and on the availability of suitable premises.

The NHS white paper makes provision for a service which is responsive to local needs and to patient demand for services. At one level, this suggests an opportunity for the expansion of complementary therapy provision. However, a service developed for a particular practice population by a GP or GPs with a particular vision of the benefits of the service will not necessarily appeal to all neighbouring practices. In principle, there is no barrier to having more than one service available within a given locality, thus offering GPs a choice of referral destinations for complementary therapies. In practice, a single centre for referral seems a more likely scenario. The semi-detached service offered by one of our study cases could be in a strong position to expand the NHS service it currently offers to one practice by substituting private work for NHS work, referred by other GPs in the locality.

The 'mixed economy' of this model may also make it more likely to survive the transition period from fundholding to PCTs as the commissioning mechanism.

Off-site examples of complementary health care services would appear to be well-suited to expanding their services within a locality. The particular focus on healing, and strong ethos of a particular type of care which characterises the first of our two off-site cases suggests that this service may be less likely to allow itself to be shaped by the demands of NHS commissioners. The independent, charitable funding basis for this service allows it the autonomy to precede according to its own ethos. In contrast, the second referral centre sampled, which is dependent on NHS funding, may be more vulnerable but ultimately more responsive to the demands of locality purchasers.

Each of the complementary health care services described in this study was unique and innovatory, and each could lend itself to changes required by locality commissioning if the provision of these therapies was perceived to be of sufficient importance at the Primary Care Trust level. In both on-site and off-site models their advantages are mediated by the level of GP involvement and commitment, the vision of integrated care held by key stakeholders, and the availability and source of funding. GPs, patients and complementary practitioners all report significant and wide ranging benefits in offering these services. If such services are to be encouraged under the new primary care arrangements, a key policy question to be addressed may be whether the way forward lies in the present ad hoc, personality-led development, resulting in a diversity of services, or whether a more standardised approach is required, offering guidelines relating to the scope, scale and purpose of these services, as well as recommendations relating to working practices aimed at facilitating the integration of complementary practitioners in the NHS.

REFERENCES

Hills D, Welford R. *Complementary Therapy is General Practice: an evaluation of the Glastonbury Health Centre*, Complementary Medicine Service, Glastonbury, The Somerset Trust for Integrated Health Care, 1998.

Hotchkiss J. *Liverpool Centre for Health: the first year of a service offering complementary therapies on the NHS*, Liverpool Public Health Observatory, 1995.

Reid T. Alternative approach. *Nursing Times* 1993;89(29):18.

Richardson J. Complementary therapies on the NHS: the experience of a new service. *Complementary Therapies in Medicine* 1995;3(3):153–7.

Smith R, Wilton P. General practice fundholding: progress to date, *British Medical Journal* 1998;48:1253–7.

Thomas K, Fall M, Parry G, Nicholl J. *National survey of access to complementary health care in a general practice*, Medical Care Research Unit, University of Sheffield, 1995.

Trevelyan J. Complementary options, *Nursing Times* 1998;94:28–9.

Secretary of State for Health. *The New NHS*, London: Stationery Office, 1998.

CHAPTER 19

HEALING IN THE SPIRITUAL MARKETPLACE

Marion Bowman

One striking feature of late 20th-century spirituality is the perception of the need for healing. As scholars such as Albanese (1992) and McGuire (1988, 1993) have indicated, the emphasis in many quarters has shifted from such questions as 'What can I do to be saved?' or 'What can I do to save the world?' to 'What can I do to be healed?' or 'How can I heal the world?'

In Britain (as elsewhere) there are a huge variety of meanings of healing and proposed means of achieving healing (see Bowman, 2000). This paper will briefly review some of the trends which are contributing to the present focus on healing and the place of healing in the spiritual marketplace, before looking at the industry which is emerging in Britain as a result of this need for healing and some of the spiritual and financial ideas underpinning it.

HEALING AND THE SPIRITUAL MARKETPLACE

The complexities of the term 'New Age' have been addressed by scholars elsewhere, most notably for the present purposes York (1995, 1997), Rose (1996) and Van Hove (1999). It is necessary to be cautious about using the label 'New Age' too broadly or indiscriminately. However, there are those who articulate a belief in their participation in, or helping to usher in, or the expected arrival of a New Age. How this New Age is to be

Edited from *Social Compass* 1999;46(2):181–9.

brought about (paradigm shift, astrological movement), when it will commence (if it has not already done so), what it will be like, and so on all remain subjects to debate.

Nevertheless, certain packages of ideas have become increasingly common both within and outside specifically New Age circles, such as the importance of the individual spiritual quest, inter-connectedness, synchronicity, a particular understanding of reincarnation, the notion that spirituality and money need not be mutually exclusive and, most significant in this context, the need for healing.

Particular stress has been laid on the role of the individual, the focus on self, and the importance accorded to individual perception and experience in the contemporary spiritual milieu. But there has always been an extent to which personal religiosity has been a very individual collage of beliefs and practices drawn from both official and vernacular traditions, influenced largely by personal experience and perceptions of efficacy (Bowman, 1992). Individuals within what might be thought of as fairly monolithic religious traditions have woven very idiosyncratic fabrics of belief. Within Christianity, for example, many have specifically believed in the importance of the individual's response to the divine (whether external or within), the individual's own understanding of scripture and contemporary events, and the authentic and authenticating nature of individual experience. The big differences nowadays can be seen in individuals' freedom to talk openly about their beliefs, the perception that there is not one version of 'Truth', the notion of serial spirituality or 'singular, serial and multiple seeking strategies' (Sutcliffe, 1997:106) and the range and availability of materials for the individual collage.

The term 'spiritual supermarket' has often been used in a derogatory fashion to describe both New Age and late 20th-century spirituality generally. However, this may well be regarded as an accurate, value-free characterisation of the contemporary situation, in which many people are experiencing greater religious consumer choice than ever before due to globalised spiritual commodification. In terms of abundance, accessibility and availability, this is a comparatively new phenomenon. The spiritual marketplace (Van Hove, 1999) is therefore a concept that is helpful and appropriate.

In the world of holistic healing there is no single paradigm of illness, healing and cure; both clients and practitioners constantly negotiate what is meant by such terms. This is not an entirely new situation. In 18th-century Britain, for example, there was a variety of paradigms or models of illness and therefore of cure. Many views of health/illness were what we would now describe as holistic. They were much concerned with balance, whether that meant the balance of the humours or whatever was considered the vital force, which might be blood, semen, or some less tangible substance. Disease as imbalance meant that there was an element of personal responsibility in maintaining the healthy balance, relating it to all aspects of life. The part could not be treated without addressing the whole. Illness was also frequently considered to contain a message; it was often seen to have a religious meaning, whether as a punishment, a warning, an ennobling experience or a test of faith. It might be potentially damning, but it might equally be positive and potentially redemptive, a timely reminder of appropriate behaviour. Illness therefore had to be considered on both the physical and metaphysical plane. (It is also worth noting that many historians locate the beginnings of 'consumer society' in Georgian England, and medical historian Roy Porter has described this period as 'an age of golden opportunity for cultivating the business side of medicine.' (Porter 1986:21))

While medical pluralism has of course continued in a variety of forms, through religious healing, homeopathy, herbalism, patent medicines and folk practices, from the latter part of the 19th century and much of the 20th century, what came to be considered 'orthodox' medicine revolved around the allopathic approach and the primacy of the germ theory. In this model, illness is seen as the indiscriminate invasion of the individual's body by germs from outside, with medicine's job being to repel or kill the invaders; alternatively, illness is seen as a breakdown in the body's mechanism or a part failure, which can be repaired or replaced. In this model of physical illness, disease is random, an alien entity which 'afflicts our "body" – which is not quite the same as our selves.' (Porter, 1987:25) Just as illness is external to us, we have come to rely on an outside agent, from the medical profession, to cure us; we are passive recipients of both disease and cure. Illness has lost its 'meaning'.

It is therefore significant that we are now seeing a large scale re-emergence of holistic ideas about health and illness, about the importance of balance, about the vital force at the base of health. What is happening in relation to healing reflects a number of social and religious trends, some of which have already been touched upon. It has, for example, been claimed that many are adopting post-material values which emphasise self-expression and quality of life, rather than simply economic and physical security, and involve a new attitude to self which takes responsibility in areas of life previously left to professionals, such as clergy or doctors. Meanwhile, the fragmentation of society experienced at the personal level might be seen to contribute to a stress on the need for wholeness and reconstruction.

Much contemporary religiosity, as I have mentioned, has been characterised as 'the spiritual supermarket' or 'pick and mix spirituality'. This characterisation would certainly fit aspects of holistic healing. The individual can choose one form of healing, or put together a package, from a huge reservoir of alternatives, according to personal choice.

> One woman told me that her mother used to treat sties by crossing them with her wedding ring (an established folk religious cure),

> crossing them with her picture of St Gerard (of whom she was particularly fond), and bathing them with boracic acid (a widely recognised folk remedy). (Bowman, 1992:16)

Nevertheless, the perceptions of available resources for healing and what needs to be healed have changed. In the present climate of enhanced consumer choice of healing predicated on a variety of worldviews, it may be both useful and legitimate to regard holistic healing as a form of non-aligned spirituality, 'believing without belonging' (Davie, 1994).

Disease is coming to be seen not simply as a powerful message for the individual, but for the universe; the need for healing is being perceived at both the individual and global levels. As a leaflet advertising healing Reiki puts it; 'Today, there is a growing awareness that each individual bears responsibility for their own health and ultimately the fate of the planet.' The publicity for a workshop on crystals claims; 'Crystals are remarkable tools for healing, personal development and planetary transformation.' Sir George Trevelyan, often described as the father of New Age in Britain, commented 'Holistic includes holiness and wholeness. Healing is the restoring of harmony to the living whole.' (The New Age, Channel 4, 1991) A key concept in such healing rhetoric is interconnectedness. Individuals may embark upon their own spiritual quest, or ostensibly seek healing for themselves, but it is ultimately seen as part of a larger whole.

HEALING AND THE SPIRITUAL SERVICE INDUSTRY

Healing can be a do-it-yourself project, embarked upon through reading within the vast range of publications on the subject. Increasingly adult and continuing education in Britain includes study relating to therapies of various sorts. The programme for the University of Bath's Community Courses, for example, always features (in addition to old favourites such as Art, Music, Literature, History and Languages) courses under the title 'Personal Skills' which include Aromatherapy, Alexander Technique, Shiatsu, Yoga and Reflexology. Throughout Britain there are innumerable healing workshops and/or holistic healers to choose from. (Bowman, 2000). In Bath the local Further Education College offers a Holistic Therapy course designed, as the course literature explains, 'to appeal to the mature student'. It includes modules in Aromatherapy, Reflexology, Advanced Massage Techniques, and 'investigative study in iridology, homeopathy, shiatsu-do, and Tai-chi'.

The dazzling range of consumer choice in the spiritual and therapeutic marketplace provides a host of job opportunities. Nowadays in management development (an area much influenced either overtly or covertly by New Age ideas) there are no problems, only opportunities. So, what might be perceived as a problem – the need for healing – presents opportunities both for the individuals who aspire to take control of this situation, to exercise their spiritual and financial autonomy to commission healing, and for the healers, who aspire to help while simultaneously making a living. Many holistic healers are female, frequently in their thirties or over, 'caring' and 'spiritual' people, whose background, education, circumstances or youthful inclinations denied them a profession, medical or otherwise, but for whom holistic healing provides hitherto unrecognised career opportunities.

For many what starts as a personal interest or spiritual quest comes to take the form of a sort of post-industrial home industry. One Bath therapist, who in the past spent time in both Buddhist and Sufi communities, is a now yoga teacher in a variety of venues, and in her home provides aromatherapy, relaxation, massage therapy, yoga therapy and stress management. She wishes to train as an interfaith minister. She is very much concerned with body, mind and spirit – ministering to physical and metaphysical needs – but rejects the title 'healer' as she sees herself merely as a facilitator, not the source of healing. The multi-skill approach of this woman, like so many of the new breed of healers, might be seen to reflect the 'bricolage' approach of much contemporary religiosity, constantly seeking new approaches and insights, both for her own benefit as well as that of her clients.

While many see the growth in holistic healing as being in tune with spiritual trends, it is not unrelated to other economic trends. In Britain, for the moment at least, National Health services are free, but holistic healing always involves charges. However, contemporary holistic healers see themselves as offering a service which should be valued in both personal and financial terms. Very much in the spirit of the New Age soteriological entrepreneur, it is thought that one can be spiritual and make money, that cash is cool, not cold. While on one level the holistic healer is trying to contribute to the paradigm shift, she or he tends to be very much in the business of consumer choice and customer care. Holistic healing is entirely client-centred, and in that respect no different to 'conventional' private medicine, which thrives on dissatisfaction with the existing system, the desire for privileged access and individual attention where the 'specialist' has time to listen. The spiritual service industry of which holistic healing is a part, alongside New Age Bed and Breakfast (Bowman, 1993: 49–54), inspirational publishing, and so on, is very much in the 'small business' ethos of the Thatcher era – although probably neither Thatcherites nor healers would be entirely happy with that thought.

The need for healing which gives rise to the healing business, in turn leads to the business of training healers. One concern raised in some quarters in relation to the explosion of alternative therapies is that of training and credentials. Very much in the New Age spirit of having to 'walk your talk', what some therapists and counsellors stress to their prospective clients is personal experience: one Bath healer's literature stresses he has trained in psychosynthesis and has more than 25 years' experience of spiritual and personal development. On the other hand, a Core Process Psychotherapist stresses her membership of the Association of Accredited Psychospiritual Psychotherapists, and her inclusion on the UK Register of Psychotherapists.

There is undoubtedly a growth in credentialism in holistic healing sector, as in society generally. This was brought home to me by a student on Bath Spa University College's New Religions course who commented, 'It's a funny thing. Have you noticed that loads of these New Age characters seem to have letters after their name?'. Professionalisation is often seen in connection with the 'angels in pinstripes' aspect of New Age, one Bath example being that of Anne Hassett the clairvoyant who became Acushia the Psychic Consultant. It is perhaps not surprising that some feel the need for diplomas and letters after their name, to assist their career and establish their credibility.

The aspiration to become a practitioner or therapist has created business opportunities for those institutions concerned with providing courses that are marketed to potential students. Diplomas in Applied Astrology will 'take you to the level of the average Astrological Counsellor', Tasseography 'can be used for personal interest or to further your development as a New Age Counsellor', while Dream Analysis is described as 'almost essential for any prospective New Age Counsellor'. The creation or moulding of the role of the 'New Age Counsellor' here is particularly interesting. BSY's advertisement in *Kindred Spirit* Issue 40, Autumn 1997, appears under the banner 'START YOUR OWN HEALTH BUSINESS' (p.63). Indeed, a brief look at the advertisements in that '10 Year Anniversary Issue' of 'The UK'S Leading Guide for Body, Mind and Spirit' demonstrates vividly the elements of variety, professionalisation, credentialism, and multiskilling in the holistic healing sector. There appear advertisements for such varied institutions as The College of Past Life Healing (p.74), the School of Channelling (p.67), the English Huber School of Astrological Counselling (p.64) and The School of Insight and Intuition (p.47). The College of Past Life Regression Studies offers individual therapy, self development courses, and a diploma for Therapists (p.74), while the Hygeia College of Colour Therapy offers 'Professional Training with Diploma' (p.74). The advertisement for the International College of Crystal Healing urges 'Train for a Professional Qualification with ICCH' (p.72), not to be confused with the International Association of Crystal Healing Therapists' offer of 'A Professional and Comprehensive Crystal Therapists' Training Course' (p.55) or the 'Crystal Healers' Certificate Courses' offered by another source (p.72). Moreover, there is a brief advertisement for a '"Promote

Yourself" Marketing Workshop for Holistic Therapists' (p.68), while Manna Management promotes a one-day seminar on 'The Business of Healing' (p.68). As Manna Management's advertising copy points out, 'The fine balance between the spirituality of healing and managing a commercial business is often a dilemma'. The day is to offer guidance on *Spirituality versus commercialism* ('How to gain the best of both worlds'), *Going it alone* and *Balancing creativity with commerce*, and is described as 'a "must" for anybody wishing to develop themselves further' (p.68).

These advertisements, along with the previous examples, tell us much about healing in the spiritual marketplace. There are books and courses which cater for the individual who becomes involved in healing therapies and techniques for her or his own interest and development. Once involved in holistic healing on a do-it-yourself or client basis, some feel moved to become providers or practitioners themselves. However, it is noticeable that many in the new healing industry feel the need for constant accumulation of new skills; they too continue to develop personally and professionally, as part of their spiritual quest, rejecting a single path or narrow specialism.

Holistic healing can be regarded as a form of non-aligned spirituality, which demonstrates a number of characteristics of late 20th-century religiosity. Among these is the motif of the individual quest, on the part of both the client and the holistic healer, and a particular attitude to money. Spiritual progress has a price, however it is measured; the idea that profit and spirituality cannot converge is rejected. Nevertheless, it is worth noting that while New Age management consultants can make hundreds (indeed thousands) of pounds a day, healers are often more of a cottage industry with comparatively modest profits. Whether this reflects the type of person drawn to healing, market forces, or the fact that so many healers are women, would be a fruitful area for further study.

Within the late 20th-century spiritual marketplace, holistic healing is perceived as a valuable commodity, both in its provision of healing and as an aid to self-development. Through healing, a variety of worldviews may be explored and experiences and insights gained, often predicated on ideas such as the individual quest, interconnectedness, reincarnation, synchronicity/meaningful coincidence and a positive view of 'spiritual materialism'. Furthermore, it has given rise to a spiritual service industry which is developing in parallel to the service industry/small business ethos of mainstream society, including a tendency towards credentialism.

The perceived need for healing and the new healing industry thus spawned are fascinating and significant aspects of late twentieth spirituality. Consumer choice has progressed from the 'corner shop' of resources previously available to the healing 'hypermarket' which is now such an important part of the spiritual marketplace.

REFERENCES

Albanese CL. The Magical Staff: Quantum Healing in the New Age. In: *Perspectives On The The New Age*, Lewis JR, Melton JG (eds). Albany: State University of New York Press, 1992.

Bowman M. *Phenomenology, Fieldwork and Folk Religion.* Cardiff: BASR occasional Papers, No 6, 1992.

Bowman M. Drawn to Glastonbury. In: *Pilgrimage in Popular Culture*, Reader I, Walter T (eds). Basingstoke: Macmillan, 1993.

Bowman M. The Need for Healing: A Bath Case Study. In: *Healing and Religion*, Bowman M (ed). Enfield Lock: Hisarlik Press, 2000; 95–107.

Davie G. *Religion in Britain since 1945.* Oxford: Blackwell, 1994.

McGuire M. *Ritual Healing in Suburban America.* New Brunswick and London: Rutgers University Press, 1988.

McGuire M. Health and Spirituality as Contemporary Concerns. In: *The Annals of the American Academy of Political and Social Sciences* 527, 1993.

Porter R. Before the Fringe: Quack Medicine in Georgian England, *History Today* 1986;36:16–22.

Porter R. *Disease, Medicine and Society in England, 1550-1860.* Basingstoke: Macmillan, 1987.

Rose S. *Transforming the World: An examination of the roles played by Spirituality and Healing in the New Age Movement* Unpublished PhD Thesis, Lancaster University, 1996.

Rose S. Healing in the New Age: It's Not What You Do But Why You Do It. In: *Healing and Religion*, Bowman M (ed). Enfield Lock: Hisarlik Press, 2000; 69–80.

Sutcliffe S. Seekers, Networks, and 'New Age', *Scottish Journal of Religious Studies* 1997;18:97–114.

Van Hove H. L'emergence d'un 'marche spirtuel, *Social Compass* 1999;46(2):161–72.

York M. *The Emerging Network: A Sociology of the New Age and Neo-pagan Movements.* Lanham, Maryland: Rowman & Littlefield, 1995.

York M. New Age and the Late Twentieth Century (Review Article), *Journal of Contemporary Religion* 1997;12(3):401–19.

CHAPTER 20

EXPANDING POLITICAL OPPORTUNITIES AND CHANGING COLLECTIVE IDENTITIES IN THE COMPLEMENTARY AND ALTERNATIVE MEDICINE MOVEMENT

Melinda Goldner

This chapter examines how collective identities change when the political opportunity structure becomes more favorable to a social movement. The chapter is based on research in the California Bay area of San Francisco and involved several stages. First, I interviewed forty individuals, three quarters of whom were practitioners who used a variety of alternative techniques, such as acupuncture, massage. Traditional Chinese Medicine, homeopathy, chiropractic, Reiki, Qigong and Rolfing. The second part of my research entailed clinical observations of a women's clinic, a solo practitioner sharing office space with other alternative practitioners, and an integrative clinic that combines Western and alternative medicine. In addition to the three clinics, I observed a professional association, with nearly 200 members, that is exploring integrative medicine. In addition to observing and interviewing members, I analyzed videotapes of eight monthly meetings and a professional symposium members had organized (Jorgensen, 1989; Van Maanen, 1982). Finally, I analyzed secondary materials such as newspaper and magazine articles, activist newsletters, event announcements, position papers and clinic handouts (Jorgensen, 1989).

Edited from *Political Opportunities, Social Movements and Democratization*, 2001;23:69–102.

Activists within the complementary and alternative medicine (CAM) movement in the San Francisco, California Bay area have traditionally competed with physicians by criticizing Western medicine and providing an *alternative* medical model for consumers. Physicians are increasingly interested in CAM given financial changes within Western medicine, and increased consumer interest and governmental recognition in CAM. Activists in the Bay area are beginning to form networks with physicians and develop an *integrative* model of medicine, which combines Western and alternative approaches. Consequently, some activists are changing their collective identity now that they are advocating an integrative, rather than alternative, model of medicine. Collective identities are usually considered to be made up of three components; boundaries, political consciousness and strategies. They transform individuals into political actors and unite activists within a movement. Taylor and Whittier (1992) define collective identity as the 'shared definition of a group that derives from members' common interests, experiences and solidarity'. Collective identities enable participants to turn their sense of who they are into a sense of 'we' tied into a movement aimed at social change (Billig, 1995; Gamson, 1992; Klandermans, 1992; Taylor and Whittier, 1992).

ALTERNATIVE ACTIVISTS

Alternative activists began by creating an alternative model of medicine intending to challenge Western medicine and influence individuals. These activists created *boundaries* that positioned themselves as an alternative to Western medicine. Alternative practitioners and their patients developed a *political consciousness* as they learned that others had the same frustrations and experiences with Western medicine. Their personal troubles became public issues that required collective, structural solutions (Mills, 1959). Activists turned their practice and use of CAM into a form of activism that *politicized everyday life* in order to improve upon Western medicine and support alternative beliefs. This collective identity, though retained by some activists today, was more prevalent at the beginning of the movement. Activists were trying to justify their place, however narrow, within the health care system. English-Lueck (1990) points out that this strategy was also advantageous because 'any alternative system must define itself as narrowly as possible outside orthodox medicine. In the beginning, this [was] a wise strategy – orthodox medicine was unmoved by the intrusion of an upstart fad'.

INTEGRATIVE ACTIVISTS

Some Bay area activists are beginning to change their collective identity from 'alternative' to 'integrative.' Activists change their *boundaries*, *polit-*

ical consciousness and *strategies* as political opportunities arise. In terms of boundaries, some activists in this study have expanded their definition of 'we' to include physicians. Physicians bring legitimacy and resources to the movement so this group of Bay area activists embrace their increasing involvement, even though they must make adjustments. For example, activists are very concerned with appearing professional since physicians are garnering more media exposure for the movement and activists are wanting to emulate physicians. Integrative activists are still critical of the way physicians practice Western medicine, especially their objectification of patients and over reliance on technology and physical processes; however, activists are less openly critical of Western techniques such as drugs and surgery. This reflects a significant change in their political consciousness. Finally, activists have developed a range of *strategies* to gain access to mainstream institutions such as hospitals. Attempting to influence existing institutions is allowing activists to extend beyond the personalized political strategies they were employing to change individuals. Activists are now seeking support from businesses and insurance companies.

Activists begin to change their collective identity as more physicians join their organizations and practices. A practitioner involved with an integrative practice says, 'I just see that there's interest in alternative medicine. For a while it didn't include many physicians, and now that seems to be one of the groups leading the way.' A physician is on staff at the integrative clinic. Physicians established the professional association, and one acts as the director. The latest figures for this organization's membership show that more than 60 of the 200 current members are physicians. This study cannot determine the extent to which physicians simply advocate CAM or actually identify with the CAM movement. Yet, as more physicians explore CAM, whether they identify or not, activists begin to change their collective identity. Activists now call their work 'complementary' or 'integrative,' rather than 'alternative.' A dance therapist says she views her work 'as complementary. Clients would agree with that. A few people wouldn't want to see a physician, but the majority combine modalities.'

Activists are willing to open the movement to physicians because they are noticing changes in physicians' attitudes toward CAM. A Rolfer says she 'noticed a change in physician's reactions... There is more popular awareness [among physicians] that alternative medicine can work in some cases, and that nothing works universally.' Another practitioner says she sees 'a lot of AMA types reaching out for holistic healing.' A client even says she has been 'moving back into including Western medicine, because it seems a little more open than it was.'

Activists are also embracing physician support because of the resources that they bring to the movement, such as increased media exposure and public support. The media have certainly covered CAM more in the past several years. Due to their credentials and respectability, physician interest in CAM is responsible for much of this media attention. In part, activists open their boundaries to physicians for the resources, such as media attention, they provide. Activists want to appear credible to these physicians and to be worthy of their participation. However, these activists also recognize that the movement receives more public exposure and support given physician involvement. As Lowenberg (1989) argues, 'once a group of physicians started advocating these themes [of holistic health], the public listened. When less powerful groups such as nursing and public health had represented the same themes, they did not have the equivalent impact on public perceptions'. Activists are even willing to make significant changes to their collective identity given the power physicians continue to hold in our society. Allowing physicians into the movement changes interactions between activists and physicians. One respondent calls herself 'an evolutionist not an activist,' because of her desire to work with physicians. She rarely attends conferences solely for alternative practitioners, nor does she join alternative organizations, because she wants to maintain her legitimacy with people in the system. Activists who are working directly with physicians are also concerned with appearing professional. To illustrate, the professional association organized a symposium to educate practitioners about alternative techniques and explore ways to integrate Western and alternative medicine. Speakers explained a range of techniques, such as homeopathy and acupuncture, and audience members asked questions as to how to incorporate these techniques into their work. Members discussed professionalism throughout the organizing stages, especially since they wanted favorable media coverage. They had a strict dress code for speakers that included specific information on how to look best on camera. A professional meeting planner asked each speaker to prepare a one minute sound bite on their presentations in order to increase the chances that the local news stations would cover their symposium.

This group had been interested in their public image long before the symposium. They have a public relations committee focused 'on maintaining our public image.' These examples illustrate how members are aware of how they need to portray themselves professionally if they want favorable media coverage. Yet, members' concern for professionalism is also tied to the fact that physicians were involved. One member said:

> [Physicians] are taking a risk [by exploring integrative medicine], and with good justification. It's not just paranoia. They know the power of the state board and what it can do to you...And they see security in numbers. If they get a movement going that's large, and therefore has political strength, they will be less susceptible to divide and conquer tactics. *So they want [the symposium] to look good* (emphasis added).

Activists use professionalism as a way to appear legitimate before the larger public and physicians within their movement.

DISCUSSION

New political opportunities are allowing activists in the Bay area to work more closely with physicians, thereby changing their collective identity. The increased complexity and scale of the medical field has led to new financial arrangements within Western medicine. Medicine has been transformed into a health care industry where profit, efficiency, financial managers and consumers take center stage. One physician suggested that people in his profession are now 'outsiders' due to changes in medical reimbursement. Given the resulting dissatisfaction, some physicians are turning to complementary and alternative medicine for a solution. Other physicians are examining these techniques given increased consumer interest and governmental research. Activists see this opening in the political opportunity structure as an opportunity to work with physicians to integrate Western and alternative medicine.

Holistic ideology states that practitioners need to use multiple therapies since they address more than physical symptoms; rather, practitioners need to examine how illness can result from emotional, spiritual and social problems, as well (Alster, 1989). Activists have an 'expanded selection of tools for helping patients' when they work with physicians. Practically, activists realize that the movement gains potential patients if they moderate their stance to advocate alternative techniques as a complement to, rather than replacement for, Western medicine. Fewer individuals are willing to use CAM if it means abandoning Western practices. Some activists alter their collective identity to bring increased resources to the movement. On a strategic level, alternative practitioners know they will gain legitimacy and possibly insurance reimbursement if they work with recognized medical professionals with more power and authority in our society. Activists within the CAM movement have started to advocate integrative medicine as a practical strategy to ensure their survival in a political climate that is more favorable, but still volatile and unpredictable.

This strategy of integration is not without drawbacks. Most importantly, co-optation is always possible once activists achieve some success and interact more closely with established actors. Physicians have already begun to co-opt alternative techniques. In their review of the literature, Astin et al (1998) found that, on average, 19% of physicians practiced massage and chiropractic, 17% offered acupuncture, and 16% used herbal therapy in their medical practices. One respondent in my research noted that, 'some [physicians] want to collaborate in group practices with a nutritionist, chiropractor, body worker, and use their knowledge. Some are doing that, but others may say I need to learn more about nutrition so I can prescribe it.' Given the diversity of techniques and practices included under CAM, physicians are more likely to co-opt some techniques than others. To illustrate, Mattson (1982) argues that techniques for stress management, such as meditation, would be the easiest to integrate into Western medicine; whereas, any form of CAM that includes a spiritual principle or practice would be much harder to incorporate. Baer et al (1997), also examining the CAM movement in the Bay area, discuss the possibility of physicians co-opting acupuncture 'not so much for philosophical reasons as fiscal ones'. Wardwell (1994), as well as Goldstein et al (1985) and Wolpe (1985), go further to suggest that acupuncture has already been co-opted to the point where it is rarely considered alternative. Much like what happened to the 'medical accommodation' of alternative birth centers, physicians could co-opt these practices based upon the need for 'medical supervision' (DeVries 1984). Activists try to achieve legitimacy by asserting their credentials, as Coy and Woehrle (1996) explain. Yet, physicians have more prestige in our society given the credentials they establish through extended medical education (Starr, 1982). This type of co-optation, where physicians usurp alternative practitioners' techniques, is particularly difficult. As my respondents noted, it confines many activists to a 'bitter role' since they 'aren't part of it' when Western medicine and CAM merge. Physicians and insurance companies 'get all the glory and control' (and financial compensation) even though activists have done all the work. In short, the opposition receives credit for the movement's ideas at the same time that they exclude activists from the process of change.

Activists are especially concerned that physicians are not adequately trained in these techniques, and that physicians will use these alternative techniques without the corresponding holistic principles. I will use acupuncture to illustrate these forms of co-optation. First, an acupuncturist without a medical degree needs 2,400 hours of clinical training and experience for a license to practice acupuncture; whereas, a physician needs only 200 hours for certification (Phalen, 1998). One acupuncturist said that you simply cannot learn the theory behind these practices in such a short time period. He adds that 'they wouldn't let me do needle biopsy' after simply reading a book on the subject. Thus, he says that 'MD's can practice acupuncture legally, but not well.' The resulting patient dissatisfaction, which acupuncturists in this study feel is inevitable, may reflect negatively on acupuncturists as a whole, however. Second, a physician may practice acupuncture, but not stress the connections between the mind and the body. By doing this, the physician is separating the technique of acupuncture from the alternative beliefs underlying this practice. This is especially likely among physicians who are motivated by financial gain, because it is time consuming (thus costly) for them to practice these techniques within the context of alternative beliefs. For example, it takes more time for an acupuncturist to ask a patient about his or her well-being and teach this patient about lifestyle changes, than it is simply to insert acupuncture needles. One respondent knew of an acupuncturist who stopped training someone for this reason. Another example he provided is that physicians may simply 'use herbs like prescription drugs.' They will be 'ineffective' if they are used in this way, though, because he believes that herbs are only effective if used in accordance with alternative principles such as lifestyle changes.

Activists are hopeful that physicians learn that integrative medicine requires the expertise of alternative practitioners given the time and effort involved in learning new techniques and altering their practices. One respondent says, 'there's a certain amount of fear by alternative practitioners that MD's will co-opt what they have, since MD's already have the credibility and following. I think it's very possible. But they don't have time to leam all these things.' An acupuncturist adds that when 'physicians see the amount of training needed for alternative techniques...they will know they can't retrain in these techniques given their full workload.'

Several players influence the eventual outcome of integrative medicine to varying degrees. I limit the discussion here to three influential groups. First, physicians retain a great deal of power to determine whether, and how, CAM merges with Western medicine. As of now, Western medicine retains the upper hand. As one acupuncturist in my study says, 'this could easily be squashed. The AMA is very powerful, and they may just decide [they] don't like this.' Second, insurance companies play a large role. One alternative practitioner said that:

> There is a push now with doctors trying to keep control. It's economic. Those doctors aren't a part of this group [the professional association]. So we need to go outside of that to the insurance companies and government. In California people have a choice. It's the law. If they get in a car accident they can come see me without a MD's referral. So I don't think it's something MD's will have complete control over. Insurance will play a role.

Third, activists also have some degree of control depending upon which strategy they emphasize. I have shown that alternative and integrative medicine are very different. Speaking of the CAM movement, Schneirov and Geczik (1996) argue that 'the extent to which it has solid roots in the lifeworld (submerged networks)' affects activists ability to resist co-optation. Alternative medicine keeps activists further away from mainstream institutions and possible co-optation, because they remain primarily within submerged networks. On the other hand, integrative medicine requires a more fundamental change in Western medicine. Integrative medicine requires the use of Western and alternative techniques within the framework of holistic ideology. Physicians would have to do more than simply provide more personal care. They would have to radically restructure their practices.

It will probably take years to determine the level of success that the CAM movement achieves with integrative medicine, because this medical model is so new. Not every activist will embrace the newer collective identity or strategy of integrative medicine; rather, some activists will hold on to the older collective identity of alternative medicine. Whether multiple identities lead to divisions or separate movements, as well as what level of success this newer strategy brings, remains to be seen. What is clear is that physicians remain powerful despite their loss of autonomy and authority. Moreover, not withstanding the recent successes of the movement, most physicians are not open to integrative medicine as activists conceive of it. Whether physicians begin to identify with the CAM movement is an empirical question unanswered in this study. Yet, changing collective identities among Bay area activists within the CAM movement may simply be the precursor to significant changes in medicine. As Phalen (1998) notes:

> The birth of integrative medicine will force the medical establishment to form previously unheard of alliances with practitioners once shunned by Western medicine. Transforming the course of our nation's curative path, our sick care system will become obsolete. New strategies, blending the spiritual, emotional, and natural with high-tech procedures, will evolve. Although it may seem overwhelming, this change is close at hand.

REFERENCES

Alster KB. *The Holistic Health Movement.* Tuscaloosa: The University of Alabama Press, 1989.

Baer HA, Jen C, Tanassi LM et al. The Drive for Professionalization in Acupuncture: A Preliminary View from the San Francisco Bay Area. *Social Science and Medicine* 1998;46:533–7.

Billig M. Rhetorical Psychology, Ideological Thinking, and Imagining Nationhood. In: *Social Movements and Culture*, Johnson H, Klandermans B (eds). Minneapolis: University of Minnesota Press, 1995.

Coy PG, Woehrle LM. Constructing Identity and Oppositional Knowledge: The Framing Practices of Peace Movement Organizations During the Persian Gulf War. *Sociological Spectrum* 1996;16:287–327.

DeVries RG. 'Humanizing' Childbirth: The Discovery and Implementation of Bonding Theory. *International Journal of Health Services* 1984;14:89–104.

English-Lueck JA. *Health in the New Age: A Study in California Holistic Practices.* Albuquerque: University of New Mexico Press, 1990.

Gamson W. The Social Psychology of Collective Action. In: *Frontiers in Social Movement Theory*, Morris A, Mueller CM (eds). New Haven: Yale University Press, 1992, 53–76.

Goldstein MS, Jaffe DT, Garell D, Berke RE. Holistic Doctors: Becoming a Nontraditional Medical Practitioner. *Urban Life* 1985;14:317–44.

Jorgensen D. *Participant Observation: A Methodology for Human Studies.* Newbury Park: Sage, 1989.

Klandermans B. The Social Construction of Protest and Multiorganizational Fields. In: *Frontiers in Social Movement Theory*, Morris A, Mueller CM (eds). New Haven: Yale University Press, 1992, 77–103.

Lowenberg J. *Caring and Responsibility: The Crossroads Between Holistic Practice and Traditional Medicine*. Philadelphia: University of Pennsylvania Press, 1989.

Mattson PH. *Holistic Health in Perspective.* Palo Alto, CA: Mayfield Publishing Company, 1982.

Mills CW. *The Sociological Imagination.* New York: Oxford University Press, 1959.

Phalen KF. *Integrative Medicine: Achieving Wellness Through the Best of Eastern and Western Medical Practices.* Boston: Journey Editions, 1998.

Schneirov M, Geczik JD. A Diagnosis for our Times: Alternative Health's Submerged Networks and the Transformation of Identities. *The Sociological Quarterly* 1996;37:627–44.

Starr P. *The Social Transformation of American Medicine: The rise of a sovereign profession and the making of a vast industry.* New York: Basic Books, 1982.

Taylor V, Whittier N. Collective Identity in Social Movement Communities: Lesbian Feminist Mobilization. In: *Frontiers in Social Movement Theory*, Morris A, Mueller CM (eds). New Haven: Yale University Press, 1992, 104–30.

Van Maanen J. Fieldwork on the Beat: This being an account of the manners and customs of an ethnographer in an American Police Department. In: *Varieties of Qualitative Research*, Van Maanen J, Dabbs J Jr, Faulkner R (eds). Beverly Hills: Sage, 1982, 103–49.

Wardwell WI. Alternative Medicine in the United States. *Social Science and Medicine* 1994;38:1061–68.

Wolpe PR. The maintenance of professional authority: acupuncture and the American physician. *Social Problems* 1985;32:409–24.

CHAPTER 21

LESSONS ON INTEGRATION FROM THE DEVELOPING WORLD'S EXPERIENCE

Gerard Bodeker

It is now recognised that about half the population of industrialised countries regularly use complementary medicine. Higher education, higher income, and poor health are predictors of its use (Astin, 1998). This growth in consumer demand and availability of services for complementary medicine has outpaced the development of policy by governments and health professions.

As Western governments grapple with policy issues entailed in integrating complementary medicine into national health services, many developing countries have long since addressed these issues. Their experience constitutes a valuable, although largely unexplored, pool of policy data.

TRADITIONAL MEDICINE

Almost 20 years ago the World Health Organisation estimated that 'In many countries, 80% or more of the population living in rural areas are cared for by traditional practitioners and birth attendants' (Bannerman, 1983).

The WHO has since backed away from the 80% estimate, settling for the safer position that most of the population of most developing countries regularly use traditional

Edited from *British Medical Journal* 2001;322:164–7.

Considerations by the Commonwealth Working Group on Traditional and Complementary Health Systems

- Policy framework, including integration of traditional and conventional medicine, regulation, and provision of services
- Training of traditional and conventional practitioners
- Development of standards of practice
- Mechanisms for enhanced sharing of experiences by countries
- Evidence based research and safety of herbal medicines and practices of complementary medicine
- Conservation of medicinal plants and related intellectual property rights

medicine in developing countries, only a minority have regular access to reliable modern medical services. Hence the formalisation of the traditional sector has implications for equity, coverage of primary health care, and financing.

Key policy issues in integration have been outlined by Commonwealth health ministers (Bodeker, 1999). Ministers established the Commonwealth Working Group on Traditional and Complementary Health Systems to promote and integrate traditional health systems and complementary medicine into national health care, giving consideration to several areas (box). Although it is not within the scope of this chapter to address all of these areas, several can be addressed by considering consumer trends, response from governments, and cost issues.

CONSUMERS

Medical pluralism – the use of multiple forms of health care – is widespread. Consumers practise integrated health care irrespective of whether integration is officially present. In Taiwan, 60% of the public use multiple healing systems, including modern Western medicine, Chinese medicine, and religious healing (Chi, 1994). A survey in two village health clinics in China's Zheijang province showed that children with upper respiratory tract infections were being prescribed an average of four separate drugs, always a combination of Western and Chinese medicine (Hesketh and Zhu, 1994). The challenge of integrated health care is to generate evidence on which illnesses are best treated through which approach. The Zheijang study found that simultaneous use of both types of treatment was so commonplace that their individual contributions were difficult to assess.

INTEGRATION

Asia has seen the most progress in incorporating its traditional health systems into national policy. Most of this began 30–40 years ago and has accelerated in the past 10 years. In some Asian countries such as China the development has been a response to mobilising all healthcare resources in meeting national objectives for primary health care. In other countries, such as India and South Korea, change has come through politicisation of the traditional health sector and a resultant change in national policy,

Two basic policy models have been followed: an integrated approach, where modern and traditional medicine are integrated through medical education and practice (for example, China, Vietnam) and a parallel approach, where modern and traditional medicine are separate within the national health system (for example, India, South Korea).

China

In China, the integration of traditional Chinese medicine into the national healthcare system began in the late 1950s. This was in response to national planning needs to provide comprehensive healthcare services. Previously, traditional Chinese medicine had been viewed as part of an imperial legacy to be replaced by a secular healthcare system. Integration was guided by health officials trained in modern medicine; harmonisation with modern medicine was the goal. This was accomplished by a science based approach to the education of traditional Chinese medicine and an emphasis on research. Both were supported by a substantial organisational infrastructure. To many observers, modern medical control over the terms and process of integration has resulted in the loss of important aspects of traditional theory and practice, issues seemingly unimportant to modern medicine. Fewer acupuncture points are taught than in the classic system, and aspects of the theory of traditional Chinese medicine have been de-emphasised. The effect of 'modernisation' resulting in a lesser system has also occurred with traditional medical education in India.

The state administration of traditional Chinese medicine now comprises nine departments and manages the entire sector, ranging from legislation, regulation, and policy through to hospital administration, drug control, and international economic and academic cooperation. Hospitals practising traditional Chinese medicine treat 200 million outpatients and almost three million inpatients annually. Overall, 95% of general hospitals in China have traditional medicine departments, which treat about 20% of outpatients daily (The State Administration of Traditional Chinese Medicine of the People's Republic of China, 1997).

South Korea

South Korea established the parallel operation of two independent medical systems in 1952. It set a goal for full integration of western and oriental medicine by the year 2001. Measures taken to improve the quality of care with oriental medicine include promotion of clinical cooperation, training of consultants, and the lifting of a ban on the employment in the public hospital sector of doctors practising oriental medicine. Most doctors practising oriental medicine are self employed at the primary care level. The profit margin on herbal medicines for oriental medicine is variously estimated to be 100–500% compared with their basic cost. Not surprisingly, two thirds of practitioners in traditional medicine do not want herbal remedies to be included within national medical insurance (Cho, 2000).

Political conflict between oriental and modern medicine has been high during the 1990s over issues of fees, the ability to sell and prescribe herbal medicines, and the licensing of practitioners in traditional medicine. As the clientele and revenues of practitioners in oriental medicine have increased, there have been moves by modern medicine to restrict the practice of specialists in oriental medicine and to ascribe their functions to modern medical practitioners trained in oriental medicine. Litigation, demonstrations and strikes, and failed government attempts at mediation were the outcome for most of the 1990s. The Korean experience highlights the difficulties when the traditional sector is not held financially accountable and when modern medical practitioners, through training, join the traditional sector and seek to dominate. The absence of a strong central control mechanism has underpinned this professional conflict in Korea.

India

In India a parallel model was adopted through the Indian Medicine Central Council Medicine Act of 1970. The council was established to oversee the development of Indian systems of medicine and to ensure good standards of training and practice. Training is in separate colleges, of which there are now over 100. These offer a basic biosciences curriculum followed by training in a traditional system. Thirty years on, however, the Department of Indian Systems of Medicine has expressed concern over the substandard quality of education in many colleges, which in the name of integration have produced hybrid curriculums and graduates, unacceptable to either modern or traditional standards. The department has made it a priority to upgrade training in Indian systems of medicine (Department of Indian Systems of Medicines and Homoeopathy, 2000).

Priorities for Indian systems of medicine include education, standardisation of drugs, enhancement of availability of raw materials, research and development, information, education and communication, and larger involvement of this type of medicine in the national system for delivering health care. The Central Council of Indian systems of medicine oversees research institutes, which evaluate treatments. The government is adding 10 additional medicines into its family welfare programme, funded by the World Bank and the Indian government. Medicines are for anaemia, oedema during pregnancy, postpartum problems such as pain, uterine, and abdominal complications, difficulties with lactation, nutritional deficiencies, and childhood diarrhoea (Kumar, 2000).

New regulations were introduced in July 2000 to improve Indian herbal medicines by establishing standard manufacturing practices and quality control. The regulations outline requirements for infrastructure, manpower, quality control and authenticity of raw materials, and absence of contamination. Of the 9000 licensed manufacturers of traditional medicines, those who qualify can immediately seek certification for good manufacturing practice. The remainder have two years to comply with the regulations and to obtain certification.

The government has also established 10 new drug testing laboratories for Indian systems of medicine and is upgrading existing laboratories to provide high quality evidence to licensing authorities of the safety and quality of herbal medicines. This replaces an ad hoc system of testing that was considered unreliable.

Randomised controlled clinical trials of selected prescriptions for Indian systems of medicine have been initiated. These will document the safety and efficacy of the prescriptions and provide the basis for their international licensure as medicines rather than simply as food supplements (Kumar, 2000).

Malaysia

Malaysia has recently adopted a coordinated approach to integration, based on self regulation by complementary professions. Malaysia's health minister, Honorable Dato' Chua Jui Meng, announced on 13 November 2000 the establishment of a council comprising five umbrella organisations representing Malay, Chinese, and Indian traditional health systems, complementary therapies, and homoeopathy. Under the new council, these bodies will recognise, accredit, and register their own practitioners while developing standardised training programmes, guidelines, accreditation standards, and codes of ethics (*Straits Times*, 2000). This sectoral development 'across the board' represents a faster track towards integration than that of Britain, where accreditation is conducted on a profession by profession basis according to the standards of training, practice, and self regulation that each profession has attained.

Africa

African countries typically utilise the parallel model. In April 2000 Ghanaian legislation established a council to regulate the practice of traditional medicine. By 2004, certified herbal medicines will be prescribed and dispensed in Ghanaian hospitals and pharmacies. Nigeria has developed guidelines for regulating herbal medicines, and draft legislation has been prepared to establish national and state traditional medicine boards for regulation of practice and to promote cooperation and research (Osuide, 1999).

FINANCE

In China, until recently, traditional Chinese medicine was centrally managed and funded. In 1980 China was the first country to negotiate a component for traditional medicine with a health sector loan from the World Bank. A recent expansion of hospital beds financed by the World Bank included provision that 20% of these be in hospitals practising traditional medicine (Hesketh and Zhu, 1997).

Through sectoral changes, resulting partly from market reforms promoted by the World Bank, services providing traditional Chinese medicine are now covered by health insurance. Only about 12% of the population has comprehensive medical insurance that covers the cost of being admitted to hospital. The proportion of uninsured may be as high as 50%. In hospitals, insured patients are more likely to receive traditional Chinese medicine. This is because one of the primary sources of a hospital ward's profit under the new market system is the 15–25% mark-up for prescribed drugs. Accordingly, the changed incentive system has become associated with increased polypharmacy. Under the market system, many hospitals in China practising traditional Chinese medicine operate at a deficit, as better equipped western hospitals attract more patients. As traditional Chinese medicine is largely an outpatient, low technology specialty, most of the income of traditional hospitals comes from the sale of traditional medicines. Even with the 25% mark-up allowed, it is hard to cover operational costs (Hesketh and Zhu, 1997). Although government subsidies currently ensure survival, there is no surplus for improving services, and further market reforms may threaten this subsidy system.

Conversely, health insurance can increase access to traditional medicine. In Taiwan, four out of five people would use traditional Chinese medicine if it were covered by national health insurance (Chi, 1994). In Australia the use of acupuncture by doctors has increased greatly since the 1984 introduction of a Medicare rebate for acupuncture. In 1996, 15.1% of Australian doctors claimed for acupuncture, with almost one million insurance claims made (Easthope et al, 1998).

Insurance schemes for traditional and complementary medicine are biased towards those with the ability to pay. An equity formula is needed if the poor are to be guaranteed access to these services.

Drawing from the Asian experience (Chi, 1994), it is clear that effective integration strategies will promote communication and mutual understanding among different medical systems, evaluate traditional medicine in its totality, integrate at both theoretical and clinical levels, ensure equitable distribution of resources between complementary and conventional medicine, provide a training and educational programme for both traditional and conventional medicine, and generate a national drug policy that includes herbal medicines.

REFERENCES

Astin JA. Why patients use alternative medicine: results of a national study. *JAMA* 1998;279:1548–53.

Bannerman RH. *Traditional medicine and healthcare coverage*. Geneva: World Health Organization, 1983.

Bodeker G. Traditional (i.e. indigenous) and complementary medicine in the Commonwealth: new partnerships planned with the formal health sector. *J Alternative Complement Med* 1999;5:97–101.

Chi C. Integrating traditional medicine into modern health care systems: examining the role of Chinese medicine in Taiwan. *Soc Sci Med* 1994;39:307-21.

Cho HJ. Traditional medicine, professional monopoly and structural interests: a Korean case. *Soc Sci Med* 2000;50:123–35.

Department of Indian Systems of Medicines and Homoeopathy. *Annual Report 1999–2000*. Department of Indian Systems of Medicines and Homoeopathy, 2000. http/mohfw.nic.in/ismh/ (Data accessed 25 October 2000).

Easthope G, Beilby JJ, Gill GE, Tranter BK. Acupuncture in Australian general practice: practitioner characteristics. *Med J Aust* 1998;169:197–200.

Hesketh TM, Zhu WX. Excessive expenditure of income on treatments in developing countries. *BMJ* 1994;309:1441.

Hesketh T, Zhu WX. Health in China. Traditional Chinese medicine: one country, two systems. *BMJ* 1997;315:115–7.

Kumar S. India's government promotes traditional healing practices. *Lancet* 2000;335:1252.

Osuide GE. *Regulation of herbal medicines in Nigeria: the role of the National Agency for Food and Drug Administration and Control (NAFDAC)*. Paper presented at the international conference on ethnomedicine and drug discovery. Silver Spring MD, Nov 3–5, 1999.

Straits Times, Kuala Lumpur, Malaysia, Nov 14, 2000.

The State Administration of Traditional Chinese Medicine of the People's Republic of China. *Anthology of policies, laws, and regulations of the People's Republic of China on traditional Chinese medicine*. Shangdong: Shangdong University, 1997.

CHAPTER 22

HOMOEOPATHY, HOSPITALS AND HIGH SOCIETY

Phil Nicholls

Homoeopathic treatment has been available to patients under the National Health Service (NHS) since its formation in 1948. Almost certainly, this would not have happened without concerted efforts, throughout the 1940s, by the British Homoeopathic Society (BHS) and the British Homoeopathic Association (BHA) – the 'medical' and 'lay supporters' wings of the movement at the time. Both organisations lobbied hard to protect the position of homoeopathy and its hospitals within the new state medical service. On a more mischievous note, it may also be conjectured that government ministers, who were well aware that members of the Royal Family had often preferred to choose homoeopathic doctors as their personal physicians, were already predisposed to support the case for the incorporation of homoeopathy into the NHS. Since 1948 homoeopathic provision within the NHS has grown, and Royal support has remained enthusiastically constant.

Co-existing with the availability of state funded services provided by medically qualified and other statutorily regulated health professionals (some of whom, of course, will also take private patients), is a burgeoning number of practitioners who, though formally trained and certified in homoeopathy, do not possess a medical qualification. These are often referred to as 'professional' homoeopaths. The Society of Homoeopaths, which is the largest organisation registering such practitioners in the UK, currently has some 936 registered and 606 licensed members.

Royal blessing of this array of homoeopathic services – or, at least, of those homoeopathic services provided by the medically qualified – has

This chapter has been comissioned by the editors for inclusion in this Reader.

come in three forms: through patronage of homoeopathic institutions, through the appointment of homoeopathic doctors to the Royal household, and through support for organisations and activities which are aimed more generally at promoting the cause of complementary medicine.

In the same year that the NHS was founded, King George VI granted permission for the London Homoeopathic Hospital (LHH) to use the prefix 'Royal' in its title, and on her accession to the throne in 1952 the current Queen became, and has remained, its patron. The Queen's personal physician, Dr R. W. Davey, is also a homoeopath. Currently, the Duke of Gloucester is the royal patron of the BHA; before him, the late Queen mother had held this position from 1982.

The Prince of Wales has shared the family enthusiasm for alternative forms of medicine. As President of the British Medical Association (BMA) (1982–3), the Prince had urged its members to take a serious interest in the more 'holistic' approaches to health care that tended to be favoured by non-conventional practitioners. The first response to the Prince's call for action was a report by the BMA's Board of Science and Education (1986) on Alternative Medicine. This report, in fact, was much less supportive of the potential value of non-conventional therapies than the Prince might have anticipated – although it was followed, in 1993, by a second report which was noticeably more sympathetic.

Although, by this time, the tide of public opinion and the level of patient interest would probably have persuaded the BMA to review its position on alternative medicine, the Prince's role as President had undoubtedly been influential in stimulating an early response. And he has continued to promote the cause of alternative medicine – most recently in the form of the Prince of Wales's Foundation for Integrated Health.

The conjunction of royal and aristocratic patronage of homoeopathy as a system of medicine with the availability of hospitals specialising in the care of patients according to homoeopathic principles is not, however, a new phenomenon. Indeed, it is a feature which has characterised homoeopathy in Britain from its first emergence as a distinctive therapeutic system in the early decades of the nineteenth century (Nicholls, 1988: chapters 8–11).

This conjunction was embodied in the career of Dr Frederick F. H. Quin (1799–1879), who was the first significant homoeopathic practitioner in Britain, and who was largely responsible for establishing the organisational and institutional infrastructure of the movement in the nineteenth century. Quin, who was very probably the illegitimate son of the Duchess of Devonshire (Cook, 1981: 146), had graduated with an MD from the University of Edinburgh in 1820. Soon after, he joined the Duchess's entourage as her personal physician during her travels through Italy. After her death in 1824, Quin became physician to Queen Victoria's uncle, Prince Leopold of Saxe-Coburg, who was later to become King of the Belgians. It was during these travels in Europe as part of aristocratic households that Quin first encountered homoeopathy. By the time he settled in London in 1832, Quin had been treated homoeopathically himself, had been practising the system for several years, had met Hahnemann, and had studied under him in Paris for a year.

Quin's wit, charm, intelligence and aristocratic connections made him a popular figure among London's social elites, and came to be an invaluable ally in building support for homoeopathy in the face of mounting medical criticism and hostility. By 1850, Quin could look back on three notable achievements. Firstly, the establishment of a medical society – The British Homoeopathic Society (BHS) – in 1844. Secondly, the regular publication of a professional journal – The *British Journal of Homoeopathy* (*BJH*) – whose first volume appeared in 1843. And thirdly, the establishment of a hospital, the London Homoeopathic Hospital (LHH) – which was founded at 32, Golden Square in October 1849.

Homoeopathy in the early decades of the nineteenth century, had some influential and powerful friends. Indeed, during the final genuinely Whig administration of Russell in 1846 no fewer than eight prominent aristocratic supporters of homoeopathy had been appointed to the royal household. Among these were the Marquess of Anglesea (Master General of the Ordnance), Lord Clarence Paget (Secretary to the Ordnance), Lord Alfred Paget (Clerk Marshall), the Marquess of Westminster (Steward), Lord Robert Grosvenor (Treasurer), Lord Kinnaird and the Earl of Albermarle (Rankin, 1988: 47). But homoeopathy also had its enemies. These came not only from the medical establishment but also, interestingly, from within the ranks of homoeopathy itself.

In one sense, Quin himself was to blame for this fissure within the emerging homoeopathic movement, as he wished above everything else to preserve the professional integrity and dignity of homoeopathic practice. This meant that those among homoeopathy's supporters who favoured a more active and intimate alliance of both its 'lay' and 'medical' protagonists soon found themselves at odds with Quin and the members of the BHS.

At bottom this split was a product of two contrasting views about the control, deployment and interpretation of homoeopathic knowledge. For Quin, the practice of homoeopathy should be properly restricted to qualified practitioners since it had to be predicated on medical knowledge and medical training. For his homoeopathic critics, however, Quin's vision was restrictive and elitist. If the 'law of similars' was God's law of cure, then it belonged to everyone, and it was therefore incumbent on its supporters to disseminate homoeopathic knowledge and to promote homoeopathic practice among the wider population. Indeed if, as Hahnemann had argued, disease consisted solely in the symptoms displayed by the patient, all the empirical evidence which was required for remedy selection was available to any careful observer.

Behind this doctrinal difference also lay issues of class and politics. Quin had moved in aristocratic circles for many years and many of his leading supporters were members of the Whig aristocracy. This was a group interested in social reform, but only as long as it was managed by the aristocracy, not the masses. This mirrored Quin's view that homoeopathy was properly to be used by 'the knowledgeable expert' on and for 'the dependent patient'. The alternative populist view of homoeopathy, on the other hand, reflected the more radical political idea that social reform should emerge from, and be informed by, the views of the population as a whole (Rankin, 1988).

These opposing tendencies in homoeopathy emerged from the very beginnings of Quin's attempt to found the BHS (Nicholls, 1988; chapter 9; Rankin, 1988; Bradford, 1897: 217–24, 239–51, 532–48). Quin, in 1845, had invited Drs Gilish, Partridge and Epps to his house for dinner, and had proposed (one can almost see it happening over the port and cigars) that the four of them should constitute the non-elected 'management' committee of the BHS. Quin, of course, would remain as President. Dr John Epps objected. At least two other prominent homoeopaths, Drs Dunsford and Curie, were absent from the gathering; and, moreover, Epps felt that the constitution of the Society, as proposed by Quin, gave the President too much power. As a result, Epps withdrew from Quin's circle and joined instead with Dr Curie, and the lay enthusiasts, Mr Sampson and Mr Heurtley, to found the English Homoeopathic Association (EHA) in 1845.

Epps himself was a radical and a democrat who was opposed to all forms of hereditary and institutionalised privilege. He was also a deeply committed Christian of – not surprisingly – non-conformist persuasion, a phrenologist as well as an ardent homoeopath, and a supporter of many popular social reforms and causes. His active endorsement of the anti-slavery movement, of the anti-Corn Law League, of movements for national self-determination in Europe (such as those in Hungary, Italy and Poland) and of moderate Chartism, is testimony to the range and strength of his libertarian convictions. In addition, Epps was an avid writer and speaker, often lecturing to audiences in working men's associations up and down the country. Indeed, where homoeopathy was concerned, Epps saw it as his particular mission – as many of his books and speeches show – to address the wider public, rather than merely medical or aristocratic audiences.

The constitution of the EHA reflected these characteristics. Membership was open for a small annual sum to all supporters of homoeopathy, whether they were medical practitioners or not. The mission of the Association was unashamedly one of disseminating homoeopathic knowledge among the general public through the production and free (where possible) distribution of popular tracts and treatises. This commitment to anti-elitist and inclusive principles was well exemplified in the Association's first major publication, 'Homoeopathy: its Principles, Theory and Practice' (1845), which was written explicitly for the general reader by one of its founding members, the banker and journalist Marmaduke Sampson.

Amongst the members of the EHA was William Leaf, a merchant and book publisher, who had been responsible for bringing Dr Paul Curie, a prominent French homoeopath, to England in 1835. Leaf's ambition had been to find ways of making homoeopathic treatment available to London's working class poor. This had begun with the establishment of a dispensary, with Curie as Medical Officer, in Finsbury in 1837. In 1839, the Dispensary moved to Ely Place in Holborn. Three years later, the Dispensary moved again to Hanover Square, opening with the addition of twenty-four beds. Leaf's desire to help fund and found a homoeopathic hospital had thus been realised. The formation of the EHA in 1845 was, then, a natural home for Leaf and, at its first general meeting in 1846, both he and Curie spoke enthusiastically of developing the existing Hanover provision into a robust therapeutic community of like-minded physicians.

None of this activity, however, was of a kind of which the BHS and Quin could easily approve. Relations between the two wings of the movement worsened as Curie began to organise exhibitions of patients cured homoeopathically at the Hanover Square Hospital. They were not helped either by the death of Mr Cordwell, one of Curie's patients, whose treatment had consisted in part of a dietary regime which, so it was argued at the inquest, had left him seriously weakened. Quin made it quite clear that he wanted nothing to do with Leaf, with Curie, with the Hanover Square Hospital, or with the EHA.

Even within the EHA, however, disagreements began to emerge. Both Sampson and Heurtley apparently argued with Curie, perhaps over his exhibitions of cured patients, and resigned. Leaf and Curie's attempt to open up the Hanover Square Hospital to other homoeopathic practitioners foundered because some of Curie's more zealous supporters tried to ensure that all such doctors would remain subject to his authority, and the hospital closed.

Just as Quin's connections with elite society had been crucial in generating the resources for the opening of the LHH, so aristocratic patronage continued to remain an important feature of the institution's success. In 1874, for example, the hospital could count among its officers the Duchess of Cambridge (patroness), the Duke of Beaufort (vice-patron), the Earl of Wilton (president) and, as vice presidents, the Earls of Essex and of Albemarle, the Viscounts Sydney and Malden, and the Lords C. A. and G. Paget, Kinnaird and Ebury (Nicholls, 2001: 172).

As was the case with most similar institutions at the time, the LHH operated on a charitable basis. In return for a donation or annual subscription, patrons had the right to nominate a certain number of individuals for in or out patient care – provided that those nominated were too poor to pay for treatment themselves. To obtain treatment from the hospital an applicant (one is almost tempted to say 'supplicant') needed to present a letter of recommendation from a governor or subscriber and be examined by the Medical Board as to her/his suitability for admission. If successful, the House Committee of the hospital would then 'sign in' the patient. This took place first thing on Tuesday mornings. Patients, unless completely destitute, were expected to bring with them a towel, cup, saucer, spoon and knife and fork. These articles would be returned to them on their discharge. Patients, too, were expected to be able to supply some kind of evidence for the Medical Board – usually a testimony from a respectable householder – relating to their financial situation and character. Not only, then, did patients need to be poor to gain access to the hospital; they also needed to behave themselves appropriately to stay there.

Hospitals, however, were not the only institutions through which the poor could access homoeopathic treatment. Numerous dispensaries were also available. These tended to operate on one of three principles. Firstly, they could be run as a 'public charity', like hospitals, with subscribers or patrons having the right to nominate patients (for example, the London Homoeopathic Medical Institute). Secondly, dispensaries could operate on the basis of 'unconditional subscriptions' where patrons had no rights of patient nomination, like those in Liverpool and Manchester. Or, thirdly, they could function as a kind of 'sick club' where, in return for a nominal fee paid each quarter, people were entitled to treatment and medicines when they became ill.

By 1874, 37 public homoeopathic dispensaries were in operation. Though much humbler institutions, these dispensaries enjoyed similar aristocratic and elite patronage as did the movement's voluntary hospitals. Three groups tended to feature in particular among the individuals who comprised these institutions' management committees or patrons: the aristocracy, the clergy and the military.

The middle decades of the nineteenth century represented the high tide of homoeopathy's institutional development in Britain. By the 1870s homoeopathy was serving the needs of three groups of clients. These were the sick poor (through hospitals and dispensaries), the aristocracy and other social and economic elites (through private practice), and the educated middle class housewife and mother concerned for the health of her family (through publication of guides to domestic practice).

As a therapeutic alternative, then, homoeopathy had succeeded in mounting a powerful challenge to orthodox medicine. It was able to do this for two main reasons. Firstly, because of the parlous condition of regular practice, and of the double-edged nature of the allopathic critique that homoeopathy was equivalent to not treating the patient. After all, it could not be disputed that patients seemed to get well treated homoeopathically at least as well as those who were bled, blistered and purged – which rather undermined the case for 'active' treatment. Secondly, because homoeopathy had the advantage of being able to mobilise the support and patronage of powerful status groups, who had adopted the system at least in part as a way of marking their 'exclusivity' through living what Max Weber describes as a certain 'style of life'. For Weber, the essence of status group membership is precisely the exercise of very particular choices in the sphere of consumption (Weber, 1922).

As the century drew to a close, however, homoeopathy was very clearly in retreat. Fewer doctors were prepared to make it their 'therapy of choice'. The institutional framework of homoeopathy in general began to weaken. This occurred for a variety of reasons. In part, it was because homoeopathy's critique of regular medicine had been too successful, and the heroic, debilitating treatments of the 1830s and '40s had been progressively replaced by regimes which left much more to the 'healing power of nature'. In part, too, it was because homoeopathy, as a 'finished' system of medicine, found it difficult to incorporate the germ theory of disease and the bacteriological revolution in medicine; while on the other hand it could not avoid adopting initiatives in hygiene, antisepsis, anaesthesia and diagnosis. In short, less and less came to distinguish the two systems of medicine in practice. And, finally, it was because homoeopaths began increasingly to argue amongst themselves over matters of dosage and potency, and over who was practising 'pure' rather than 'bastard' homoeopathy (Nicholls, 1988). Such internal schisms are, in fact, quite typical of social movements in their period of decline.

But homoeopathy never lost its appeal to the aristocracy, the Royal family and to other social elites. The doctors who comprised the BHS, and the lay supporters who formed today's BHA in 1902, were fewer in number, and increasingly resembled little more than 'a rich man's talking shop' – as one disgruntled lay practitioner, Ellis Barker, put it – for much of the last century (Nicholls and Morrell, 1996: 204). The positive side of such insularity, however, was the continued sustenance of social exclusivity and social prestige. On the day of George V's funeral, for example, Dr Weir was fond of recounting that he wrote prescriptions for three kings and four queens. George VI named one of his racehorses after a homoeopathic remedy (*Hypericum*), and was attended by Dr Weir during his decline. Weir was also present at the birth of both Princess Anne and Prince Charles. The present Queen, like many of her ancestors, has tended to carry with her a small box of homoeopathic remedies on her many ceremonial travels (Anon, 1987: 19–21). Prince Charles, too, has clearly signalled his interest in and support for alternative or complementary therapies through a variety of initiatives, pronouncements and appointments.

The tradition of royal favour, then, stretches back many years. Whether this continues will probably depend on two things – the future of the monarchy and its commanding constitutional position in British society, and the survival of homoeopathy itself in the face of the continued drive for scientific validation of its mechanisms and mode of action.

REFERENCES

Anon. 'The Prince of Wales Launches NHS Centre for Integrating Complementary and Orthodox Medicine' and 'Extracts from Speeches by HRH the Prince of Wales and Dr David Reilly', *Homoeopathy*, 1998;48(2):28, 29–31.

Anon. 'Homoeopathy: the Royal Key', *Homoeopathy*, 1987;37(1):18–21.

Anon. 'Homoeopathic Medicine, Pharmacy and Lay Organisations: Their Relationship to the Monarchy', *Homoeopathy*, 1984;34(11/12):158–9.

Anon. 'Brief History of the Royal London Homoeopathic Hospital', *Homoeopathy*, 1979;29(9/10):95.

Anon. 'Editorial Comment', *The Lancet*, 1834–5;1:932.

Anon. 'Intercepted Letter', *The Lancet*, 1834–5;1:359.

Atkin G (ed). *The British and Foreign Homoeopathic Medical Directory and Record*. London: Aylott & Co, 1853.

Bayes W (ed). *The London and Provincial Homoeopathic Medical Directory*, London, 1866.

Blackley JG (ed). *The Homoeopathic Directory of Great Britain and Ireland and Annual Abstract of Literature*, London, 1874.

Bradford TL. The Pioneers of Homoeopathy, Boericke and Tafel, Philadelphia, 1897. See the entries on Paul Curie pp 217–24; John Epps pp 239–51; and Frederick Quin pp 532–48).

British Medical Association. *Complementary Medicine – New Approaches to Good Practice*. London: BMA, 1993.

British Medical Association. *Alternative Therapy*, BMA, 1986.

Cook TM. *Samuel Hahnemann: the Founder of Homoeopathic Medicine*, Wellingborough: Thorsons, 1981.

Fisher P et al. 'The Royal London Homoeopathic Hospital: 150 Years of Homoeopathy', *Homoeopathy*, 1999;49(6):123–7.

Nicholls PA. The Social Construction and Organisation of Medical Marginality – the Case of Homoeopathy in Mid Nineteenth Century Britain. In: *Historical Aspects of Unconventional Medicine: Approaches, Concepts, Case Studies*, Jutte R, Eklof M, Nelson MC (eds). European Association for the History of Medicine and Health Publications, Sheffield, 2001, 163–81.

Nicholls P, Morrell P. Laienpraktiker und haretische Mediziner: Großbritannien. In: *Weltgeschichte der Homoopathie*, Dinges M (ed). Munchen: CH Beck, 1996, 185–213.

Nicholls PA. *Homoeopathy and the Medical Profession*, London: Croom Helm, 1988.

Rankin G. Professional Organisation and the Development of Medical Knowledge: Two Interpretations of Homoeopathy. In: *Studies in the History of Alternative Medicine*, Cooter R (ed). New York: St Martin's Press, 1988, 46–62.

Sampson MB. *Homoeopathy: Its Principle, Theory, and Practice*. London: The English Homoeopathic Association, 1845.

Weber M. Wirtschaft und Gesellschaft, translated as *Economy and Society: An Outline of Interpretative Sociology*, New York: Bedminster Press, 1968 (translated by G Roth and G Wittich), 1922.

SECTION 4

REGULATION, PROFESSIONALISATION AND EDUCATION: CHANGE AND DIVERSITY

INTRODUCTION

Geraldine Lee-Treweek

CAM is under great pressure to standardise, to develop education and regulatory structures and to provide protection for users against substandard or frankly fraudulent practice through these mechanisms. This pressure comes from a number of directions: from the state, from orthodox health care professions, and from the general public (who may well be confused at the array of CAM available). This group of readings focus upon the question of providing safeguards within CAM. Such safeguards include the provision of thorough and competent education, the development of regulation through professional bodies, and the momentum towards professionalisation and the cultivation of professionalism. It can also be said that whilst such processes are often managed by the state, they are also often driven by the will, enthusiasm and vision of individuals and groups of individuals within CAM.

The set of readings begins with a reading by Roy Porter that provides a historical context for understanding regulation and protection of the public. Porter demonstrates that the notion of CAM is fairly new in the sense that prior to the rise of biomedicine in the eighteenth century, health care was provided in an open market place of equals. Anyone could practise medicine and indeed there was little to differentiate medical 'quacks' from lay people and their various remedies, medical contraptions and ideas. Porter provides a vivid description of an equal playing field in health care provision, with plenty of charismatic individuals selling their wares to a public eager for respite from the ills of the eighteenth century. His work serves to remind us of the need to attend to the historical context of health care and recognise that complementary and alternative medicine as a label does not really make sense until (after the rise of biomedicine) there was something to be complementary or alternative to.

The role of will and enthusiasm in creating change and development within CAM is illustrated in Sarah Cant's reading. She traces the history of education and training in homoeopathy and chiropractic and shows how charismatic (rather than formal) educational methods were pivotal to the development of these modalities. Whilst discussing these issues in historical context, Sarah Cant's reading directly addresses issues that affect many contemporary CAMs that, at present, are still taught by enthusiastic individuals in cottage industry style private colleges or even in private homes.

In contrast to Sarah Cant's reading, Constance Park's contribution demonstrates the extent to which CAMs are being integrated into medical education as part of the medical curriculum. The reading illustrates the growing appetite from within orthodox health care for CAMs courses and the demand for familiarisation of medical staff in this area. Constance Park elaborates on some of the features within complementary and alternative medicine that people who are learning to become orthodox health care practitioners could do well to learn. This includes an appreciation of uncertainty, understanding wider concepts that relate to different types of knowledge and experience, and a healthy questioning of biomedical reductionism.

Simon Mills' reading begins a series of three readings that examine regulation in the UK. Mills' work provides a basic understanding of the context of regulation and of the patterns of regulation in the UK. Then Clive Standen's reading focuses upon the Osteopaths Act (1994) and the impact that this has on education and regulation of osteopaths. The osteopaths were the first CAM group in Britain to get their own statutory act that, for instance, prevented the unqualified from calling themselves osteopaths. In many ways this has served as a model for other CAMs aspiring to statutory self-regulation. Clive Standen considers the effects of the act upon the status and standing of osteopaths, their relationship with patients and the effects upon the provision of continuing professional development in osteopathy. He also looks forward to the possibilities opened up by the act, such as the raising of the profile of the modality and the way that the act might allow it to be perceived as its founder Andrew Still intended – as an all-encompassing form of treatment, rather than as a modality that is only associated with treating 'bad backs'. The third reading in this cluster, which is by Mike Saks, discusses regulation as applied to one of the most controversial of the 'big five' CAMs. The reading's focus is on acupuncture in the UK and Saks argues that the nature of this CAM, involving the insertion of needles into users of the therapy, necessarily has led to public and medical calls for stringent regulation. This historical approach taken by Mike Saks also indicates that notions of regulation are a fairly modern issue in CAM and reminds us that CAMs arriving from other cultures bring with them divergent ideas about whether CAM should be regulated and how this should be done. Regulation is a controversial issue that often divides practitioners of particular modalities, whilst some wish for a regulation route that mimics the path of orthodox health care groups, for others regulation smacks of control and the quashing of creativity and spontaneity. Mike Saks' reading brings these issues to life around the contemporary case of acupuncture.

Ursula Sharma's reading examines an issue rarely discussed in academic considerations of how professions develop and change – the way that professional communities built from the aspirations and beliefs of individuals and small groups. The work indicates that a professional community does not arise overnight and indeed is fraught with micro politics around knowledge, how practitioners should be taught and what kind of values the profession should embody. Her work demonstrates the way that professional groups in CAM are constantly changing and emerging through the input of grass roots practitioners. This reading raises pertinent questions about why some CAM modalities are able to develop professional profiles and why others do not.

The final reading by Geraldine Lee-Treweek and Hilary Thomson addresses an issue that is of equal importance to the CAM practitioner community, policymakers, and users of CAM services – fraud and the existence of those who would seek to deceive members of the public through feigning CAM skills. In particular, it explores the issue of fraud in energy healing through a case study of an individual, Accora, who made claim to healing abilities to some people and yet to others emphasised the opportunistic and business side of her work. Many forms of CAM operate on the basis of trust, that is to say, it can be hard for the user to know if the therapy is helping (rather than some other factor like coincidence or a placebo effect), or if the person treating them is competent or trained in the modality they offer. The issue of fraud and the possibilities of individuals choosing to offer therapies for their own gain but with no healing ability represent an enormous challenge to the integrity of CAMs.

CHAPTER 23

QUACKERY

Roy Porter

Quackery was a bad thing, as everybody in pre-modern England knew, and the quack was a wretch – a 'turdy-facy, nasty-paty, lousy fartical rogue', in Ben Jonson's definitive phrase (Jonson B, 1908). Quacks, mountebanks, charlatans, and the like were the sweepings of the gutter, mere scum 'bred up to a Mechanic Employment', as Daniel Turner commented – illiterate, ignorant, often foreign, commonly Jews (Turner D, 1718). They possessed no medical abilities. Their much-trumpeted arts and arcana, pills and potions, were at best worthless, and, all too often, positively deadly draughts. They laid claims to miraculous powers, encyclopaedic learning, wonder cures, stupendous successes, the patronage of popes, princes and people, and universal applause. But all this was utter bunkum. For they were nothing but liars, cheats, and impostors. Above all, quacks were other people. Everybody felt happy in execrating the quack, because, everybody could agree, the quack was someone else.

Nobody ever called himself a quack. Unlike the (in some ways comparable) terms 'witch' or 'heretic', the label 'quack' was never pinned upon oneself, but always hurled against others. It always conveyed insult and abuse, always meant a bad, base doctor – indeed, in Thomas Beddoes's apt phrase, the 'bastard brethren' of the healing profession (Beddoes T, 1802–3). Most commonly, of course, the action of quackery issued from the mouths of those blessed with the attributes – or at least the reputation – of being regular doctors, and was targeted against those lacking them. But by no means always. All manner of itinerants and nostrum-vendors – precisely those themselves accustomed to being lashed as quacks

Edited from Porter R. *Quacks, Fakers and Charlatans in English Medicine.* Strand: Tempos Publishing, 2001.

– energetically returned the compliment, calling each other names, ferreting out quacks from amongst their own ranks, or detecting charlatanism in high places. And even the very scions of the profession felt few inhibitions about occasionally accusing each other of gross quackery.

Thus, when in 1788 the esteemed West Midlands practitioner William Withering – pioneer of digitalis therapy – seemed to Dr Erasmus Darwin to be poaching clients from his son, Robert Waring Darwin, the senior physician indicted Withering of the 'solemn quackery of large serious promises of a cure' (King-Hele D, 1977). 'Quack' was thus the ubiquitous swearword of an occupation many of whose terms were smeared with dubious connotations (consider the verb 'to doctor'). The quack was to the physician what the hack was to the poet, and the pretender to the king. But as well as being a multipurpose idiom of abuse, the label of quack was also, with some consistency, pinned upon a particular genre of medical operator – those who cried up their goods in the market, surrounded by zanies and monkeys, jokes and buffoonery, those who pasted bills upon walls, who puffed their wares in newspapers, who circuited the nation, who mass-marketed cure-alls and catholicons. What exactly was wrong with such operators?

Certain fusillades fired off against them – for example, aspersions against their social origins – were part of the common coin of insult in a society eager to right itself, after having just been turned upside-down in the Civil War. [The] specifically medical capacities of the quacks were impugned, too. For one thing, they were not qualified to practise. They had not been to university, or even undergone proper apprenticeship. They had no medical degrees, diplomas, or certificates; they were not enrolled in medical colleges or corporations, or licensed to practise.

For another – and this followed as the night the day – quacks were know-nothings; they had, judged the surgeon Daniel Turner, but a 'pitiful stock of knowledge' (Turner D, 1718). They had mastered none of those approved continents of learning, from Greek and Latin to botany and anatomy, which every erudite practitioner required. Their books, bills, and patents bulged with grotesque blunders – of grammar, pharmacology, and diagnosis – which exposed them as arrant sciolists. How (thundered James Makittrick Adair, self-appointed late eighteenth-century Quack-Finder General) could Godbold's nostrum possibly be sovereign (as claimed) both for asthma and for consumption? – anyone but a blithering idiot knew these were utterly diverse disorders requiring clean contrary therapeutics.

The consequence of this ignorance (the charge continued) must be that quacks were peddlers not of panaceas but of poisons. Worse still, they revelled in the unethical trick of marketing their nostrums as secrets, so the public could not even tell what dross they were swallowing. In claiming spectacular cures, quacks made a great hullabaloo about testimonials, reporting the miraculous recovery of Lady A and the Revd Z; but all of these were bogus. It was lucky for quacks, claimed the good Dr Adair, that 'dead men tell no tales' (Adair JM, 1790).

These ignoramus empirics further attempted to mask their ineptitude behind a rhetorical phantasmagoria, trading upon esoteric words and pretentious pseudotechnicalities. They were thus all mouth, slick-talking, smart operators, adepts in sleight-of-hand and showmanship, spouters of what Ned Ward called 'senseless cant' (Ward N, 1955).

Most damning of all, it was said that these masters of mendacity were callous conmen, cruelly fleecing the public, exploiting illness and trust. Indeed, for many contemporaries, imposture was the heart of the matter. In his *Dictionary* (1755), Samuel Johnson was to build a fraud charge into the very definition of the quack, regarding the creature as

1. A boastful pretender to arts which he does not understand.
2. A vain boastful pretender to physic, one who proclaims his own Medical abilities in public places.
3. An artful, tricking practitioner in Physic.

In short, the appellation 'quack' marked out a man as Mr False Pretences.

Public opinion during the 'long eighteenth century' was especially nauseated by the odour of deceit. In the mood of reaction triumphant after the Restoration, particular store was set by preserving the social order, so easily threatened by the seductive wiles of spellbinding rabble-rousers and zealot false prophets. Apologists warned of extremists and subversives and the spread of such evils as fashion, paper money, newspapers, the masquerade; novelty in religion, in taste, in natural philosophy; and the machinations of projectors, jobbers, bubblers, speculators, prophets, enthusiasts, etc. – all of which between them were creating a crazy fantasy world of false appearances, tinsel illusion, and Mandevillian hypocrisy. Medical quacks were not the least villains in this assault on four-square truth, reason, and common sense launched by the forces of fiction and trumpery, illusion and delusion. The triumph of quackery seemed as imminent as the empire of Dullness.

May the historian then assume, as a working definition, that the quack may thus be told apart from the authentic doctor by virtue of such attributes – by his being an ill-bred, uneducated, ignorant, inept impostor? The answer, quite obviously, is no – and for all the good reasons that contemporary quacks themselves never tired of pointing out. For one thing, the various elements in the Identikit definition do not, in fact, perfectly tally with those operators who were habitually branded as quacks. For instance, so-called quacks not infrequently possessed some authentic, formal medical or academic qualification, or an official diploma that licensed practice. In post-Restoration London, John Pechey, for example, was widely accused of quackish practices. He advertised his cures by handbills, through which he offered his services cut-price: 1s a consultation, 2s 6d a visit, the parish poor free. Yet he was a graduate of Oxford University, who, after receiving a medical apprenticeship from his father, became a licentiate of the College of Physicians. He dismissed the accusations of quackery levelled against him as nothing but sour grapes, contending how 'Many Men make it their business to ridicule the Public Way of Practice, because it thwarts their Private Interest'. In Pechey's polemic – one destined to run and run – self-publicizing, far from being arrant quackery (which, of course, he abominated with all his heart) was the very apex of public spirit.

Quacks who had never paced the quadrangles of a college were condemned for their unlettered 'empiricism', that is, practice by trial and error, with no formal theoretical grounding. But they had their answer. What value were the arid doctrines of the schools when compared to the university of life? They had travelled, sat at the feet of the famous adepts, winkled out medical secrets, if not from China to Peru at least from Turkey to Italy and Muscovy to France. In many of the authentic arts of medicine – not least such surgical techniques as tooth-drawing or bone-manipulation, which formed the staple of many an itinerant's livelihood – it was practice, not theory, which made perfect. Who dared belittle empiricism in physic, when, from Bacon to Locke, the empirical philosophy was being celebrated as the key to progress in scholarship and science? Indeed, precisely because they set such store by experience, rather than hide-bound authority, quacks often laid claim to pioneering innovation and experiment in therapeutics. Many of the most prominent late seventeenth-century quacks, such as John Case, boasted of their skills in 'spagyrick chemistry', rather as eighteenth-century operators championed medical electricity.

Quacks further denied the charge that their therapeutics were rash, dangerous, and outlandish. It hardly held water. Even Dr Adair, in the end, decided that the worst that could be said against most quack remedies was that they were 'pilfered... from regular practice', being the standard materia medica of the pharmacopoeia – above all, opiates, mercurials and antimoniacs – dolled up in fancy dress (Thompson CJS, 1928). Likewise, a glance at quack pamphlets shows that they typically shared the *Weltanschauung* of regular physic, embracing its disease language and its doctrines of solids and fluids, humours and complexions. Novel disease categories (for example, the idea of 'nervous' conditions), and innovations in treatments (for example, the use of medical electricity) were shared by faculty and quacks alike. One index of this convergence is the fact that it was regular doctors, such as David Hartley, who sanctioned the parliamentary purchase (at a cost of £5000) of the secret of Mrs Joanna Stephens's empiric stone-dissolving medicine.

Thus, most of the litmus tests that might be proposed to divide quacks from pukka doctors in the event confuse rather than clarify the issues. This applies, above all, to the charge that quacks were incompetent impostors, cynically intent from mercenary motives upon rooking the public. But who is to judge their motives? And what criteria would one use? The question is as sterile – and irrelevant – as asking whether late medieval pardoners believed in the efficacy of relics, or (that long-running Enlightenment debate) whether Mahomet, or Moses, was an impostor. Some empirics, we may surmise, merely plied a trade in pills; others, such as the pioneer sex therapist, James Graham, were – so far as one can judge from their careers and writings – obsessional enthusiasts, hooked on their own ideas.

In any case, if historians are to put quacks under the microscope and scrutinize their credentials, should not we do the same for the regulars? Thus ran, of course, the thrust of the quacks' counter-accusations. The faculty excoriated quacks for their patter, showmanship, and egoism. But who could match the princes of the profession in ostentatious ritual and self-advertisement? Augustan satire teems with caricatures of pompous physicians, mumbling their dog-Latin mumbo jumbo, garbling tags from Hippocrates and Galen, swanking around in their grand carriages decked out with running-footman ('a travelling sign post', snarled Smollett, 'to draw in customers') – and all to drum up custom and amaze the world (Smollett, 1971). Of course, when a scion of the faculty relieved a patient by his skill with soothing words, that was not quackery but a good bedside manner. Or when a regular larded his speech with polyglottal polysyllabics unintelligible to his patients, this was not quackish mystification, but science (*we* might say it was blinding the sick with science).

Likewise with therapeutics. Regulars praised their own treatments as safe and successful. As Dr Walter Harris (1982) contended, towards the close of the seventeenth century:

> The difference between a *Real Physician*, and a *Quack-Pretender*, does commonly appear in this, that the first is *Cautious*, *Deliberate*, and *Prudently Timorous* in all *Doubtful* cases, or *Dangerous* circumstances, generally to others, in their several degrees, as he would be content to be dealt withall himself under the same circumstances; the *Latter* is *Rash*, *Inconsiderate*, and stifly *heady* in every thing he does, his *Ignorance* makes him *Daring*, and he always ventures to Promise *Infallible success*, from the *nicest, most uncertain, and most Desperate Remedies* that are known in *Nature*, or contrived by Art.

But what did this really mean? After all, quacks themselves often accused regulars of reckless recourse to desperate remedies – for example, excessive dosing with mercurials in venereal cases. Likewise, what the likes of Harris would laud as 'prudently timorous' procedures, might, from another viewpoint, be condemned as culpably timid. Were not what Harris damned as the 'daring' and 'desperate remedies' of the irregulars the very lifeblood of innovation and improvement? 'In physic, all changes... have been forced on the regulars by the quacks', opined Isaac Swainson (1790) late in the eighteenth century: 'and all the great and powerful medicines are the discoveries of quacks. The introduction and improvements of inoculation: the use of mercury, antimony, opium, and the bark; like all the bold innovations in religion and policy, are owing to quacks. Benefits produce the bitterest ingratitude. The regulars adopted the discoveries, and persecuted their benefactors.' Swainson thus countered the standard charge: 'In the administration of remedies, there is this difference between the regulars and irregulars. The latter always attempt a cure, sometimes desperately. The former perpetuate diseases, to perpetuate a profitable attendance. This is the general fact, to which there are honourable exceptions.' (Swainson I, 1790:9) Swainson's notion that 'quackery' was the engine of invaluable innovation, was grudgingly accepted even by Dr Adair.

Thus the quacks' critics seemed guilty of the very atrocities they blamed on others. The point was not lost on the public. Indeed, a genre of works exposing the 'quackery of the medical profession' cascaded from the press, some written by empirics, others by journalists and critics, all accusing the medical profession itself of the vices and vanities it anathematized in others. Many noted that it was not only itinerants and tradesmen who were involved with nostrums. Scores of perfectly orthodox practitioners also cashed in on patent medicines or even proprietary pills prepared to secret formulae. Nehemiah Grew, MD, FRS, patented 'Epsom Salts'; a century later, Dr Thomas Henry, the eminent Manchester chemist and founder member of the Manchester Literary and Philosophical Society, patented antacids and medicines for nervous diseases. Many other leading regulars attached their names to cures in such a way that, even if they did not directly profit from their sales, their public fame was blazoned forth. Thus that giant of the Augustan faculty, Dr Richard Mead, had his name attached to a rabies powder, Mead's 'Pulvis Antylisus'; Dr Hans Sloane promoted medicinal chocolate; Dr Paul Chamberlain, FRCP, marketed teething necklaces; and so forth. Making money out of nostrums and engaging in self-publicizing, activities the Victorians deemed obnoxious to professional ethics, were regarded as marks of a good business nose – rational self-interest – by the Georgians. Quacks were guilty of sharp practice; but who was not? Early modern commentators were sceptical about the professions in general; from Ben Jonson, through Butler, Gay, Swift, and Pope to Henry Fielding and Tobias Smollett, it was 'a world of quacks', in which all professions were conspiracies against the laity. 'How flourishes *Health and Peace*?, inquired a correspondent in the *Tory Tatler* for Friday 8 December 1710:

> All's one, I answer'd; *Never a Barrel the better Herring*. Poor *Health* must needs be in a fine Condition, when so many Physicians, Quacks, Surgeons, and Apothecaries are her sworn Enemies, and whole Magazines of Pills and Drugs lie in wait for her Destruction. It is indeed often ask'd, what Disease a Man died of. Fever, Pleurisie, or the like;

> but properly speaking, the Question should be, not what Distemper, but what Doctor did he die of: Distempers seize Men, but the Physicians execute 'em.... For my part, I never hear an Apothecary's Mortar ringing, but I think the Bell's a tolling; nor read a Doctor's Prescription, but I take it for a Passport into the next World...

In short, the Georgian public was inclined to hear the faculty arraign quackery and retort, 'if the cap fits, wear it'. When quacks accused regulars of pursuing a quackery of their own, and public spokesmen hinted that irregulars and regulars were like as two peas in a pod, the constitution of a quack was far from a cut-and-dried matter.

BIBLIOGRAPHY

Adair JM. *Essays on Fashionable Disorders*. London: Bateman, 1790.

Beddoes T. *Hygeia*, 3 vols. Bristol: Phillips, 1802–3.

——— *A Letter to the Right Honorable Joseph Banks*. London: Phillips, 1808.

Hambridge, R. 'Empiricomany, or an infatuation in favour of empiricism or quackery. The socio-economics of eighteenth-century quackery', in S. Soupel and R. Hambridge, *Literature and Science and Medicine*, Los Angeles, Clark Memorial Library, University of California Press, 1982, pp.47–102.

Jonson, Ben, *Volpone*, ed. by P. Brockbank. London: 1908.

King-Hele, D. (ed), *The Essential Writings of Erasmus Darwin*. London: MacGibbon & Kee, 1968.

———, *Doctor of Revolution: the Life and Genius of Erasmus Darwin*. London: Faber & Faber, 1977.

Smollett, T. *Ferdinand Count Fathom*, ed. by D. Grant. London: OUP, 1971.

———, *Launcelot Greaves*, ed. by P. Evans. Oxford: OUP, 1977.

Swainson, I. *Direction for the Use of Velno's Vegetable Syrup*. London: Ridgeway, 1790.

Thompson, C.J.S. *Mysteries of History*. London: Faber & Gwyer, 1928.

———, *The Quacks of Old London*. London: Brentano, 1928.

[Turner, D.], *The Modern Quacks*. London: Roberts, 1718.

———, *Vindication of the Noble Art of Chirurgery* London: Whitlock, 1695 .

Ward, N. *The London Spy*, ed. by K. Fenwick. London: Folio Society, 1955.

CHAPTER 24

FROM CHARISMATIC TEACHING TO PROFESSIONAL TRAINING: THE LEGITIMATION OF KNOWLEDGE AND THE CREATION OF TRUST IN HOMOEOPATHY AND CHIROPRACTIC

Sarah Cant

INTRODUCTION

This chapter attempts to account for the shift from the charismatic transmission of knowledge to the development of professional educational practices through an examination of the pressures placed upon alternative therapists to establish external legitimacy and acquire societal trust for their practice.

Weber's (1978) concept of charisma will be used to comprehend ethnographic and historical data on homoeopathy and chiropractic. Weber argued that charisma is an extraordinary quality that is possessed by an individual who, on that account, is then treated as a leader. In this analysis such qualities equip the leader with authority and the power of domina-

Edited from an article in Cant S, Sharma V (eds). *Complementary and Alternative Medicines: Knowledge in Practice*. London: Free Association, 1996.

tion. In this chapter I want to show that the knowledge base of the therapies alone was not enough to explain their revival; rather, the enthusiasm of a select number of teachers created and sustained, for a time, collective excitement about alternative medical ideas. In particular, the early students trusted that their teachers were providing them with a radical new set of ideas. Weber predicted that charismatic authority would be short-lived and that groups/individuals would tend to claim legitimacy and authority on the basis of rationality and legal/state support. Certainly, throughout the 1980s and 1990s new methods of legitimation for alternative medical knowledge were required.

HOMOEOPATHY AND CHIROPRACTIC

Homoeopathy was founded by Samuel Hahnemann in the late eighteenth century and is based on principles that are contrary to orthodox medicine. The basic idea is that 'like cures like', that is, the prescription of a remedy to a healthy person would produce the same symptoms as those from which a sick person suffers. The homoeopaths also prescribe highly diluted doses of a remedy, so much so that the original substance is undetectable. The underlying philosophy is that of the vital force, which is conceived as an abstract form of energy which sustains life but may produce illness if weakened. The choice of remedies depends on the specific characteristics of the patient rather than a link to a disease classification and consequently prescribing is highly individualized.

Homoeopathy is practised in Britain by medically and non-medically qualified (NMQ) or lay homoeopaths. The medically qualified homoeopaths have altered the way that they have practised homoeopathy to sustain the respect of the remainder of the medical profession (Nicholls, 1988). In this chapter, I focus on one group of NMQ homoeopaths, represented by the Society of Homoeopaths and who currently have 360 licensed members.

Chiropractic is the third largest primary health care profession in the world after medicine and dentistry (Wardwell, 1992) and is widely used in the UK (Hansard, 1994). As a form of healing it was discovered serendipitously in 1895 by Daniel Palmer who adjusted the vertebrae in his janitor's neck and allegedly cured his long-term deafness. Palmer then developed a theory of disease that suggested misalignment of the vertebrae impinges on the transmission of nerve energy to the vital organs causing organic disease, as well as producing musculo-skeletal problems. Chiropractors locate these misalignments or 'subluxations' and palpate the spine to remove them. Chiropractic was imported to Britain in the 1920s and was practised by a group represented by the British Chiropractic Association. The operation of Common Law in Britain has meant that other practitioners have emerged and there are two other associations currently in existence. The McTimoney Chiropractors, represented by the Institute of Pure Chiropractic and with a membership of 188, is one of these groups and the focus of this chapter.

The data was collected between 1992 and 1994. Forty-one qualitative interviews were conducted with college tutors and representatives from the two professional associations.[1] In addition, six in-depth interviews were undertaken with the first British students in the 1970s' revival of the therapies.

CHARISMATIC REVIVAL

Following Weber (1978), charisma can be said to exist when a person is treated as a leader and has extraordinary qualities that inspire enthusiasm in his/her followers. Someone with charisma thus engages in relationships that are direct and interpersonal (Gerth and Wright Mills, 1986). Using such a definition, we can show the NMQ homoeopaths and McTimoney chiropractors had charismatic revivals in the UK, but that this charisma could only sustain *internal* legitimacy and trust from the followers.

Within homoeopathy, two Druids, Da Monte and Maughan, independently incorporated homoeopathic healing practices into their Druidic philosophy and attracted a dedicated following from their students:

> 'Each had a small group of students who were attracted by affinity. And you did not just get homoeopathy but a whole point of view. You just knew that you were getting a huge well of knowledge just by attending his classes. He taught us about the meaning of life and many of us became druids.' (Student)

There was no structure to the teaching or a curriculum; rather, these two men would talk about homoeopathy alongside other bodies of knowledge that were far removed from the teachings of medical homoeopathy. There was a great emphasis upon the spirituality of homoeopathy, the vital force and constitutional/individualized prescribing and the students felt they had discovered something that would revolutionize medical practice.

> 'We wanted to spread this to people because we saw [homoeopathy] having inestimable value and wanted to get people out of the allopathic straitjacket. So the motivating force was love ... we were very euphoric, shall I say about homoeopathy and idealistic. I wanted to shout from the rooftops.' (Student)

The homoeopathy that was taught was very different from that practised by medically qualified doctors in Britain, who had taken short, structured and examinable courses by the Faculty of homoeopathy. Medical homoeopaths were using the remedies alongside allopathic medicine and were more likely to use pathological prescribing, where a remedy is chosen on the basis of the disease category from which the patient suffers rather than the patient's individual constitution. Lay homoeopathy thus re-emerged as a highly individualistic movement and the teachings further placed great emphasis upon an interactive and non-hierarchical relationship with the patient. There were no stipulations about who could study as it was felt that the best way of expanding the popularity of the approach was to train as many people as possible.

John McTimoney had not had any official tutoring in chiropractic despite its established schools in the US and Bournemouth. After a back complaint of his own in the late 1950s he became fascinated with chiropractic and gradually developed his own techniques. He became a very popular practitioner, with patients apparently queuing down his path in Oxford and who also 'begged' him to teach them his skills. During the 1970s he started to 'pass on' his ideas. Again, there was no systematic teaching.

> 'McTimoney used to go off at tangents and different people were coming in at different times and saying, "train me", and so it went on. There would be people who had done twelve months and then someone else would join and so everyone was at different levels.'
>
> 'So how long did the training take?'
>
> 'As long as it took.'

Even if some of the students were discouraged by the haphazard organization they were convinced of the value of chiropractic.

In both cases, the teaching was unstructured. The students, drawn by both the teacher and the knowledge that was offered, gained great confidence and dispatched themselves, following a form of apprenticeship, to operate in a 'cottage'[2] industry of medical practice. The teachers emphasized openness and commitment, being less interested in a codified and structured form of knowledge. In turn, these tutors were respected for their wisdom and the students personally trusted their teacher's qualities and abilities to pass on this knowledge. Thus, charisma enabled these therapies to get off the ground.

However, in both chiropractic and homoeopathy, the teachers died and left the students without a knowledge base that could be reproduced. The death of these 'leaders' coincided with pressures from external bodies for the legitimation of homoeopathic and chiropractic knowledge claims and calls for the groups to establish their trustworthiness.

EXTERNAL PRESSURES FOR LEGITIMACY

The last decade has seen mounting external pressures to alter the practice of complementary medicine and an internal recognition by the practitioners of the need to establish boundaries between the qualified practitioner and lay person, to organize internally and to make alterations to the codification and transmission of their knowledge. For example, the government, which took an ambivalent stance towards alternative approaches to health care for many years,[3] has now required that all natural therapies 'get their act together' and has stated that they will contemplate statutory regulation if the therapies prove themselves to be united and well trained.

The influence of the dominant medical profession in the occupational development of allied groups has been extensively documented (Donnison, 1977; Larkin, 1983; Willis, 1992; Witz, 1992). Until recently the BMA's reaction to complementary medicine has been unfavourable. This was most clearly exhibited in the 1986 BMA report which attempted to discredit the health 'alternatives' as phoney and pseudo-scientific. The latest BMA report (1993) is, however, more favourable and refers to non-orthodox medicine as 'complementary'. The shift in label from alternative to complementary signifies an acceptance that the approaches are no longer antithetic but rather 'can work alongside and in conjunction with orthodox medical treatment' (BMA, 1993: 6). The BMA has used the report (BMA, 1993) as a forum publicly to make demands that the knowledge of complementary therapists be subject to scientific scrutiny, transmitted through proper courses and contain medical science and that orthodox practitioners should retain responsibility for the patient.

Moreover, the consumer through the Association of Community Health Councils (1988) has called for better training and the standardization of curricula and skills. Practitioners were also concerned to increase the popularity of their approach and could see the advantages of colleges and credentials. Importantly, these external pressures have served as a catalyst for change.

TRANSFORMING THE PRODUCTION AND TRANSMISSION OF KNOWLEDGE

The death of the leaders of these two groups of alternative practitioners signified a crisis for the legitimacy and future direction of their knowledge and practice. In both cases, it was increasingly recognized that the groups must respond to the demands from the public and the state and protect themselves from European Union rulings and the medical profession. There was a realization that the groups needed to distinguish themselves from the lay public and the criticism that they were untrained and unsafe. To be able to make such a case for their legitimacy required that changes be made to their knowledge. Specifically, it was important that they could be clear about what constituted and demarcated homoeopathic and chiropractic knowledge. Thus, both groups independently came to the decision that their teachings had to acquire an 'authenticity'. The changes made to the knowledge can be divided into four areas: codification and accreditation, tempering of knowledge claims, alignment to science, and the creation of boundaries around who can exercise the knowledge. The alterations resemble the professionalization process of orthodox medicine undertaken in the late nineteenth century.

Codification and accreditation

The most immediate concern for the students of homoeopathy and chiropractic was to ensure that the knowledge they had acquired would not be lost. In both cases a college and professional association was established with the aim to establish a curriculum and an educational institution that would be attractive to a wider body of students. McTimoney chiropractic still has only one college, whilst NMQ homoeopathy has expanded greatly and currently has 21 colleges. Whilst there are some differences amongst the colleges, the Society of Homoeopaths, established in 1981, has stipulated the prerequisites of a core curriculum, will only recommend to students courses that meet these criteria and has ensured the systematization of the teaching.

Naturally the knowledge base of these therapies did not become coterminous with the core curriculum, but there have been serious attempts to codify the knowledge so that it can be passed on in a structured way. The retention of the principle that patients be seen as individuals now sits alongside the systematic teaching of the repertory and the organon, in the case of homoeopathy, and the mechanics of the body in the case of chiropractic. Moreover, students who successfully complete the courses receive qualifications and can join a register of qualified practitioners that is guaranteed by the professional association. The chiropractors successfully gained statutory regulation in 1994, whereby only properly qualified practitioners are allowed to call themselves chiropractors, and this provides their training with legal status.

Tempering of knowledge claims

The early teachings within both groups alerted students to the wideranging potential of their discipline. There was an espousal of the holism of their 'art' and a suggestion that other forms of medical care, particularly orthodox medicine, would gradually become redundant. Within chiropractic it was believed that the manipulation of the spine had the potential to cure the whole range of mechanical and organic problems, and the Druidic homoeopaths stressed the danger of orthodox medicine, the spirituality of the vital force and the ability of homoeopathy to deal with all medical problems. However, throughout the 1980s we have witnessed the gradual curtailment of these ideals.

Within homoeopathy, the Druidic and esoteric components of the teaching have been largely jettisoned in the public portrayal of the therapy. Chiropractic had attracted a great deal of scepticism because of the original broad scope of practice. However, during the last ten years, we have seen the group emphasise and develop the musculo-skeletal side of their therapy. Moreover, both groups publicly state that their practice should not be regarded as alternative but, rather, complementary to orthodox medicine.

Alignment to scientific paradigm

In homoeopathy and chiropractic, the legacy of broad claims for their therapies, and the inconsistency of their knowledge base in comparison to orthodox medical sciences has had the potential to stand as an obstacle to recognition. Thus, both groups have made consistent efforts to attach their knowledge *publicly* to the scientific paradigm. These efforts have operated at three levels. First, all the colleges have incorporated medical science into their curriculums and conceive of biology, pathology and physiology as constituent parts of their knowledge system.

Second, the groups have attempted to use scientific theories to try and explain why their therapy works. This has been less successful for the homoeopaths, who despite attempts to use biophysics as an explanatory framework, have yet to produce an agreed theory of the law of similars.[4] Chiropractic has, however, had more success, in particular through the application of orthopaedic principles to explain the operation of chiropractic.

Third, the chiropractors and medically qualified homoeopaths have used scientific procedures, particularly randomized control trials to establish that their therapy works in practice (Meade et al, 1990; Reilly et al, 1986).

Boundary construction

Originally, as we have seen, both forms of medical practice were very open. As one homoeopath stated:

> 'We had discovered and had been part of a system that was truly wonderful, really and truly wonderful and the fire was there, we wanted to get it to others ...'

However, both groups recognized the need to close off their knowledge. Such closure is made possible by higher entry requirements and longer training programmes (Weber, 1968). In homoeopathy, the courses now run over four years part-time with a fifth year of supervised clinical practice, and the McTimoney chiropractic course lasts three years. Recommendations have also been made about entry requirements; homoeopath students should ideally possess two A levels.

The establishment of registers of qualified practitioners has also served to demarcate the 'authentic' practitioner from one that simply calls him/herself a chiropractor or homoeopath as permitted by the conditions of Common Law. Once on the register, the practitioners have proved that they have passed their examinations and supervised practice and that they have agreed to conform to a strict code of ethics.

CONCLUSION

During the last twenty years the homoeopaths and chiropractors have engaged in alterations to their knowledge production and transmission. The codification of knowledge, the abandonment of informal modes of knowing and learning, the limitation of access and the alignment to the scientific paradigm have provided the groups with an external legitimacy based on their professionalism. Yet, this shift from charismatic leadership and teaching, which inspired commitment and following, to professional training has been in direct contradiction to many of the original principles of these therapies. Moreover, it was these early principles that made homoeopathy and chiropractic attractive to patients and students in the 1970s. Evidence about the use of alternative medicine suggests that some of the attraction for the therapies comes from a desire for increased participation in the healing process and greater attention to the social and spiritual dimensions of health care (Bakx, 1991; Cant and Calnan, 1991; Sharma, 1992), as well as more pragmatic demands for more time from the practitioner and less interventionist methods (Thomas et al., 1991). It is possible then that such transformations may serve to reduce the appeal of these healing approaches.

NOTES

1. The project was generously funded by the Economic and Social Science Research Council. The project was undertaken with Ursula Sharma and I am grateful for her extensive support and encouragement.
2. The practitioners tended to work alone and survive by attracting their own local and often dedicated patients.
3. Evidenced by the operation of Common Law in the UK. The government has

not always acted in the favour of the medical profession, spiritual healers were allowed to work in the NHS in the 1970s and 1991 saw the clarification that GPs could purchase the services of complementary therapists.

4. Sharma in this volume shows that internally there are many more various efforts to make sense of homoeopathy.

REFERENCES

Association of Community Health Councils. *The State of Non-Conventional Medicine – The Consumer View*. London: ACHC, 1988.

Bakx K. 'The Eclipse of Folk Medicine in Western Society'. *Sociology of Health and Illness*, 1991;13(1):20–38.

BMA. *Complementary Medicine. New Approaches to Good Practice*. Oxford: Oxford University Press, 1993.

Cant S, Calnan M. 'On the Margins of the Medical Marketplace? An Exploratory Study of Alternative Practitioners Perceptions'. *Sociology of Health and Illness* 1991;13(1):39–57.

Donnison J. *Midwives and Medical Men*. London: Heinemann, 1977.

Gerth H, Wright Mills C. 'Bureaucracy and Charisma'. In: *Charisma, History and Social Structure*, Glassman R, Swatos W (eds). London: Greenwood Press, 1986.

Hansard. 'Chiropractors Bill', 18 February 1994.

Larkin G. *Occupational Monopoly and Modern Medicine*. London: Tavistock, 1983.

Mease TW, Dyer S, Browne W et al. 'Low Back Pain of Mechanical Origin: Randomised Comparison of Chiropractic and Hospital Out-Patient Treatment'. *BMJ* 1990;300(2):1431–7.

Nicholls P. *Homoeopathy and the Medical Profession*. London: Croom Helm, 1988.

Reilly DT, Taylor MA, McSharry C, Aitkinson T. 'Is Homoeopathy a Placebo response? Controlled Trial of Homoeopathic Potency, with Pollen in Hayfever as a Model'. *Lancet* 1986;287:337–9.

Sharma U. *Complementary Medicine Today. Practitioners and Patients*. London: Routledge, 1992.

Thomas K, Carr J, Westlake L, Williams B. 'Use of Non-orthodox and Conventional Health Care in Great Britain'. *BMJ* 1991;302:207–10.

Weber M. *Economy and Society*. Roth G, Wittich C (eds). New York: Bedminster Press, 1968.

Weber M. *Economy and Society*. London: University of California Press, 1978.

Willis E. *Medical Dominance*. Sydney: Allen and Unwin, 1992.

Witz A. *Professions and Patriarchy*. London: Routledge, 1992.

CHAPTER 25

DIVERSITY, THE INDIVIDUAL, AND PROOF OF EFFICACY: COMPLEMENTARY AND ALTERNATIVE MEDICINE IN MEDICAL EDUCATION

Constance M Park

THE MISSION OF MEDICAL PRACTICE

Biomedical research and medical student education often occur side by side, and sometimes intertwined, in academic medical centers. It is clear, however, that the concerns of biomedical research and of medical practice, although related, are not the same. As in the case of engineering and architecture, the discoveries and principles of the first expand the options for the practice of the second. But drawing *only* on biomedical knowledge in medical practice can lead to mechanical, uncaring, unethical, and ineffective health care just as surely as drawing *only* on engineering knowledge in architectural design can lead to aesthetically, functionally, and socially unacceptable structures built to the wrong scale, in the wrong places. In both cases, there is a failure to serve individual and community needs.

The goal of medical practice is to maintain and improve the health of individuals and populations, and the goal of medical education is primarily to train practitioners, albeit with an interest in research for its own sake as well as for the benefit of patients. To better meet the needs and expectations of patients, the concept of health has evolved in recent years

Edited from an article in *American Journal of Public Health* 2002;92(10).

to include the interrelated concepts of physical health and emotional health, as well as spiritual health.

Successful clinical practice involves not only skilled interpretation and application of medical data with all its uncertainties, but also the ability to care about and care for individual patients as unique, total people in social and cultural contexts. Patient education, patient advocacy, and the incorporation of the patient's values and preferences into jointly made decisions are all part of the clinician's work. Thus, medical school curricula now present the practice of medicine as a complex activity drawing on emotional and interpersonal processes as well as cognitive processes, which themselves require a broad range of knowledge bases, including biomedical, epidemiological, psychosocial, cultural, economic, and ethical (Association of American Medical Colleges, 1999).

The views expressed above are fundamental to the integrative medicine (Gaudet, 1998; Snyderman and Weil, 2002) movement, and are widely prevalent in CAM and conventional medicine communities. It serves no useful purpose to overlook this commonality. Rather, we should develop curricula in which the contributions of each group are acknowledged and combined to further the common mission. Ideally, this collaborative effort would include CAM practitioners familiar with current teachings in biopsychosocial medicine (Engel, 1977), medical anthropology (Carrillo et al, 1999; Eisenberg, 1977; Kleinman and Eisenberg, 1978), patient-centered medicine (Balint et al, 1970; Laine and Davidoff, 1996; Yeheskel et al, 2000), psychiatry, and public health as well as conventional practitioners aware of what can be learned from the rich diversity of healing traditions that address the totality of the human condition (Hellman, 1997; Sargent and Johnson, 1996).

UNCERTAINTY AND MEDICAL PRACTICE

To practice joint clinical decision making with patients, health care practitioners, whether regarded as conventional providers, CAM providers, or integrative medicine providers, must be able to share their 'ways of knowing' and the levels of uncertainty in the data they draw on, especially as applied to individual patients. Curricula on the nature of evidence, taught by members of all these provider groups, would increase everyone's ability to think critically about all therapies – those considered proved and unproved, conventional and alternative. These discussions are crucial to any consideration of CAM in an academic context. Fortunately, students report to us that while it can be difficult to focus on discussions of epistemology and epidemiology, carrying these discussions out in the context of exploring CAM therapies makes them immediate, relevant, and interesting. Thus, the scholarly consideration of CAM-related topics creates, as an important byproduct, students better able to think about the rules of evidence and the nature of proof.

Origins and limits of different types of knowledge

Conventional medicine, like CAM, is fraught with uncertainty. Discussions of CAM provide regular opportunities for considering the evidence for all therapies and showing that there is a spectrum of certainty, with no absolute standards for what therapies should be considered proved and unproved.

Health professionals must understand how each of their knowledge bases attempts to establish 'facts,' and they must feel comfortable with the levels of ambiguity and uncertainty inherent in various types of knowledge. Students would benefit from a basic background in epistemology, highlighting the scientific method, statistics, and causal inference, thus allowing them to appreciate the limitations of all types of data. This curriculum should be broad enough to include the various ways of knowing we draw on in daily practice.

Different aspects of the practice of medicine depend on different knowledge bases, and the data they contribute to diagnosis and treatment differ in method obtained, ease of testing, and level of certainty. For example, current case presentations of a chronically anxious, hypertensive cardiac patient might well discuss not only medications and cardiac procedures but also behavioral, psychological, and cultural issues. The 'objective' blood pressure readings, the 'subjective' symptoms, and the patient's observed anxiety would all be conditionally accepted as data, although they carry varying degrees of certainty and are arrived at by different means. Implicit in the case presentation would be questions of knowing, evidence, and uncertainty, even before the management discussion of the possible merits of various forms of psychotherapy or CAM mind–body stress reduction programs. But, despite these uncertainties in the data and despite the relatively unproved status of many conventionally accepted psychotherapies, it is the proposal of the controversial mind–body therapies that is most likely to provoke discussions of evidence.

Much of the data we use in conventional clinical practice, such as our perception of a person's mood, and many tools we bring to the encounter, like empathy, and even many therapies, like psychiatry, involve extremely complex processes much harder to define, study, or monitor than blood pressure, which is itself a challenge. It is important for students, who may be attracted to the more certain data of 'hard science,' to understand that the relative certainty of biochemical data compared with physiological data, or of physiological data compared with psychosocial data, is a natural consequence of statistical realities – such as the complexity of the study objects, the number and similarity of the objects available for study, and the difficulty of controlling experimental conditions. These differences in certainty are not an indicator of comparative merit, intellectual legitimacy, or relevance to medical practice. The proper use of the more complex and uncertain data that identify patients as total persons in social and cultural contexts can be crucial to the health care of the patient.

The framework outlined above illustrates that conventional medicine and CAM must both draw on diverse knowledge bases with varying levels of certainty and different ways of knowing. It would be a welcome development if practitioners of CAM and conventional medicine had open, respectful discussions of what criteria they use to accept data as fact and why. Conducting such explorations in the context of the medical school curriculum would enrich the dialogue between current practitioners and help develop an open-minded generation of physicians better able to assess all therapies that might help individual patients.

The uniqueness of individuals: 'N-of-1' in epidemiological perspective

The scholarly investigation of various CAM therapies presents a humbling opportunity to reflect on what we believe will help a particular patient and why. These reflections should be brought to all therapies, not just to those treatments deemed 'alternative.'

Evidence-based medicine uses the methodologies of clinical epidemiology to identify and compare the health outcomes of various interventions (McAlister et al, 2000; Ray, 2002; Sackett et al, 1996). A fundamental fact of clinical practice is that we are applying data gained from populations to one person, without knowing how these probabilistic data relate to this one unique individual (Goodman, 1999). If a therapy is the best choice for 7 out of 10 people, how do we predict whether our patient is in that 70% or is in the 30% of exceptions? This inevitable uncertainty is often called the N-of-1 problem, referring to the fact that we can never do clinical trials on large numbers of patients identical to the one before us because that patient is unique. Progressively larger studies, with statistical power for deeper levels of subgroup analysis, can provide us with progressively more textured information on how the study results apply to patients resembling our single individual patient. But no matter how large the study and how detailed the subgroup analysis, we will never have data detailed enough to provide with absolute certainty the answer for our one unique patient.

It is instructive to consider how this reality of evidence-based medicine may affect patient and practitioner behavior, and the patient–practitioner relationship, in various types of therapeutic interventions. For some interventions, like choosing one toxic drug over another or surgery over radiotherapy in cancer treatment, the patient and the disease process may change substantially with the passage of time or with each intervention, and there is no second chance to go down the road not taken. In such cases, practitioners may treat all patients with the 70% effective treatment, the best-documented strategy for maximizing group outcome. At other times, however, practitioners may want to rely on unproven, difficult-to-codify clues, personal experience, or even feelings (their own or the patient's) to choose the other therapy (Cranney et al, 2001; Mayer and Piterman, 1999). It is likely that most patients want their physicians not only to be well informed about evidence-based medicine (Carter and Spink, 2001) but also to have this individualizing option in clinical decision-making and to know individual patients well enough to exercise that option meaningfully.

Given this N-of-1 problem, it is likely that many patients seek additional complementary therapies not only to feel more comfortable or more generally in control (Astin, 1998) but more specifically to take part in the search for a package individualized to their unique needs. The fact that many CAM hands-on therapies appear to be based on the immediate perception and treatment of 'findings' (e.g., muscle spasms, subluxed joints, or blocked energy), present at that time in that patient, probably increases the patient's sense of being treated as a unique individual, a sense often missing in evidence-based medicine. If this therapy conveys an underlying message with personal meaning that speaks to that patient's sense of self, it may prove particularly attractive (Kaptchuk and Eisenberg, 1998; Kaptchuk, 2002; Moerman and Jonas, 2002). And if the therapy is understudied and considered unproved, but appears safe and feels good, it may be attractive exactly because it is not overtly associated with statistics, leaving freer reign for the patient's imagination and sense of hope, both factors that may themselves have positive physiological as well as psychological effects.

A variety of therapeutic interventions in both conventional medicine and CAM do allow for serial trials with an individual patient over time, such as an internist trying out various antihypertensives or an acupuncturist trying out related acupuncture points on a given patient. There is a set of epidemiological rules for evaluating the observed results in so-called 'N-of-1 experiments' (Sackett et al, 1998). Despite problems of proving causation, it is likely that these trials provide patients with therapies more suitable to their needs, as well as a comforting sense of being respected and cared for as unique individuals.

In cases in which they are feasible, therapeutic trials with individual patients play an important role in helping clinicians deal with the N-of-1 problem present in both conventional and CAM interventions. But these sequential trials regard the patient as effectively being the same person despite the passage of time. It is important to note that some traditional medicine systems do not accept this approximation under any circumstances and see themselves as always providing each individual with the most effective treatment possible at each point in time. Discussing, this stance in an academic setting clearly provides an opportunity to question how any practitioner can claim to know for sure what is best in a unique case. It also provides an opportunity to note and probe the therapeutic power of a conveyed sense of certainty and respect for the ever-changing individual. What is the nature of this appeal, which exists even when the patient's cognitive processes dictate that such certainty is an extraordinary claim requiring extraordinary evidence?

Because of the complexity of total patient care and the individual needs of each unique patient, there is more to the practice of both conventional medicine and CAM than the information emerging from clinical trials. To address the N-of-1 problem, both conventional and CAM practitioners operate outside the bounds of evidence-based medicine, at least some of the time. A discussion of this reality and how practitioners and patients cope with it, conducted by practitioners of CAM, integrative medicine, and conventional medicine, would help students deal with uncertainty as they care for each individual patient.

DIVERSITY AND CULTURAL COMPETENCE: N-OF-1 IN SOCIOLOGICAL AND PSYCHOLOGICAL PERSPECTIVE

Gaining perspective on how information about aggregates relates to an individual member therein is a fundamental challenge from sociological and psychological perspectives as well as from the purely statistical perspective above. Societies are struggling with ways to be responsive to culturally based needs without cultural (ethnic, religious, etc.) profiling. Similarly, individuals themselves feel a tension between their unique identity and their desire to identify with groups. Patients want to be recognized as individuals, but many are vocal about wanting also to be recognized and respected as members of various groups from which they gain a sense of identity.

Good medical practice requires seeing each patient as a unique individual and avoiding stereotyping, while acknowledging and respecting the sociocultural identities that help give meaning to the patient's life. A number of organizations recommend or mandate the teaching of cultural competence in medical school (Health care rx, 2002; Lum and Korenman, 1994; US Dept Health and Human Services, 1998; Welch, 1998; Whitcomb, 2002). There is a natural role for CAM teaching in this endeavor since the practice of culturally sensitive health care clearly requires an awareness of and respect for cultural traditions and practices, especially those related to health and healing. It could be argued that CAM curricula are important here, not only because they provide information on traditional and folk health care systems but also because the growth of CAM in the developed world itself reflects new, or newly blended, cultural ideas and themes. Medical anthropology and medical ethics would provide conceptual frameworks for such a curriculum, which would be taught by faculty as well as by providers of CAM and conventional medicine and by patients themselves.

CAM-RELATED RESEARCH DEVELOPMENTS

The inclusion of CAM in medical education encourages ongoing research in CAM-related areas, and vice versa. CAM has already increased interest in the exploration of possible new therapies and contributed to the development of new areas of inquiry (Straus, 2000). In addition, there is growing recognition of the difficulties in understanding the full impact of complex therapeutic regimens by isolating their constituent parts. The current research interest in botanical products, dietary supplements, micronutrients, and special diets is an example of this. Basic and clinical science reach a point in their own development when it becomes clear that micronutrients exist and that the presence of one ingestant may influence the absorption and metabolism of another. Thus, interest grows in whole foods and in the dietary and botanical knowledge acquired over centuries by various healing traditions. This interplay between planned scientific inquiry and sociocultural folk knowledge helps drive both basic and CAM research.

Similarly, with the explosion of interest in the association between illness and stress (Angerer, 2001; Krantz et al, 2000; McEwen, 1998; Matthews and Gump, 2002; Miller et al, 1996; Peters et al, 1996; Rozanski et al, 1999) and with recent advances in mind–brain–body research, the Cartesian mind–body duality is losing its grip on medical thinking. It is not surprising that there is increasing interest in CAM therapies based on conceptual frameworks that posit connections between the mind and the body, thus enabling the mind to affect bodily health and vice versa. Research in neuroendocrinology (Chrousos and Gold, 1992), neuroimmunology (Sternberg, 1997a, b), and the autonomic nervous system (Sloan, Shapiro and Bigger, 1994) have identified many humoral and neurological systems that could take part in mediating such mind–brain–body connections. With a number of recent studies on the placebo effect involving CAM therapies and their related therapeutic tools, such as the power of suggestion, CAM is playing a role in directing parts of this research agenda (Petrovic et al, 2002).

It is intriguing that the placebo effect, long invoked to downplay patients' positive responses to CAM, is coming to be understood as a complex and powerful therapeutic tool as well as a confounder of scientific inquiry (Kaptchuk and Eisenberg, 1998; Kupfjer and Frank, 2002;

Moerman and Jonas, 2002). The emerging vision of medicine is one in which mental and bodily functions cannot be cleanly separated. Studying the placebo effect may provide insights into how the brain functions and into the fundamental nature of health and healing. Thus, popular therapies, which have survived over centuries but remain unproved, may ultimately help elucidate the complexities of human beings – the very same complexities that we may in future years invoke to critique our current understanding of proof in medical practice.

ACKNOWLEDGMENTS

This work was funded in part by the Russell Berrie Foundation, the National Institutes of Health's National Center for Complementary and Alternative Medicine (grant P50-AT00090) and the Centers for Disease Control and Prevention (grant U48/CCU209663-08).

REFERENCES

Angerer P. Social support, hostility, and other psychosocial conditions in coronary heart disease. *Cardiovasc Rev Rep* 2001;22:332–333.

Association of American Medical Colleges. Learning objectives for medical student education – guidelines for medical schools: report 1 of the Medical School Objectives Project. *Acad Med* 1999;74:13–l8.

Astin JA. Why patients use alternative medicine: results of a national study. *JAMA* 1998:279:1548–1552.

Balint M, Hunt J, Joyce D, Marinker M, Woodcock J. *Treatment or Diagnosis: A Study of Repeat Prescriptions in General Practice*. Philadelphia, Pa: J.B. Lippincott; 1970.

Carrillo JE. Green AR, Betancourt JR. Cross-cultural primary care: a patient-based approach. *Ann Intern Med* 1999;130:829–834.

Carter M, Spink JD. Consuming the evidence: consumers and evidence-based medicine. *Med J Aust* 2001:175:316–319.

Chrousos GP, Gold PW. The concepts of stress and stress system disorders. *JAMA* 1992;267:1244–1252.

Cranney M, Warren E, Barton S, Gardiner K, Walley T. Why do GPs not implement evidence-based guidelines? A descriptive study. *Fam Pract* 2001:18:359–363.

Eisenberg L. Disease and illness. Distinctions between professional and popular ideas of sickness. *Cult Med Psychiatry* 1977:1:9–23.

Engel GL. The need for a new medical model: a challenge for biomedicine. *Science* 1977:196:12936.

Gaudet TW. Integrative medicine: the evolution of a new approach to medicine and to medical education. *Integrative Med* 1998:1:67–73.

Goodman SN. Probability at the bedside: the knowing of chances or the chances of knowing. *Ann Intern Med* 1999:130:604–606.

Health care rx: access for all. Barriers to health care for racial and ethnic minorities: access, workforce diversity and cultural competence. A report prepared by the Department of Health and Human Services and the Health Resources and Services Administration for the Town Hall Meeting on the Physician's Initiative on Race. Boston, Mass. July 1998. Available at: http://www.hrsa.gov/NRredesign/testimony.htm. Accessed July 14, 2002.

Hellman GC. *Culture, Health and Illness: An Introduction for Health Professionals*, 3rd ed. Oxford. England: Butterworth-Heinemann; 1997.

Kaptchuk TJ. The placebo effect in alternative medicine: can the performance of a healing ritual have clinical significance? *Ann Intern Med* 2002;136:817–825.

Kaptchuk TJ, Eisenberg DM. The persuasive appeal of alternative medicine. *Ann Intern Med* 1998;129;1061–1065.

Kleinman A, Eisenberg L, Good B. Culture, illness, and care. *Ann Intern Med* 1978.88:251–258.

Krantz DS, Sheps DS, Carney RM, Natelson BH. Effects of mental stress in patients with coronary artery disease. *JAMA* 2000;283:1800–1802.

Kupfjer DJ, Frank E. Placebo in clinical trials for depression: complexity and necessity. *JAMA* 2002;287:1853–1854.

Laine C, Davidoff F. Patient-centered medicine: a professional evolution. *JAMA* 1996;275:152–156.

Lum CK, Korenman SG. Cultural-sensitivity training in US medical schools. *Acad Med* 1994;69:239–241.

Matthews KA, Gump BB. Chronic work stress and marital dissolution increase risks of posttrial mortality in men from the Multiple Risk Factor Intervention Trial. *Arch Intern Med* 2002;162:309–315.

Mayer J, Piterman L. The attitudes of Australian GPs to evidence-based medicine: a focus group study. *Fam Pract* 1999:16:627–632.

McAlister FA, Straus SE, Guyatt GH, for the Evidence-Based Medicine Group. Integrating research evidence with the care of the individual patient: user's guide to the medical literature. *JAMA* 2000;283:2829–2836.

McEwen B. Protective and damaging effects of stress mediators. *N Engl J Med* 1998;338:171–179.

Miller TQ, Smith TW, Terner CW, et al. A meta-analytic review of research on hostility and physical health. *Psychol Bull* 1996;119:322–348.

Moerman DE, Jonas WB. Deconstructing the placebo effect and finding the meaning response. *Ann Intern Med* 2002:136:471–476.

Peters RW, McQuillan S, Resnick SK, et al. Increased Monday incidence of life-threatening ventricular arrhythmias. Experience with a third-generation implantable defibrillator. *Circulation* 1996;94:1346–1349.

Petrovic P, Kalso E, Petersson K, Ingvar M. Placebo and opioid analgesia: imaging a shared neuronal network. *Science* 2002;295:1737–1740.

Proceedings of the National Conference on Cultural Competence and Women's Health Curricula in Medical Education, October 1995. Washington, DC: US Dept of Health and Human Services; 1998.

Ray JG. Evidence in upheaval: incorporating observational data into clinical practice. *Arch Intern Med* 2002;162:249–254.

Rozanski A, Blumenthal JA, Kaplan J. Impact of psychological factors on the pathogenesis of cardiovascular disease and implications for therapy. *Circulation* 1999;99:2192–2217.

Sackett DL, Haynes RB, Guyatt GH, Tugwell P. *Clinical Epidemiology: A Basic Science for Clinical Medicine*, 2nd ed. Boston, Mass: Little Brown & Co; 1998:223–244.

Sackett DL, Rosenberg WMC, Muir Gray JA, Haynes RB, Richardson WS. Evidence-based medicine: what it is and what it isn't. *BMJ* 1996;312:71–72.

Sargent CF, Johnson TM. *Medical Anthropology: Contemporary Theory and Method*, Rev ed. Westport, Conn: Praeger; 1996.

Sloan RP, Shapiro PA, Bigger JT. Cardiac autonomic control and hostility in healthy subjects. *Am J Cardiol* 1994;74:298–300.

Snyderman R, Weil AT. Integrative medicine: bringing medicine back to its roots. *Arch Intern Med* 2002;162:395–397.

Sternberg EM. Emotions and disease: from balance of humors to balance of molecules. *Nat Med* 1997;3:264–267.

Sternberg EM. Neural-immune interactions in health and disease. *J Clin Invest* 1997;100:2641–2647.

Straus SE. Complementary and alternative medicine: challenges and opportunities for American medicine. *Acad Med* 2000;75:572–575.

Welch M. Required curricula in diversity and cross-cultural medicine: the time is now. *J Am Med Womens Assoc* 1998;53(suppl):121–123.

Whitcomb ME. Assisting medical educators to foster cultural competence. *Acad Med* 2002;77:191–192.

Yeheskel A, Biderman A, Borkan JM, Herman J. A course for teaching patient-centered medicine to family medicine residents. *Acad Med* 2000;75:494–497.

CHAPTER 26

REGULATION IN COMPLEMENTARY AND ALTERNATIVE MEDICINE

Simon Y Mills

Complementary and alternative therapies have became more widely used over the past two decades, but many practitioners in the United Kingdom are largely unregulated. One of the recommendations of last year's report on complementary and alternative medicine by the House of Lords Select Committee on Science and Technology was that 'in order to protect the public, professions with more than one regulatory body make a concerted effort to bring their various bodies together and to develop a clear professional structure' (House of Lords Select Committee on Science and Technology, 2000). That some health professions remain unregulated in a developed country seems extraordinary, and I shall review how this situation has arisen before considering the prospects for change.

In the United Kingdom the common law right to choose one's own treatment for illness has been barely constrained by law (Stone and Matthews, 1996). It is thus legal for practitioners to set themselves up in a wide variety of healthcare professions, as long as they do not claim to be registered medical practitioners and do not practise protected disciplines such as dentistry, midwifery, and veterinary medicine or supply medicines limited to prescription. By contrast, in most other European Union countries, as well as the United States, there are few healthcare activities that are allowed without state authorisation. Acupuncturists, herbalists, osteopaths, and naturopaths have been prosecuted for practising without medical qualifications, and the technical illegality of much complementary practice has

Edited from an article in *British Medical Journal* 2001;322:158–60.

meant that it has been pursued informally and disparately, with less opportunity for professional organisations to develop, The increasing demand for alternative health care across the developed world has, therefore, sometimes been met by practitioners outside the law and without recognisable training qualifications, professional standards, or insurance.

In the United Kingdom, the lack of proscription has meant that there are few formal obligations to meet any particular standard, and individual practitioners have been able to pursue their own path, even set up their own training programme or professional body, without sanction. They do not have to submit to authority, building their base on their ability to please their market – their patients. On the other hand, a benign legal climate has also allowed enlightened responses to increasing public demand. The natural instinct for self enhancement of professional status has led most practitioners to subscribe to organisations overtly raising standards. In 1997 and 2000 the Centre for Complementary Health Studies reported the results of surveys of about 140 professional bodies representing about 50 000 practitioners working in up to 30 complementary or alternative therapies (Mills and Budd, 2000; Mills and Peacock, 1997). Professional standards varied widely. In part to reflect this diversity, the House of Lords report classified complementary and alternative therapies into three groups (see box) and related many of its recommendations to this classification.

Two disciplines, osteopathy and chiropractic, have moved along the path of self regulation and now have acts of parliament that protect their titles and provide additional external and orthodox regulation of their activities. Both the General Osteopathic Council and the General Chiropractic Council have opened their statutory registers. Once the process of registering existing practitioners is complete, it will be a criminal offence to practice as an osteopath or chiropractor unless you are registered with the appropriate council.

The House of Lords also identified acupuncture and herbal medicine as two therapies ready for moves towards statutory regulation under the Health Act 1999 and considered such moves might later be appropriate for non-medical homoeopaths.

CODES OF PROFESSIONAL CONDUCT AND PUBLIC ACCOUNTABILITY

Most complementary medicine organisations are run as conventional professional bodies; they publish formal codes of ethics and practice, and registers of their members are available to the public. Almost all subscribe to insurance schemes that provide professional indemnity and public liability cover for their members (the cost of cover is generally not high, reflecting the lack of litigation so far in this area). However, the opportunity

Categories of complementary and alternative therapies (House of Lords Select Committee on Science and Technology, 2000)

Group 1: Professionally organised alternative therapies
Acupuncture
Chiropractic
Herbal medicine
Homoeopathy
Osteopathy

Group 2: Complementary therapies
Alexander technique
Aromatherapy
Bach and other flower extracts
Body work therapies, including massage
Counselling stress therapy
Hypnotherapy
Meditation
Reflexology
Shiatsu
Healing
Maharishi Ayurvedic medicine
Nutritional medicine
Yoga

Group 3: Alternative disciplines
3a: Long established and traditional systems of healthcare
Anthroposophical medicine
Ayurvedic medicine
Chinese herbal medicine
Eastern medicine (Tibb)
Naturopathy
Traditional Chinese medicine
3b: Other alternative disciplines
Crystal therapy
Dowsing
Iridology
Kinesiology
Radionics

for the public to pursue complaints against practitioners, and the provision of formal disciplinary codes, sanctions, and procedures and published complaint procedures was notably patchy, even among well established organisations. Given the moves to increase professional accountability in the medical profession, complementary and alternative medicine organisations will need to increase public scrutiny of their affairs, regardless of whether they get statutory regulation.

EDUCATIONAL STANDARDS

Little external pressure has been put on practitioners of complementary and alternative medicine to reach any particular educational standard. Those professional organisations that have attempted to raise standards have been self motivated. The House of Lords report, however, recommended that regulatory bodies set objectives of training and define core competencies. Such objectives will clearly depend on the extent to which a profession claims that its members see patients independently of the family doctor. The Centre for Complementary Health Studies found that most practitioners of complementary or alternative medicine were likely to do so (Mills and Peacock, 1997; Mills and Budd, 2000). On the other hand, much anecdotal evidence, supported by at least one systematic study (Thomas et al, 1991), has suggested that most patients consult complementary practitioners concurrently with conventional medical doctors.

Practitioners of many therapies – for example, those classified as complementary therapies in the box – are unlikely to tackle critical diagnostic issues or face the prospect of serious interaction with medical treatment. Nevertheless, other therapists may see patients who choose not to consult a doctor, and some practitioners may even encourage such independence. This uncertainty needs to be clarified: if complementary and alternative medical professions claim therapeutic autonomy then they are vulnerable to the charge that only a full medical education can equip them to work independently of doctors (Ernst, 1995).

It could also be argued that all practitioners of complementary or alternative medicine should show that they are aware of potentially dangerous situations and know the contraindications for their practice, possible adverse effects, and mechanisms of referral to medical treatment (Mills, 1996). As complementary medicine grows the public may become more careful of its claims. The current position whereby organisations can happily operate at almost any level they want may not be tenable. Organisations should develop realistic strategies to justify how they would handle patients who have not already been assessed by a doctor. Such progress is most likely through more rigorous educational curriculums – for example, imbuing the new generation of practitioners with the necessary culture of inquiry. This will lead to better articulation of limits to practice (and efficacy) and encourage fruitful debate with other health professionals.

Progress has been made. Leading groups of complementary and alternative practitioners have established degree courses at, or validated by, universities (this is particularly notable among therapies in group 1). Other professional groups are considering the precedent set by the British Acupuncture Accreditation Board. The board, which has an independent chair and a majority of non-acupuncturists, was established by leading acupuncture professional organisations and colleges as a forum to assure the public that subscribing colleges are meeting self imposed criteria for educational achievement and to formally engage the public in the overall debate (Shifrin, 1993).

ROLE OF ORGANISATIONS REPRESENTING OTHER HEALTH PRACTITIONERS

The position of organisations which represent doctors, nurses, midwives, physiotherapists, chiropodists, and other registered health professionals who practise complementary therapies is bound to be different from that of organisations principally concerned with representing complementary specialists. There may, for example, be a view that what is being practised is a 'technique' rather than a wider encompassing 'therapy,' with the corresponding assumption that training standards need not be particularly rigorous. However, the House of Lords report took a firm view on the standards that such bodies need to apply: 'We recommend that if CAM [complementary and alternative medicine] is to be practised by any conventional healthcare practitioners, they [patients] should be treated to standards comparable to those set out for that particular therapy by the appropriate (single) CAM regulatory body.'

PROSPECTS FOR PROFESSIONAL INTEGRATION

The surveys by the Centre for Complementary Health Studies confirmed that there is no immediate prospect of a concerted move for wholesale integration of complementary and alternative medicine with the wider medical community (Mills and Budd, 2000; Mills and Peacock, 1997). In both accomplishment and aspiration, the groups are too disparate to be considered as one movement. Indeed it is misleading to view them as such.

In the 1980s, as complementary therapies became more widely used, many practitioners pressed for the development of complementary medicine as a whole. It soon became clear, however, that it would be more feasible for the various professions to develop at different paces, to reflect the variety of their characteristics and aspirations. Nevertheless, because many practitioners use more than one therapy it may be too complicated and expensive for individual practitioners to belong to separate registers for each therapy, This leads to the argument that legislation should be essentially unitary, with something resembling a Council of Professions Complementary to Medicine.

The Lords report concluded that the best prospects for coordination are likely to come from each discipline setting its own standards and competence. There is an obvious benefit for the public as well as the practitioner in agreeing what a particular therapy actually entails. The final, and most appropriate, shape of any statutory regulation could then emerge more clearly once individual standards have been set.

In 1997 the Foundation for Integrated Medicine published a discussion document on the way forward for integrated medicine after wide consultation across conventional and complementary medicine (Foundation for Integrated Medicine, 1998). The document set out the work of four expert working groups on research and development, education and training, delivery mechanisms, and regulation. It also made important recommendations for regulation of complementary medicine, including criteria for any system of self regulation. The foundation has encouraged integration among complementary medicine professions and has recently received a grant from the King's Fund to help it to work towards forming central regulatory bodies.

CONCLUSIONS

Public demand for complementary medicine has grown to a level where communication and cooperation with orthodox health services is necessary (Dickinson, 1995). Many patients see complementary practitioners concurrently with their doctor. However, they often do not tell their doctor about it, perhaps because they fear a negative response. Evidence that professionals from all parts of the healthcare spectrum were engaging in constructive debate about their relative roles would encourage greater communication between all practitioners and their patients.

Competing interests

SYM is a former director of the Centre for Complementary Health Studies and was a specialist advisor to the House of Lords Select Committee on Science and Technology report on complementary and alternative medicine. He is co-chair of the regulatory working group of the Foundation for Integrated Medicine.

REFERENCES

Ernst E. Competence in complementary medicine. *Complementary Therapies in Medicine* 1995;3:6–8.

Dickinson DPS. Complementary therapies in medicine: the patient's perspective. *Complementary Therapies in Medicine* 1995;3:9–12.

Foundation for Integrated Medicine. *Integrated healthcare: a way forward for the next four years?* London: FIM, 1998.

House of Lords Select Committee on Science and Technology. *Complementary and alternative medicine: session 1999–2000, 6th report.* London: Stationery Office, 2000.

Mills S. Safety awareness in complementary medicine. *Complementary Therapies in Medicine* 1996;4:48–51.

Mills S, Budd S. *Professional organisation of complementary and alternative medicine in the United Kingdom 2000: a second report to the Department of Health.* Exeter: Centre for Complementary Health Studies, University of Exeter, 2000.

Mills S, Peacock W. *Professional organisation of complementary and alternative medicine in the United Kingdom 1997: a report to the Department of Health.* Exeter: Centre for Complementary Health Studies, University of Exeter, 1997.

Shifrin K. Setting standards for acupuncture training – a model for complementary medicine. *Complementary Therapies in Medicine* 1993;1:91–5.

Stone J, Matthews J. *Complementary medicine and the law.* Oxford: Oxford University Press, 1996.

Thomas K, Carr J, Westlake L, Williams BT. Use of non-orthodox and conventional health care in Great Britain. *BMJ* 1991;302:207–10.

CHAPTER 27

THE IMPLICATIONS OF THE OSTEOPATHS ACT

Clive S Standen

INTRODUCTION

The Osteopaths Bill, which passed its third reading in the House of Commons on 7 May, was described by parliamentarians as the largest private Member's Bill ever to be brought to a successful conclusion. This is a reflection of the comprehensive way in which it approaches the regulation by statute of a profession which has been voluntarily self-regulating since it failed in a previous attempt to obtain parliamentary regulation, as far back as 1935.

THE NEW GENERAL OSTEOPATHIC COUNCIL

The major change resulting from the Bill will be that osteopaths no longer practice under Common Law; from the date on which the Act becomes law the practice of osteopathy will be controlled by a new General Osteopathic Council, established under the auspices of, and responsible to, the Privy Council. It will then be an offence for any person to 'describe himself as an osteopath, osteopathic practitioner, osteopathic physician, osteopathist, osteotherapist, or any other kind of osteopath ... unless he is a registered osteopath', thus granting the profession the effective closure of title.

Edited from an article in *Complementary Therapies in Medicine* 1993;1:208–10.

Perhaps the most important effect of this measure will be to reassure members of the public who consult anyone using the title 'osteopath', that their practitioner is 'properly trained, and trustworthy', bound by standards prescribed by a governing body that is answerable, ultimately, to the Privy Council under an Act of Parliament. In order to do this the Act lays down a comprehensive set of committees and criteria within which the profession will be self-regulating. There will initially be four 'statutory committees' – Education, Investigating, Professional Conduct and Health, and the Council has the power to establish others.

The junior health minister, Tom Sackville, who guided the Bill through the Commons, has said that it embodies the most up-to-date thinking on professional self-regulation, and regards it as a model for others to follow. Under this system the General Osteopathic Council will have the power to scrutinise the health and fitness to practise of osteopaths, and to suspend them if it believes this is necessary in order to protect the public. John Warden, parliamentary correspondent of the *British Medical Journal* 1993; 306: 608, points out that, unlike the powers currently available to the General Medical Council, the Act will enable the General Osteopathic Council to cite 'incompetent practice' as an explicit reason for disciplinary investigation, and goes on to speculate that this may have significant implications for the medical profession, given that the Medical Act is due for amendment in the not too distant future.

HEALTH INSURANCE

In terms of gaining access to osteopathic treatment, it will be interesting to see whether the Act has any effect on the policies of private health insurers. Some schemes presently pay for subscribers' treatment at the hands of osteopaths, but BUPA has been reviewing its policy for more than a year and has yet to include osteopathy within its benefits framework. It is, of course, impossible to predict what other changes may occur, but what can be foreseen is the attention osteopathy will attract as a result of the Act; there will be increased interest in research into all aspects of the work of osteopaths, no doubt including its efficacy in various situations, how it achieves results, and so on. As well as originating in academic inquiry, such interests will also have much to do with the application of clinical audit to osteopathy as it is to other forms of health care. There are already examples of osteopaths being recruited and financed by NHS budget and fund-holders to treat their patients.

An intriguing and important side issue for osteopaths will be this potential tension inherent in having a patient's costs met by a third party who may seek the power to determine the number of treatments given in order to stay within budgetary limits. Until now osteopaths have in most instances worked within the framework of a direct relationship with the patient, and either of the two could suggest that treatment cease. A third party who holds the purse strings will complicate matters. As this becomes more widespread the need for an effective method of auditing osteopathic practice will therefore become more pronounced. This is something that is already under consideration but, as many potential researchers have found, establishing valid and effective criteria for the selection of patients and assessment of outcomes is far from straightforward.

PROFESSIONAL IMPLICATIONS

It is also possible to foresee that the Act has significant implications for the osteopathic profession itself. Osteopaths are frequently associated, in the minds of the public and other professions, with the treatment of low back pain. Given current concern over the enormous level of suffering caused by low back pain, and the working days lost because of it, osteopaths have to anticipate being put under the spotlight, as I suggested above. However, important as this may be, studies have shown that osteopaths spend only 50% of their time treating patients who complain of low back pain. They also deal with other spinal problems, and have considerable expertise in the treatment of shoulders, elbows, knees and feet – in fact any pathophysiological situation in which there is a musculoskeletal component It seems likely that the profession will have to seek a means of promoting awareness about the contribution its members can make to the management of these patients.

I believe this is particularly significant when considered in conjunction with the new arrangements for care in the community. Osteopaths have a great deal to offer in the treatment of the elderly, the house-bound, and people with a variety of handicaps and disabilities. Osteopathy demands low levels of capital investment and is applicable to many of the patients who might be described as currently being 'in the twilight' of the existing system.

As an example of how the osteopathic profession might widen its contribution in this respect, the British School of Osteopathy has made a commitment to improving access to members of the local communities who suffer from a disability. This has involved considerable structural work to the entrance of its premises, and the employment of a project co-ordinator to liaise with key workers in local authorities and voluntary groups. This not only benefits those in the locality unable to reach a clinic without assistance, but serves to widen the experience of the students, which we hope will make them more flexible in their approach to practise when they graduate.

In other respects, osteopathic education is unlikely to change radically as a result of the new Act. In fact it can be argued that it was the objective improvement in education that was the first factor in setting the profession on the road to statutory regulation. The success of the British School of Osteopathy in securing validation of its course by the Council for National Academic Awards demonstrated the profession's commitment to entering the mainstream of the higher education community, and to offering itself for outside scrutiny and review. The confirmation that the profession is capable of maintaining an autonomous institution which is able to offer education to degree level marked the attainment of a significant professional maturity. The new education committee will be called upon to determine the requisite standard for recognition of courses but it is unlikely, given the prevailing models of medical education, that there will be any significant departure from the present system.

Perhaps more interesting is the provision for the Council to introduce compulsory postgraduate education as a condition for continuing registration. This is again something which other professions will look at with interest, since the legislation has government support. It is another aspect of the Act which the profession has anticipated, having already been under active consideration for some years, and likely to be welcomed by all existing osteopathic groups.

CONCLUSION

In conclusion, it is interesting to dwell on the potential contradictions inherent in the process of regulating and bringing within 'the establishment' a profession that has generally been regarded as 'alternative' or 'unorthodox' in this country since the beginning of the century. I am not yet certain whether it is possible to be both established and unorthodox at the same time. I wonder whether, as time passes, we will notice a change in the people who consider osteopathy as a career. In the past, a proportion of students have been attracted by its 'alternative' status and the freedom which that seemed to confer to pursue a role on the fringes of the system. It must be said that being answerable to the Privy Council is just about as far as it is possible to go in the opposite direction. Will future generations of osteopaths therefore consist of those who by inclination favour a contrasting role which reflects the profession's new-found position? The corollary of this question must also be posed: can true scientific or epistemological orthodoxy be conferred simply by parliamentary statute? We shall have to wait and see.

CHAPTER 28

REGULATING COMPLEMENTARY AND ALTERNATIVE MEDICINE: THE CASE OF ACUPUNCTURE

Mike Saks

REGULATION AND COMPLEMENTARY AND ALTERNATIVE MEDICINE

Regulation has become an important topic in health care in the UK at a time when there is increasing government concern to protect the public, especially as ever more health scandals come to light in medicine and related fields (Allsop and Saks, 2002). There is also a particular need to examine regulatory mechanisms in complementary and alternative medicine (CAM), as rapidly growing numbers of people are now using such therapies (Saks, 2003). This is underlined by the fact that presently there is a wide diversity of regulation of CAM, with most therapies being largely unregulated. Such a position certainly applies to self-help where the public engage in a relatively unfettered manner in everything from the use of crystal therapy to the purchase of over the counter homoeopathic preparations. Even here, though, there are boundaries – as, for example, those imposed by laws variously restricting the availability and consumption of a range of foods and medicines (Fulder, 1996).

A similar pattern applies in relation to CAM practitioners, on which this piece focuses. Currently, and unusually in a European context, people can practise most forms of CAM under the Common Law – even without any form of training or qualification (Saks, 1999). Having said this, there are

This chapter has been commissioned by the editors for inclusion in this Reader.

some restrictions, including on the types of conditions that practitioners can claim to treat, with areas such as cancer, epilepsy and glaucoma being legally off limits (Larkin, 1995). Forms of self-imposed regulation – whilst not yet completely the norm – have also increasingly emerged in the CAM field. This is well illustrated by the Society of Homoeopaths that has established a voluntary register and an ethical code for its members, as well as accreditation arrangements for training (Cant and Sharma, 1996). However, by definition, such arrangements are not comprehensive in their coverage – and do not prevent non-members of such bodies in specific areas from working independently, outside of these boundaries.

This contrasts with the position of the orthodox health professions, such as nursing, physiotherapy and medicine. These bodies are based on statutory as opposed to voluntary regulation – with those whose names do not appear on legally underwritten registers being excluded from practice in the fields concerned. This applies as much to the operation of the recently reformed Nursing and Midwifery Council and Health Professions Council as that of the much longer established General Medical Council (Allsop and Saks, 2002). To be sure, the precise form of regulation of the orthodox health professions has changed over time and there is a fair amount of variability in regulatory mechanisms between professional groups. However, typically regulation now covers everything from registration for eligible practitioners to the development of prescribed education for the profession in question and disciplinary procedures for errant professionals (Saks, 1998).

Interestingly, two groups of CAM practitioners – the osteopaths and chiropractors – broke the mould in gaining statutory regulation in the first half of the 1990s (Saks, 2002). Like more orthodox health professions, they won the right to establish their own registers, with protection of title and self-regulatory powers. However, they have not yet gained comparable access to orthodox health professions to financial support from the National Health Service. Nonetheless, this still puts them at the vanguard of CAM practitioners – ahead of groups like the acupuncturists and herbalists that have the most advanced forms of voluntary self-regulation in CAM (Cant and Sharma, 1999). In order better to understand the issues associated with the regulation of CAM, this contribution focuses on the case of acupuncture, where still stronger forms of regulation are currently being sought. This case study is dealt with from the perspective of the past, present and future.

REGULATION AND ACUPUNCTURE: THE HISTORICAL CONTEXT

To understand the position of acupuncture in Britain in terms of regulation, some knowledge of its history is helpful. In this respect, acupuncture is taken primarily to involve the insertion of needles into the body for therapeutic purposes, although there are variations in practice as to how it is used and the theories that lie behind it (Saks, 2001). As such, its origins go back some two and a half thousand years to China where classically it was employed to balance the polar forces of yin and yang by inserting and manipulating needles on points on the meridians – channels linking the twelve vital organs of the body along which the life force (Qi) was held to flow. Knowledge of the practice spread from China to other countries in the Far East, eventually reaching Europe by the seventeenth and eighteenth centuries. A vogue for the method developed in much of the Western world in the first half of the nineteenth century (Lu Gwei-Djen and Needham, 1980).

This early nineteenth-century interest in acupuncture was reflected in this country where members of the Royal College of Surgeons and the Royal College of Physicians employed it pragmatically for conditions such as rheumatism and injuries to the muscular fibre of the body. Rival non-medical practitioners often used acupuncture more widely, as a panacea for all ills (Saks, 1996). At this time, though, there was little knowledge of the classical Oriental theories of acupuncture and no systematic training in this therapy. Traditional acupuncture needles were not normally available. A good deal of improvisation therefore took place with the use of sewing needles and the development of spring-loaded needles to create artificial eruptions on the skin. Needles were also typically inserted at the site of the complaint, as opposed to at a distance as in classical acupuncture (Saks, 1995). From a regulatory viewpoint there was an open field at this time with few restrictions, in which practitioners of acupuncture and other health providers competed freely for business in the marketplace (Porter, 2001).

This changed, however, with the rise of the medical profession in the mid-nineteenth century. With the establishment of the 1858 Medical Registration Act, which created a national register of medical practitioners policed through the General Medical Council, the profession increasingly closed ranks behind the newly developing biomedical paradigm based on drugs and surgery (Waddington, 1984). This induced doctors – with their newfound monopoly over medical practice – progressively to abandon the practice of acupuncture by the turn of the century and to stigmatise those who continued their association with it within the profession. It also led medical bodies to marginalise non-medical practitioners of acupuncture and other CAM therapists through attacks in professional journals and other means; while such practitioners were still able to operate under the Common Law, their wide-ranging, empirically based practice created a threat to the income, power and status of doctors who were seeking to establish a more theoretical, biomedical foundation for their work (Saks, 1995).

The marginalisation of acupuncture and other CAM therapies increased in regulatory terms with the passing of the 1911 National Health Insurance Act and the 1946 National Health Service Act. These added far greater state financial underwriting as well as legitimacy to orthodox medicine and the growing numbers of allied health professions – from nursing and midwifery to physiotherapy and occupational therapy (Saks, 1999). This legislation was complemented by laws restricting claims to be able to treat a range of more serious conditions to doctors in the 1930s and 1940s (Larkin, 1995). It is not therefore surprising that the use of acupuncture by medical and other practitioners declined to virtually zero by the mid-twentieth century. However, a revival began in the 1950s that culminated in the founding in the early 1960s of the Medical Acupuncture Society, which provided a base for the medical practice of acupuncture. The College of Traditional Chinese Acupuncture and the British College of Acupuncture were also established at a similar time, offering programmes of training largely for non-medical practitioners that were substantially longer than those provided by the Medical Acupuncture Society (Saks, 1996).

ACUPUNCTURE: THE CURRENT REGULATORY POSITION

Having said this, acupuncture was still marginalised both inside and outside the medical profession. This position, however, shifted from the 1970s onwards in the wake of the development of a strong counter culture – especially with the reopening of political relations with China in the period of ping-pong diplomacy in the mid-1970s (Saks, 1995). Since then acupuncture has become one of the most accepted CAM therapies in orthodox health care, in National Health Service pain clinics and elsewhere. In medicine this has been epitomised by the rise in the numbers of items on the subject in professional journals, increases in officially sponsored research and expanding training and education at ever-higher levels (Saks, 1996). It has also been reflected in the growing membership of the reconstituted British Medical Acupuncture Society to over one and a half thousand by the end of the millennium – with an equivalent figure for the Acupuncture Association of Chartered Physiotherapists and some two hundred and fifty for the nurse membership of the British Academy of Western Acupuncture (British Medical Association, 2000).

This has more than been matched by the growth of non-medically qualified acupuncturists. The members of the voluntarily established British Acupuncture Council now exceed two thousand (British Medical Association, 2000). This has built on the initial formation of the Council for Acupuncture in 1980, which – paralleling a number of other CAM therapies – sought to unite previously divided groups of practitioners. In the case of non-medical acupuncturists, it brought together a myriad of bodies including the British Acupuncture Association and Register, the Chung San Acupuncture Society, the International Register of Oriental Medicine, the Register of Traditional

Chinese Medicine and the Traditional Acupuncture Society (Saks, 1995). This grew into the British Acupuncture Accreditation Board and the British Acupuncture Council – which respectively sets minimum standards of education and holds a register of practitioners with an agreed code of ethics – with the power to discipline those who do not conform to these.

In terms of regulation, the British Acupuncture Council and its predecessor body has worked with government in drawing up guidelines on acupuncture, not least in face of concerns about outbreaks of AIDS and hepatitis B (Saks, 1996). The relationships between medically and non-medically qualified acupuncturists have not always been positive in this and other contexts, in part because of potential competition for services in the private market (Saks, 1995). However, it is now possible for medical referrals to be made as a result of the General Medical Council ending its longstanding ethical prohibition on collaboration between doctors and non-medically qualified CAM therapists in the mid-1970s – a position that was finally recognised by the British Medical Association over a decade later (Saks, 1999). Despite more constructive medical attitudes to acupuncture, though, a recent study showed that, while over half of general practitioners had arranged acupuncture for their patients, in the vast majority of cases this was provided by another doctor or a physiotherapist – as distinct from a non-medical CAM practitioner (British Medical Association, 2000).

This may reflect conflicting interests between the two groups because of the continuing challenge to orthodox doctors from the more traditional and widely applied Oriental practice of acupuncture by non-medical practitioners. Doctors tend to favour a more limited model of acupuncture compatible with orthodox biomedicine. This has three main dimensions: application to a restricted range of areas such as pain and addictions, a formulaic approach based on points to be needled in given conditions, and a desire to explain the *modus operandi* of acupuncture in terms of orthodox neurophysiological theorising – such as through the release of endorphins (Saks, 1995). There seems therefore to be a desire by orthodox medical practitioners to incorporate acupuncture into their repertoire on their own terms in face of growing public demand for this and other CAM therapies. This is far less challenging to the income, power and status of doctors than sanctioning broad based, individually tailored, traditional acupuncture, centred on balancing the yin and the yang, in which their non-medical competitors have the strongest profile (Saks, 1992).

ACUPUNCTURE: THE POTENTIAL REGULATORY FUTURE

This leads on to the potential regulatory future for acupuncture. The House of Lords Select Committee on Science and Technology (2000) argued that there should be a more coherent regulatory framework in CAM, with single lead bodies for particular therapies. It was felt that the education of health professionals should familiarise them with acupuncture and other CAM therapies and that there should be more dialogue between medical and non-medical CAM practitioners. Education and training courses should also be more standardised, with accreditation in association with higher education institutions. The report argued that in some cases voluntary self-regulation alone would be sufficient for practice. However, for acupuncture – like herbal medicine – it was felt that the time was ripe for statutory regulation. The reasons include the risks to patients of not so doing, the well-organised voluntary system of regulation that already exists, the wish of most CAM therapists to move in this direction, and the degree of development of a research base.

These conclusions were underlined by the publication of a subsequent report by the Prince of Wales's Foundation for Integrated Health (2003) commissioned by the Department of Health and other bodies on the regulation of acupuncture. This report notes that acupuncture in this country is currently remarkable for its diversity and the wide range of contexts in which groups spanning from traditional practitioners to doctors, physiotherapists, nurses and other CAM therapists use it. It advocates the statutory regulation of acupuncture – aimed at protecting the public from the untrained and incompetent, while preserving the broad range of practice of acupuncture. This involves setting up a common register and initiating further work developing equivalence in the different styles in which acupuncture is practised, based on National Occupational Standards. This would entail some seven thousand practitioners being on the register, with other arrangements for the remaining five thousand practitioners who employ acupuncture on a more limited basis to ensure that they have adequate training.

This report clearly points the way towards collaboration between orthodox and CAM practitioners who use acupuncture. This integrated approach – whilst still not providing an entirely level playing field between orthodox medicine and CAM – prompts reflection on the position in China where acupuncture is not an alternative medicine as it has been in the West, but an integral part of its tradition along with other elements of Traditional Chinese Medicine (Saks, 1997). As such, it forms an important strand of medicine in its own right. The education and training of doctors and other grades of health personnel also typically includes both traditional and modern medicine, such as the use of acupuncture, herbs and Western drugs. There have of course been periods in China when acupuncture has been marginalised, as in the 1920s and 1930s when it was banned along with other elements of Traditional Chinese Medicine as the Kuomintang sought to modernise China in face of Western imperialism. However, acupuncture is now extensively used as a mainstream therapy in China in both its classical and modern Western forms (Saks, 1995).

In conclusion, the most appropriate forms of regulation of acupuncture in Britain remain subject to further debate. One of the key advantages of statutory professional regulation is that it positively protects the public against the effects of untrained practitioners using an invasive method like acupuncture. The need for such regulation is illustrated by the case of the hepatitis B outbreak affecting thirty-five patients in Birmingham in 1977 as a result of the failure of a non-medical acupuncturist to sterilise his needles (McDonald, 1982). Another argument for such statutory regulation is that it helps to provide an evidence base for acupuncture practice through higher education qualifications – in a field where research is currently fast developing (see, for example, Ernst et al, 2001). It also secures a strong ethical framework for practice. Whilst there are benefits from voluntary regulation, they are not as all encompassing as statutory regulation as far as public protection is concerned.

Against this, the merits of such regulation depend on the sensitivity of any legislation that is enacted. The extent to which statutory regulation encompassing diversity is desirable is related to the research evidence that exists for different types of acupuncture. This was a source of controversy in the House of Lords Select Committee on Science and Technology (2000) that clearly differentiated the 'big five' disciplines – including acupuncture, chiropractic, herbal medicine, homoeopathy and osteopathy – from Traditional Chinese Medicine, in which statutory regulation was seen as less justified in terms of its evidence base. There are ongoing debates too as to whether it is wise to place control of referral to acupuncturists in the National Health Service in the hands of orthodox medical practitioners as advocated by the House of Lords Select Committee on Science and Technology (2000). This is because they may not be best placed to make judgements about what will be of most help to patients in this broad ranging and complex field. Whatever the outcome, though, acupuncture provides a fascinating case study in the regulation of CAM.

REFERENCES

Allsop J, Saks M (eds). *Regulating the Health Professions*, London: Sage, 2002.

British Medical Association. *Acupuncture: Efficacy, Safety and Practice*, Amsterdam: Harwood Academic Publishers, 2000.

Cant S, Sharma U. 'Demarcation and transformation within homoeopathic knowledge: A strategy of professionalization', *Social Science and Medicine* 1996;42:579–88.

Cant S, Sharma U. *A New Medical Pluralism? Alternative Medicine, Doctors, Patients and the State*, London: UCL Press, 1999.

Ernst E, Pittler M, Stevinson C, White A (eds). *The Desktop Guide to Complementary and Alternative Medicine*, London: Mosby, 2001.

Fulder S. *The Handbook of Alternative and Complementary Medicine*, 3rd edition. Oxford: Oxford University Press, 1996.

House of Lords Select Committee on Science and Technology. *Report on Complementary and Alternative Medicine*, London: The Stationery Office, 2000.

Larkin G. State control and the health professions in the United Kingdom: Historical perspectives. In: *Health Professions and the State in Europe*, Johnson T, Larkin G, Saks M (eds). London: Routledge, 1995.

Lu Gwei-Djen, Needham J. *Celestial Lancets: A History and Rationale of Acupuncture and Moxa*, Cambridge: Cambridge University Press, 1980.

Macdonald A. *Acupuncture: From Ancient Art to Modern Medicine*, London: George Allen & Unwin, 1982.

Porter R. *Quacks: Fakers and Charlatans in English Medicine*, Manchester: Manchester University Press, 2001.

Prince of Wales's Foundation for Integrated Health. *The Statutory Regulation of the Acupuncture Profession: The Report of the Acupuncture Regulatory Working Group*, London: PoWFIH, 2003.

Saks M. The paradox of incorporation: Acupuncture and the medical profession in modern Britain. In: *Alternative Medicine in Britain*, Saks M (ed). Oxford: Clarendon Press, 1992.

Saks M. *Professions and the Public Interest: Professional Power, Altruism and Alternative Medicine*, London: Routledge, 1995.

Saks M. 'Educational and professional developments in acupuncture in Britain: An historical and contemporary overview'. *European Journal of Oriental Medicine*, 1996;Winter:32–4.

Saks M. East meets West: The emergence of an holistic tradition. In: *Medicine: A History of Healing*, Porter R (ed). London: The Ivy Press, 1997.

Saks M. Professionalism and health care. In: *Sociological Perspectives on Health, Illness and Health Care*, Field D., Taylor S (eds). Oxford: Blackwell Science, 1998.

Saks M. 'The wheel turns? Professionalisation and alternative medicine in Britain', *Journal of Interprofessional Care* 1999;13:129–38.

Saks M. Acupuncture. In: *The Oxford Companion to the Body*, Blakemore C, Jennett S (eds). Oxford: Oxford University Press, 2001.

Saks M. Professionalisation, regulation and alternative medicine. In: *Regulating the Health Professions*, Allsop J, Saks M (eds). London: Sage, 2002.

Saks M. *Orthodox and Alternative Medicine: Politics, Professionalization and Health Care*, London: Sage, 2003.

Waddington I. *The Medical Profession in the Industrial Revolution*, Goldenbridge: Gill & Macmillan, 1984.

CHAPTER 29

BUILDING A PROFESSIONAL COMMUNITY; COLLECTIVE CULTURE IN A GROUP OF NON MEDICALLY QUALIFIED HOMOEOPATHS IN BRITAIN

Ursula Sharma

The literature about professionalisation is full of references to 'strategies', 'projects' (e.g., Witz, 1992). Yet who or what are the agents who entertain these projects, seek to carry out strategies? According to this literature they are groups of would-be professionals organised into associations which then act corporately on behalf of the emergent profession.

For an association to develop in the first place there must be networks of practitioners with established patterns of interaction and some sense of common cause. To develop effective strategies there needs to be some degree of consensus about means and ends, about how members communicate with each other and with agencies outside the profession, i.e., there must be some degree of common political culture, as well as common occupational skills and knowledge.

The ways in which such cultures develop among professions has been given little attention. Where orthodox medicine is concerned, quite a lot of research has been done on the ways in which professional education helps to generate certain attitudes of mind (e.g., Becker et al, 1961; Good, 1994). And prior to the experience of education there is the process of selection of candidates for that education. Consciously or otherwise, prior

Edited from an article in Høg E, Olesen SG (eds). *Studies in Alternative Therapy, Communication in and about alternative therapies.* Denmark: Odense University, 1996.

to the introduction of equal opportunities policies (and possibly even then), they were selecting people who could be presumed to have a fair degree of cultural community already, excluding ethnic minorities, women, working class candidates, those with recent background in humanities etc.

Where complementary therapy in Britain is concerned, however, one of the major problems in unifying a community of practitioners so that a national organisation can be formed has been the divisive effect of training having been given in highly diverse establishments, often founded by influential and charismatic practitioners, with their own distinctive ethos and version of the therapy. Many of these training establishments had already set up professional associations exclusively for their own alumni, and sometimes it proved hard to integrate all these into one.

The Society of Homoeopaths, which I shall consider here, did not have this particular problem but originated in a group of people who had common experience of being taught informally by two influential and charismatic teachers in the late sixties and early seventies (Cant, forthcoming). I have conducted research on this organisation for several years, attending its conferences and gatherings, interviewing local members and officers and scanning its journals and publications. I present here some observations based on this fieldwork.[1]

THE SOCIETY OF HOMOEOPATHS; HISTORICAL BACKGROUND

In Britain homoeopathy is practised by two main kinds of practitioner, doctor homoeopaths and non-medically qualified homoeopaths (NMQ homoeopaths).[2] The Faculty of Homoeopaths provides postgraduate training in homoeopathy for people who are already qualified in medicine. Until recently the courses provided by the Faculty constituted the only formal homoeopathic education available in Britain. In the seventies, two NMQ homoeopaths – John Da Monte and Thomas Maughan – taught groups of students, probably mostly ex-patients, in their homes. The two were friends, though their study groups were run separately. Homoeopathic knowledge therefore seems to have seeped out of the medical academy. In spite of these informal links, the doctor homoeopaths of the Faculty did not, and still do not, recognise the NMQ homoeopath as equal in competence to the doctor homoeopath. This exclusion, and the general contempt in which the medical profession as a body held practitioners of complementary medicine in general no doubt contributed to a sense of solidarity within the group, a sense of campaigning for the virtues of homoeopathy from a beleaguered position.

Da Monte and Maughan died within a few months of each other in 1975/6. The Society of Homoeopaths was founded by their pupils in 1978 to help encourage the development of NMQ homoeopathy in Britain, and a new college, the College of Homoeopathy, was founded in London in the same year. The only other association of NMQ homoeopaths had its origin in a more direct leakage from medical homoeopathy. Its members were mainly drawn from graduates of the Hahnemann College of Homoeopathy, founded by an Indian doctor. Dr. Pyara Singh, in 1980. This college provides training mainly, though not exclusively, for people who have some professional qualification in a field such as nursing or dentistry. The United Kingdom Homeopathic Medical Association was founded in 1985, originally primarily as a professional association for graduates of the Hahnemann College.

These two organisations started out quite separately and with rather different kinds of membership and orientation, although there has been a good deal of rapprochement in recent years, and some considerable overlap of membership. However, what made the Society of Homoeopaths quite distinct, and the factor which has shaped a good deal of its development (though some would say has caused it problems), was the fact that both Da Monte and Maughan were active Druids, also keenly interested in esoteric and Eastern philosophy, and they evidently mixed these interests in their teaching of homoeopathy to their pupils in the late sixties and seventies.

DEVELOPING A POLITICAL CULTURE; BASIC ASSUMPTIONS AND STYLES OF ACTION

To develop a project and to pursue it consistently, the members of an association must already share to some extent, or else must develop, a political culture. By this I do not mean that they must actually agree on all political matters, simply that they must share some dominant values and notions about the proper way to go about getting things done, including the right way to resolve disagreements. The Society of Homoeopaths, like many similar professional organisations in the field of complementary medicine, has had to make the transition from a coterie of inspired activists to a formally constituted public group, capable of being taken seriously as a proper professional association, with all that this implies in terms of being capable of enforcing ethical codes, guarantee competence of registered members etc. On the whole it has done this remarkably rapidly and successfully.

The Society has a formal constitution which gives a good deal of discretion to an elected Board of between six and nine Directors. With the growth of membership and functions the Directors initiated a review of management in 1992 which resulted in (amongst other things) the setting up of various working groups dealing with specialised areas, to which ordinary members were invited to offer their services (Society of Homoeopaths Newsletter June 1993: 8). The Society certainly sees itself explicitly as 'non-hierarchical and democratic' (Society of Homoeopaths Newsletter March, 1994: 5).

On the whole there appears to have been few fundamental disagreements about the constitution of the Society and its formal working (I am not speaking here of substantive differences about how homoeopathy itself should be practised or taught, of which there have been a few, some quite important). However, from a number of sources (comments made in interviews, letters and articles in the Society Newsletter etc.) one picks up certain underlying political tensions, or perhaps one should say ambivalences. These are not to do with the organisation of the Society as such, but they do surface in relation to particular issues which the Society has to tackle. These are in the nature of felt contradictions between different but related goals rather than conflicts between identified factions or groups of people.

For example, there is the anxiety which was, and to some extent still is, frequently voiced in the complementary therapy movement (not just among homocopaths) between the need to professionalise in order to be 'respectable' and accepted, and the fear that once NMQ practitioners become a profession they will act in the self-serving way attributed to the medical profession, losing their idealism. Statutory regulation is widely held to be an important goal for NMQ homoeopaths. Yet Pauline Price, herself a doctor studying to become a homoeopath, voices the worry that whilst homoeopaths ought to be striving for a professional approach to their work,

> 'Devious means can be used to achieve a given end. Concern can be professed for the people when the profession is really self-serving. So the danger of a profession is that its members become self-serving' (Society of Homoeopaths Newsletter December, 1995: 13).

Secondly, there is the tension between an ethos of cooperation and mutual support in a beleaguered group, and the realisation that once the supply of homoeopaths reaches a certain level, practitioners are actually competing with each other for a living in a market which is not unlimited. (This is a problem for many complementary practitioners, not just homoeopaths; see Sharma, 1995: 159.) On the one hand, members of the Society have worked hard at building up local networks of homoeopaths who provide support for each other and share information. On the other, the directorate has had to recognise that from the patient's point of view the various homoeopaths in an area are in competition for his/her patronage; what etiquette should be inscribed into the code of ethics to deal with the situation when a patient transfers from one homoeopath to another (Society of Homoeopaths Newsletter September, 1993: 3)?

To illustrate the way in which such emergent tensions have surfaced, I will describe only one such issue in detail, that of gender equality.

GENDER AND THE POLITICAL CULTURE OF THE SOCIETY

A feature of the Society's meetings which I noticed very early on was the predominance of women. This reflects the composition of the membership at the present time (less than a third of the 360 odd registered members are men, a gender imbalance which seems to be reproduced in the current student body also, judging by class lists of homoeopathic colleges which I have come across). Whether as a cause or a consequence of this 'feminisation' of the professional group, there seems a fair degree of gender consciousness reflected in publications and activities. A creche is a regular feature of the conference and larger gatherings. In January 1980 a note in the Newsletter announced that an explanatory leaflet produced earlier was being revised so that all reference to 'he' was being replaced by 'he or she' throughout when both sexes were intended.

More controversial was the decision to hold women only conferences, the first of several being held in 1991. A letter to the Society's Newsletter from one of the participants hailed the conference as a useful new departure which would do something to redress the disproportionate practical dominance of men in the Society (disproportionate that is in relation to the feminine nature of the membership already remarked upon). This letter produced uncomprehending responses in the following issue from two other members, who evidently could not see the necessity for a women only conference when women actually predominated in the Society, and felt uncomfortable about what they perceived as a too militant style of ensuring gender equality:

> 'I, being a person first and also a woman, don't want to be included as a participant in a crusading march and banner parade to save downtrodden Homoeopathic womanhood – no such thing really exists in this country'.

And from a (male) founder member:

> 'Is it only a matter of numbers?. . . I would like to divert the talk about male/female numbers on the Board of Directors to that of suitability for the job' (Society of Homoeopaths Newsletter 31,1991).

The women's conference seems to have become an accepted feature of the Society year in spite of this reaction, and the controversy consequent upon this first conference was to become drowned in a wider controversy that broke out over the nature of homoeopathic prescribing, which was to prove far more divisive. However, the incident is worth mentioning to illustrate the fact that common commitment to homoeopathy and broadly similar cultural background does not in itself ensure that the members of an emergent professional group have the same ideas about the kind of political practices that are normal and acceptable, or the kind of political language which should be used within the group.

THE EMERGENT PROFESSION; COLLEGES AND NETWORKS

The emerging public culture of the group as I have described it so far is based on a number of ingredients: the familiarity and friendship which obtained among the founding group and is reproduced among cohorts of new students, the solidarity engendered through the perception of being a threatened group, some deliberate decisions made as a matter of public relations policy with regard to style and design of publications, members' notions about the kind of profession homoeopaths should aspire to be and about the proper way to achieve it, their ideas and feelings about different styles of activism and their experiences of activism in other contexts.

In the end the dominant and enduring culture of NMQ homoeopathy will be made primarily in the colleges. Common experience of training (whatever the form it takes) with its rites of passage, its trials and solidarities, is an important basis for the formation of professional identity – whether we are dealing with healing professions or any other.

Professional education is more than the ingestion of certain information required to do professional work. It involves the adoption of certain ways of thinking and communicating and interacting with others through the practices of the professional academy, whatever the nature of that academy may be. Thus, Good describes how medical students at Harvard learn medicine through the acquisition of a particular way of constructing the human body, learnt through experiences such as the dissection of a cadaver, use of slides in lectures etc. (Good, 1994: 73).

They also learn certain forms of communication, such as the writing up of case notes. A good write-up of a case establishes the student as someone who has learnt what is relevant to pick out from the interview, experienced as an event, to communicate to colleagues and to put on the record.

I never interviewed students themselves. However, from interviews with recent graduates, study of material put out by colleges etc., we can get some hints.

The founding generation of homoeopaths created a group culture based on the way they had developed as a very informal group of friends and fellow students. Informality still seems to be a characteristic of education with the frequent use of forenames which I noted earlier. Most of the original group is still involved in homoeopathic education in some way. Many founded colleges of which they are now principals, and there is much mutual visiting; members of the original group often give guest lectures in each others' colleges, and act as each others' external examiners.

Most colleges work with small groups, largely because they are still relatively small institutions. However, smallness and intimacy have also been perceived as a positive virtue by some educators. One school even called itself for some time the Small School of Homoeopathy (as in 'small is beautiful' – I thought at first it had been founded by a person with the surname of Small). But whilst professionalisation does not require size, it does require a degree of formalisation of the educational process, if only in the sense that a respectable professional course must have recognised forms of validation, transparent criteria for assessment of performance, a proper system of external examiners etc. Interviews with college principals showed that whilst the impetus for this kind of development came as much from the educators as anyone else in the homoeopathic world, they did not always find it easy to move from the informal/charismatic mode of transmission of knowledge through discipleship to the formal/bureaucratic mode of the publicly legitimated modem professional academy. Many were concerned as to how they should move to the latter without losing some of the inspiration and personal care they saw as characteristic of the former.

Another salient aspect of homoeopathic education is that it is largely part-time at the moment. The students are mature men and women (mostly the latter) who have typically had some other career. That is, they will already have been inducted into some other profession before coming to homoeopathy; they are less 'raw material' than the typical medical student who proceeds straight to training from high school, and their sense of professional identity will not be forged in the same way. They prepare to be homoeopaths by attending courses of (usually) four years, studying intensively at monthly weekend sessions.

It would seem that the sense of solidarity which develops among a cohort of students is very strong.

A good number of graduates evidently enter into professional cooperation of one kind or another with former classmates, perhaps in the form of some kind of joint practice. Setting up in practice on one's own is often a very difficult and isolating experience and the Society has recognised the need for ongoing professional contact through support groups, or local supervision groups, in which an established homoeopath holds sessions for recently graduated homoeopaths practising in a certain area to come together, discuss problems and seek advice on specific cases. The relative structural isolation of the homoeopathic student or the newly qualified homoeopath is therefore balanced by existence of informal regional or local networks which mostly have an established homoeopath at their centre.

The shape of the collective professional culture and community that emerges will depend much on the ethos of the colleges, the kind of interaction favoured between staff and students, the kind of values and attitudes cultivated in students.

CONCLUDING REMARKS

I have dealt with styles of communication and interaction rather than the substantive issues which homoeopaths communicate about or the details of the formal politics of the group. I have not touched upon debates about classical versus 'not-so-classical' homoeopathic prescribing, debates about the structure of the Society, or the nature of homoeopathic education. Rather, I have concentrated on the informal and the implicit, the apparently trivial and the assumed . . . but as any anthropologist will tell you, it is these apparently trivial aspects of everyday communication which you notice when you come into another culture – most of the time the members of the group do not have to notice it; it is part of the cultural air they breathe, and as such is as important to communication and solidarity as air is to life.

REFERENCES

Becker H, Geer B, Hughes E, Strauss L. *Boys in White: Student Culture in Medical School*, Chicago University Press: Chicago, 1961.

Cant S. From charismatic teaching to professional training: the legitimation of knowledge and the creation of trust. In: *Complementary Medicines; Knowledge in Practice*, Cant S, Shanna U (eds). Free Association Books: London, forthcoming.

Good B. *Medicine, Rationality and Experience. An Anthropological Perspective*, Cambridge University Press: Cambridge, 1994.

Maceoin D. The choice of homoeopathic models: the patient's dilemma. *The Homoeopath*, 1993;51:108-15.

Sharma U. *Complementary Medicine Today. Practitioners and Patients*, Routledge: London, 1995.

Witz A. *Professions and Patriarchy*, Routledge: London, 1992.

NOTES

1 Some of the interviews on which I have drawn in this paper were carried out by Sarah Cant as part of a wider project on the professionalisation of complementary medicine, funded by the Economic and Social Research Council. I

acknowledge both this funding support and Sarah's practical and intellectual contribution to the development of my ideas. I also acknowledge the help of the Society itself in permitting the research and of those individual directors, administrators and members who gave specific help.

2 I use the term 'NMQ' in preference to the term 'lay', which as NMQ homoeopaths themselves point out, suggests a less than professional command of knowledge.

CHAPTER 30

ACCORA THE HEALER: A CASE STUDY OF DECEPTION AND FRAUDULENT IDENTITY IN HEALING

Geraldine Lee-Treweek and Hilary Thomson

INTRODUCTION

This paper would appear from the first clause of its title to be about healing, but in fact it is about deception, or more precisely, claims to healing that involve deception. Defining healing is difficult but Benor (2002), on his online holistic healing research network, argues it can be defined as, 'practitioners who claim to be, (1) shifting biological energies manually (either between themselves and healees or within healees) and/or (2) influencing health through meditation/intent/prayer.' It would be fair to say that the majority of people who practice healing have positive intention and believe in what they do. This paper is not an attack on healing or an attempt to say that all healers are frauds. What it does serve to demonstrate is the ways by which overt deception may be perpetrated by some who would use the name of CAM for their own ends. It also identifies some of the mechanisms that seem to make such deception believable. Many of these mechanisms relate to a recipient's wish to believe and to social notions of what a healer is. Accora[1] is a real person and the situations described involved both of the authors, however, some details have been changed to protect the anonymity of all involved.

This chapter has been commissioned by the editors for inclusion in this Reader.

IDENTITY, PERFORMANCE AND FRAUD

The social sciences have much to say about the nature of social interaction and how individuals present their identities and selves to others (Cicourel, 1973; Denzin, 1992; Giddens, 1991; Goffman, 1972). Symbolic interactionist theorists argue that social life has a performance element to it; that is individuals, as cognisant and reflective beings, are able to recognise the impact their actions and behaviour have upon others (Denzin, 1992; Goffman, 1972). In recognising this they are also able to 'act up' or present themselves in particular ways in specific settings in order to control the outcome of social interactions. From this point of view there are set roles that are socially expected from say the doctor, the bus driver, the estate agent and indeed the complementary medicine practitioner. There are also roles associated with parts played in society in general, i.e. father, customer, passer-by in the street. Individuals are constantly moving between different roles to deal with the situations they experience. This ability to present oneself in particular ways is also related to the capacity to put ourselves in the shoes of another person, to quite literally understand how others may be seeing us and modify our behaviour accordingly. This is what the social psychologist Erving Goffman (1972) called the 'presentation of self' and according to him we all engage in this every day. These skills (usually) allow people to interact with each other in the world in a predictable and orderly way; without them it would be difficult to get on with any kind of business without confusion over who was doing what.

However, there are individuals who use social expectations and roles in a deceptive manner. They are happy to take on the performance of a role fraudulently in order to make a living. The skills that according to Goffman enable everyday life to go smoothly also enable the fraudster to be someone else, to take on a role and give people what they expect. Whilst there have been some studies of tricksters and fraudsters that have looked at how they manage to convince others of their 'taken on' identity (Hyde and Zanetti, 2003; Maurer, 2000), there is very little written about deception and CAM (for an exception see Randi, 1989). Some historical work has looked at so-called 'quacks' and the various remedies and treatments they peddled prior to and during the rise of biomedicine. However, it is unclear whether these people were just misguided or openly deceptive and fraudulent. It is also the case that during this time there was not a clear-cut division between the quacks and 'genuine' healthcare providers as many types of practitioners were involved in peddling unhelpful and bizarre treatments and ideas. A case in point is Dr Elisha Perkins who worked in Plainfield, Connecticut in American in the 1700s (Gevitz, 2000:4). He believed he had discovered a way of removing pain by touching muscles with metal rods. Belief in his discovery, which became known as tractorization, led to articles in newspapers, lecture tours and followers of this new technique in America and Europe. His discovery was, of course, incorrect and, a

Dr John Haygarth of Bath England, was able to prove that rubbing patients with rods other than metal ones had a similar effect, if they believed it would help them (Gevitz, 2000:6). Dr Haygarth put the efficacy of tractorization down to the placebo effect. This is a good illustration that when something appears to work it is easy for a practitioner to believe that the healing must be related to the particular therapeutic technique being used. But the critical practitioner must always be aware that the wish to believe is very powerful and discernment is needed (combined with research) to uncover the exact processes that heal.

The media often uncovers CAM fraud that involves deception on the part of the practitioner (as can be seen in the popularity of rooting out fraud through programmes such as the BBC's 'Kenyon Confronts'). Another arena from which many such claims are made is from 'fraud-busting groups' such as QuackWatch and the National Council Against Health Fraud (both sited in the USA). In the case of these groups identifying fraud has to some extent become intertwined with presenting most CAM as non-scientific and therefore (by the standards of these groups) fraudulent. For many CAMs there is little evidence of efficacy and a paucity of methodologically sound research. Moreover, in marketing speak, CAMs are services that by their very nature are 'intangible' (Berry and Parasuraman, 1993); it is difficult for the consumer of these to know exactly what they are getting and whether in the long run it will do them any good. It is, for instance, very difficult to show in a tangible way what has happened in a healing session and whether the recipient is in fact receiving any healing at all. In such a climate where the user or client is reliant upon a practitioner to be what they say they are deception becomes possible.

The discussion of Accora below is made up of two accounts. Whilst one is of a healer, the other is of a businesswoman or entrepreneur who is very aware of her performance of a role. Whilst Accora is the focus of the piece, key players are the social expectations of the two authors.

ACCORA THE HEALER – GERALDINE'S ACCOUNT

On joining the introduction to CAM therapies class Accora struck me as someone who appeared already skilled and knowledgeable about the subject area. Well liked, she appeared a charismatic person who had a big personality. It was common to see her making positive comments about group members and she seemed to always be listening and being supportive to others. Accora was also extremely open to others about her personal life. It appeared that she had experienced a lot of difficulties but she was adamant that these had made her stronger and better able to connect with other people. Accora would often be seen during lunchtime sitting outside with other students with her hands on or near them. This did not surprise me as Accora had already told me that she was a healer.

I was fascinated by the idea that Accora was a professional full-time healer and talked to her on many occasions at length about what she did. Accora said she had been born with special healing abilities. Although at points in her life she had tried to reject them she felt there was little she could do as it was 'in the blood'. By her account she had been brought up in rural Wales within a family in which psychic skills and healing abilities were not only the norm but also part of their cultural heritage as Romany gypsies. Having 'the gift' had provided a natural way to financially provide for her family and also fitted in with her idea that to help others was ultimately to help oneself. Although healing was 'in the blood' it was not a totally natural progression to go onto being a healer. It was Accora's belief that experiencing suffering in her own life had brought her closer to understanding and being able to use her gift properly. In particular, suffering she argued had brought her closer to a more spiritual way of understanding other people and to the spiritualist church.[2] She attended such churches on a regular basis as she felt that the spiritualists were good people with 'a lot of love'. Another of the reasons she gave for attending was that such places offered a supportive arena in which her skills were seen as both acceptable and indeed special. Accora gave the impression that she was proud of her lifestyle and drawn to it by a sense of it being part of both her heritage and her destiny. She said she was doing quite well in her field and had built up a regular group of clients as well as attracting new ones through the churches. Accora said she felt that I was a very sensitive person who probably would benefit from spiritualism.

On the second of the classes I had an extremely bad muscle spasm in my back. Accora offered to help, although highly sceptical I appreciated that she was putting herself out and I also felt that I would be glad for any relief from anywhere. When we went outside she began scanning my back with her hands. She stopped suddenly and looked straight at me, 'I can tell you have been through a lot, a lot of pain and worry, your energy is very low just here (pointing to my middle). This imbalance is not going to help you recover at all', she continued 'scanning'. After the treatment Accora went on to interpret the energy pattern she had found in my body. Some Chakras (energy centres believed to be sited in the torso of the body at various points) she said related to confidence and belief in myself. Around my neck areas there was a weakness, which indicated a need to deal with my self-confidence problems and put myself forward more – a strange comment given my personality and general attitude to life. Accora then told me that she also felt there was a message from the spirit world for me. The message was that my health would definitely improve and that I was to stop worrying as I was a 'worrier'. Finally, Accora said I should see if I felt better after the treatment and if not she would treat me the next day. She then said that it would benefit me greatly to see her in her professional capacity at her caravan for some more healing, this of course would be proper healing sessions and not free. Healing with other people around and other eyes upon you was not easy Accora argued, whereas healing worked much better in the privacy of the caravan. I said I would think about it, and indeed curiosity and the possibility of relief tempted me. However, I pointed out that it was unlikely that I would be able to travel to her as she lived some distance away. As it turned out, no further treatment was offered the next day and Accora did not even ask how I was. I thought perhaps I had offended her somehow as she breezed past me and began speaking to another member of the introduction to CAMs class. It was this student who was chosen to receive healing at lunchtime.

In the meantime I tried to make sense of what had happened during the healing session. Many of the things said to me could have related to anyone. For instance, being told that you need more confidence could relate to many people – we all need this at different points in our lives. And did I get well? I did feel better at the end of the day's training, however, most research on chronic back pain shows that symptoms tend to come and go. Doubtless reassurance and personal attention does contribute to relaxing and feeling more positive about symptoms too. However Accora's account of herself was compelling and believable.

ACCORA THE ENTREPRENEUR – HILARY'S ACCOUNT

My initial contact with Accora was being paired up to work with her at the classes. At first it seemed that she did not wish to speak much, she just introduced herself to me as a healer who was also training in aromatherapy. I was interested in this combination of CAMs and asked Accora when she had realised that she had 'the gift'. This seemed to give her much amusement and she laughed as she replied, 'you can call it that if you want', she went on to add that she did the work, 'purely as a business'. As she expanded on her attitude to her work she noted that much of what she did involved telling people what they wanted to hear and it was a good living. I was quite shocked at the openness with which she was able to discuss what essentially seemed to me to be a fraudulent attitude to healing. As the group work went on and I chatted to her more and watched her interacting with others it became very clear to me that she had what one might term, 'the gift of the gab' and she seemed comfortable speaking to anyone in the group.

During one lunch break I saw Accora leave with Geraldine to do a healing treatment. They returned sometime later and Accora begin to discuss attending spiritualist churches with Geraldine. I realised that what I was watching was the drumming up of business. During these discussions Accora was unwavering in her concern; she sympathetically nodded and maintained eye contact throughout. To all intents and purposes she presented herself as an empathetic and caring ear, but at the end of her conversations the offer was always there of more healing. I began to watch Accora carefully throughout the class. It was clear that she was a people person. She tended to listen intently to what people said and would very often feed back to them what they had said. On one occasion a new member of the class revealed himself to be a successful businessman. Accora having been told by others of his accomplishments went up and introduced herself. Taking his left hand in both hers she clasped it and said, 'I can tell from your energy that you are a very forthright person who does well in the world'. After a short conversation and introductions she walked back to her chair rejoining the group she was working in with a flourish, 'you can just feel that he has success, you can feel it in his whole aura'. Accora gave the impression that she had picked up on this man's success through some kind of sixth sight. Later that day she tried to sell, with some success, special necklaces that she said she had channelled energy into. The introduction to CAMs class certainly proved itself to be a means of wealth-generation. The next week she confided in me that she felt that attending the course would provide, as she put it 'more scams' to add to her portfolio of activities.

You may be wondering why Accora let me into her secret about her occupation. Later in the course Accora confided in me that she thought I was distantly related to her. I was left wondering if this was the reason that I did not receive her account of herself as a genuine healer. There were some other reasons why I was probably not chosen to receive the story of Accora as a healer. It seemed that many people Accora spent time with in breaks were, for various reasons, in some state of need. One day it would be a woman with a migraine and on another, a man who was, by his own admission, very stressed. In Geraldine's case there was pain and her constant moving around during the class and her remedial seat cushion indicated that she may be a possible client. In other words those who were chosen for special attention were also those who would most 'benefit' from Accora's healing – people who were ill, stressed or anxious.

DISCUSSION: BUT WHY DID PEOPLE BELIEVE ACCORA?

Accora provides an uncommon example of deception in healing; we simply do not know enough about this phenomenon in CAM because of its secrecy and the tendency of fraudsters to protect their fraudulent identities. As noted earlier, it is not the purpose of this article to say that all healing is fake or deceitful. Whether or not research will eventually show healing to work Accora, by her own admission, set out to deceive and make a living out of pretending to have healing abilities. What is different about Accora is the openness she displayed to Hilary about her wish to make a living in this way. So why do people pay £30 an hour for her services, often at times in their lives when they are quite vulnerable? Accora reported that people went back time and again and referred other people, therefore something was happening – whether a placebo effect or the fulfilment of other needs, curiosity, the need for comfort/reassurance or linking into their wish for a spiritual worldview more generally.

Accora's main client group can be said to be people who were vulnerable in some way, through illness, worry and anxiety or some critical life event. The people she chose to work on at the class fitted this category. She also sought clients at spiritualist churches where she knew people would be open to the idea of energy healing. Accora's story of her background, family and 'gift' added to this image of someone whose healing role in life had been chosen for her – almost out of her control. One of the most fascinating issues is the sense of connection that Accora was able to create between other people and herself. Many of the linguistic skills she demonstrated are common ones used in deception. In particular Accora used what psychologists call Barnum statements – statements that could apply to anyone (Dickson and Kelly, 1985). Often these statements also have on the recipient what is termed 'the Forer effect' (Marks, 2000:274); that is, many people will tend towards believing the statements are a true and accurate description of themselves because of their vague nature. For instance, in her treatment of Geraldine Accora's reference to 'having been through a lot of pain and worry' would probably resonate with many people with long-term health problems. Accora's use of the message that Geraldine was 'a worrier' again is a term that has been found to be easily accepted by many people. Other similar statements could include, 'you have a good sense of humour', 'you can be really good fun but also serious when you want to be', 'you like to be with others but also sometimes like to be alone' and so on. The plausibility and confidence of a fraudster is often reliant upon the person's wish to believe and the way that individuals often will try to piece information together to make sense and to find meaning in disparate ideas or notions (Lee-Treweek, 2002). Therefore, Accora used known methods to induce an impression that she had great insight into the individual she was 'healing'. Similarly the recycling of information that Accora displays – finding something out and then using it to demonstrate her deep knowledge of a person – is also a common method used by those involved in deception across a number of areas (Maurer, 2000).

For genuine healers who have worked in this area a long time, or perhaps who are registered with the Federation of Spiritual Healers or a Reiki organisation, Accora's story must raise difficult issues about routing out deception and fraud in their own fields. For instance, what does Accora's story mean in relation to the public trust of healers? After all, when someone places their hands upon another person for healing purposes nothing can be seen to be happening and the person may not always get better. Most genuine forms of healing recognise that healing is not about curing; sometimes the experience is about changing one's perspective or beginning to accept illness or disability. These different notions of what healing may entail could make claiming a healing ability easier for someone like Accora and clearly she had worked at a 'presentation of self' that fitted with clients notions of what a healer should be like. This has ramifications for the important issue of protecting consumers of CAM from the unscrupulous; Accora, and others like her, demonstrate the problems of regulation and authenticity in the world of CAM and the 'intangible services'.

REFERENCES

Benor D. Numbers of Healers in the United States of America. http://www.wholistichealingresearch.com/Projects/HealerNos.htm#top Accessed 07/04/04, 2002.

Berry LL, Parasuraman A. Building A New Academic Field – The Case of Services Marketing, *Journal of Retailing*, 1993;Spring:13–60.

Cicourel AV. *Cognitive Sociology: language and meaning in social interaction.* London: Penguin, 1973.

Denzin NK. *Symbolic Interactionism and Cultural Studies: the politics of interpretation.* Oxford: Blackwell, 1992.

Dickson DH, Kelly IW. The 'Barnum Effect' in Personality Assessment: A Review of the Literature, *Psychological Reports*, 1985;57:367–82.

Gevitz N. *Other Healers: unorthodox medicine in America.* USA: Johns Hopkins, 2000.

Giddens A. *Modernity and Self-identity: self and society in the late modern age.* Cambridge: Polity Press, 1991.

Goffman E. *The Presentation of Self.* London: Penguin, 1972.

Hyde S, Zanetti G. *Players, Con Men, Hustlers, Gamblers and Scam Artists.* New York: Thunders Mouth Press, 2003.

Lee-Treweek G. Trust in complementary medicine: the case of cranial osteopathy. *Sociological Review*, 2002;50, No.1, February.

Marks D. *The Psychology of the Psychic.* London: Prometheus Press, 2000.

Maurer D. *The Big Con.* London: Arrow, 2000.

Randi J. *The Faith Healers.* New York: Prometheus Books, 1989.

NOTES

1 Accora is a pseudonym.

2 It is important to note here that healing is not necessarily associated with spiritualism or any other religious perspective. There is often confusion, for instance, between spiritual healing and spiritualism. However, the one does not assume the other and to be a spiritual healer only requires a belief in the idea of a person having a spirit or ethereal body that can be rebalanced through healing. It is not, therefore associated with any one set of religious beliefs. Some spiritualists though do also practise spiritual healing.

SECTION 5

EVIDENCE AND EFFICACY

INTRODUCTION

Hilary MacQueen

This section of the Reader looks at the analysis of complementary and alternative therapies from a scientific standpoint. This is a relatively new approach for much of the CAM community, with many users and practitioners remaining sceptical about the value of applying a rational, scientific approach to modalities which influence emotions, body energies and well-being factors that are difficult to quantify. Nevertheless, such analysis is increasingly important, to allay fears about efficacy and safety, and indeed is essential if CAM is to be integrated formally into mainstream health care provision. Conventional medicine is becoming more and more evidence-based, and this change is driven to no small extent by the prevailing economic, legislative and retributive social culture. Similar constraints increasingly apply to CAM, and indeed the modalities whose professional bodies are most interested in becoming more integrated have been the most responsive to demands for an evidence base. The selected readings address various aspects of CAM research.

The issue of how to test whether CAM really works is addressed by Marja Verhoef, Ann Casebeer and Robert Hilsden in their reading 'Assessing efficacy of complementary medicine: adding qualitative research methods to the "gold standard"', first published in full in 2002, and reproduced in an edited form here. In this reading the authors consider the relative importance of randomised, controlled trials (RCTs) and other, qualitative research methods, in CAM testing. They make the point that many types of trials can have merit for CAM research.

This point is also made by Janet Richardson in her attractively titled reading, 'Evidence-based complementary medicine: rigour, relevance, and the swampy lowlands'. Richardson looks at the widespread rise of evidence-based medicine, and considers the kinds of research that might be applied to CAM to provide it with the evidence base it needs. She discusses concerns that can arise when applying reductionist thinking to holistic phenomena.

The reading by Edzard Ernst, 'The evidence for or against common complementary therapies' summarises the evidence available in 2003 relating to three popular modalities: acupuncture, herbal medicine and homoeopathy. This evidence has been gathered together from a variety of sources, using the powerful tools of systematic review and meta-analysis. Evidence relating to both efficacy and safety is presented and discussed.

A reading by Joanne Barnes, edited from a fuller reading published in 2003, considers in some depth the large amount of evidence relating to the safety of herbal medicines. 'Quality, efficacy and safety of complementary medicines: fashions, facts and the future. Efficacy and safety' makes the point that even when herbal remedies have a clean bill of health in their own right, the large differences in product quality and the possibilities of interactions between different remedies can sometimes lead to unexpected adverse reactions that may actually be life-threatening.

The last reading in this section, 'The crack in the biomedical box: the placebo effect' by Zelda Di Blasi, explores the importance of belief for the healing process. Much research specifically excludes contributions made by placebo, and there are concerns that this could mean that much of the therapeutic benefit of CAM, particularly that relating to feelings of well-being, is being ignored and discounted by the design of research trials.

CHAPTER 31

ASSESSING EFFICACY OF COMPLEMENTARY MEDICINE: ADDING QUALITATIVE RESEARCH METHODS TO THE 'GOLD STANDARD'

Marja J Verhoef, Ann L Casebeer and Robert J Hilsden

INTRODUCTION

The strengths and limitations of the use of randomized controlled trials (RCTs) to assess the efficacy of complementary and alternative medicine (CAM) have been widely debated in the literature (e.g., Nahin and Straus, 2001; Vickers et al, 1997) and this debate continues. Adaptations to RCTs that have been suggested increase the potential of RCTs to assess the efficacy of CAM. However, despite these adaptations to RCTs, many questions remain regarding the usefulness and effectiveness of CAM that are not easily addressed using these strategies.

In this paper we argue that although RCTs have an important place in the assessment of the efficacy of CAM, the addition of qualitative research methods to RCTs can greatly enhance the understanding of CAM. Such additions have the potential to improve CAM interventions, and, thus, health care delivery.

Edited from an article in *Journal of Alternative and Complementary Medicine* 2002;8(3):275–81.

LIMITATIONS OF RCTS

An RCT is a study design in which individuals are randomly allocated to at least two groups, usually called the 'study' and the 'control' group. One group is subject to a standardized experimental intervention, while the other group receives placebo or standard treatment. The results are assessed by rigorous comparison of the outcome(s) in the study and control groups respectively. In order to limit bias, group allocation may be concealed to participants (i.e., blinding). RCTs are generally considered as the most scientifically rigorous method of assessing the efficacy of an intervention and, thus, represent the 'gold standard.'

Challenges to RCTs of CAM interventions are various and include the following. First, CAM interventions are often complex and use multiple modalities (e.g., naturopathy and Traditional Chinese Medicine). Second, CAM treatments are frequently not standardized, but individualized and flexible, adjusting treatment as needed for the individual patient. In addition, there are wide variations in practice. Third, CAM interventions often apply to nonspecific, multifactorial conditions (e.g., stress, lack of energy) or patients with complex, chronic conditions (Walach et al, 2002). Thus, defining clinical problems (and treatment) may be very difficult. In addition, the focus is often on restoring balance rather than treating specific symptoms. Fourth, recruitment and randomization can be problematic because of participants' beliefs, practices, and preferences. Fifth, identification of appropriate placebo treatment (e.g., acupuncture, massage therapy) is often difficult or impossible, which results in difficulty blinding patients and practitioners. Finally, RCTs generally try to minimize or exclude the impact of the patient–provider relationship (nonspecific effects) on the outcomes, while in CAM the therapeutic effect of the patient–provider relationship is considered a crucial part of the intervention. It is important to understand that many of these challenges are not unique to CAM and apply equally to several conventional interventions, such as physiotherapy, psychotherapy, surgery, and nursing care.

A challenge of a different nature is related to limitations to the type of information that can be generated from RCTs. Mostly knowledge generated from RCTs is general and in aggregate form and answers questions about frequencies and strength of association. Qualitative research, however, is designed to generate specific information regarding the why and how of individual experiences and, therefore, should be considered as an addition to RCTs.

QUALITATIVE RESEARCH AND ITS PURPOSES

Qualitative research consists of the investigation of phenomena in their natural context, in an in-depth holistic fashion through the collection of rich narrative data. As such it does not seek quantified answers. Its goal is the development of concepts, which helps us to understand social phenomena in natural (rather than experimental) settings, giving due emphasis to the meanings, experiences, and views of all the participants (Pope and Mays, 1995). Research purposes for which qualitative studies are especially suited include the following (Green and Britten, 1998; Maxwell, 1996). The first purpose is gaining an understanding of an intervention by identifying the meaning of the intervention for participants in the study, of the events, situations, and actions in which they are involved. The second purpose involves understanding the particular (natural) context within which the participants act, and the influence that this context has on their actions. An important part of this is identifying the role of patient–provider interaction in the intervention. The third purpose is understanding the process by which events and actions take place, and the fourth, assessing how perspectives of reality of different stakeholders (patients, practitioners, and researchers) on interventions differ. In the process of conducting qualitative research it is common that unanticipated phenomena and influences emerge that have the potential to formulate new research questions and to improve health care practice.

As in quantitative research, there are multiple strategies to ensure rigor in qualitative research (Mays and Pope, 1995). Although these strategies are different, there is no reason to assume that qualitative research in itself is not rigorous.

RELEVANCE OF ADDING QUALITATIVE METHODS TO RCTS

Understanding the meaning of the intervention

RCTs can establish whether an intervention works by means of a strong, highly controlled design in which two or more groups are randomized to rule out confounding variables. However, just as there are intervention studies that generate statistically significant results that have no clinical significance or substantive or real-life importance either to patients or to their caregivers, it is also possible to find nonstatistically significant results that have important implications for individual patients. If an RCT shows no treatment effect, it cannot tell us whether the intervention worked in ways other than expected or whether some specific individuals benefited from the intervention. Although less dramatic, this may also apply to RCTs that do show a treatment effect.

Although such issues have been addressed in disciplines such as nursing and education, medicine is slower to follow, and information has appeared in abstracts and/or is as yet unpublished. Becker et al (2001) conducted a controlled intervention study aimed at evaluating the effects of *qigong* lessons on performance, social behavior, and health in school children. While improvements were found with respect to several outcomes, no significant differences were found between the two groups in quality of life using a validated quality-of-life scale. However, data collected in qualitative interviews with teachers illustrated a calming and relaxing effect of *qigong*, as well as a decrease in complaints for some children. These elements were not part of the quality of life scale. Pope found several significant outcomes following an RCT of a mind–body intervention for patients with a chronic disease, however no improvement was found in the amount of personal stress (cited in Verhoef et al, 2001). In qualitative interviews, participants described a personal growth process, which they felt was moving them toward improved well-being. They spoke about gaining self-awareness, which they viewed as a positive outcome, even though their reaction to this awareness was not always positive. How an intervention works has also been addressed by Alraek and Baerheim (2001) who qualitatively assessed participants' subjective experiences in a trial of acupuncture in the prevention of recurrent cystitis. This trial has not yet been published. The qualitative study was based on the investigators' experiences in their practice that patients often described changes in their health in addition to curing the problem they came for, which seemed to reflect going from disharmony to harmony. The results demonstrated experiences related to changes in urinary habits, more energy, reduced stress level, better sleep, better digestion, and reduced pain from headaches, back pain and joint pain.

These examples show that an intervention may result in meaningful and desirable changes to patients that may not be apparent as improvement on instrumental measures designed with a specific conceptualization of normal, average, or optimal functioning. In order to assess such changes, research needs to address the individual experiences of people receiving the intervention. Qualitative research as opposed to quantitative research is case-oriented rather than variable-oriented and is more suitable to detecting subtleties in the intervention process that account for the research findings (Sandelowski, 1996).

Outcomes of an intervention

The above examples illustrate that available outcome measurements do not always address all potential benefits of CAM interventions. Cohen and Mount (1992) found that the tendency of most instruments to weigh their questions toward the physical while ignoring issues related to meaning, purpose, and spirituality renders them invalid in the palliative care setting. We would argue that this also applies to many CAM interventions that frequently are holistic in nature and are based on a strong belief in the mind–body connection. In addition, the previous examples identified that we do not always know what potential benefits of interventions are. Levin et al (1997) describe that according to the literature on Bach Flower remedies, treatment with the water violet formula is said to restore serenity. Most likely, available outcome measurements will not assess this quality, and thus, may conclude that this remedy has no effect. In such cases it is useful to conduct qualitative research before the start of the trial, to assess what relevant outcomes are, in order to develop appropriate measures.

To increase sensitivity, outcome measures need to be valid, reliable, specific, amenable to change (long- or short-term) and have a range of scores that allow detection of change (Stewart and Archbold, 1992, 1993).

Context

For the purposes of research and analysis, interventions in RCTs are studied in isolation, whereas in clinical practice any intervention is but a part of a treatment approach. van Weel (2001) indicated that 'nonspecific effects work through their integration into the overall treatment approach, which is an essential way into which context effects differ from specific effects.' The value of context effects is in their enhancement of specific interventions, so that efficacy is maximized. RCTs are not the ideal design for assessing context effects. Therefore, exploring the unique physical and psychosocial context in which an intervention takes place is an important added value of qualitative research.

One of the most frequently discussed nonspecific effects is the patient–physician relationship, which is often seen as an integral part of treatment by complementary practitioners. Di Blasi et al (2001) have conducted a systematic review to examine whether there was any empirical evidence to support the therapeutic effects of the doctor–patient relationship. Their results showed much inconsistency regarding these effects and the only relatively consistent finding was that physicians who adopt a warm, friendly, and reassuring manner are more effective than those who keep consultations formal and do not offer reassurance. Systematically and rigorously conducted qualitative research might lead to deeper insight and, thus, allow building theoretical models that can be tested in quantitative research. Similarly, Jobst (2001) comments that 'while it may be well said that good bedside manners work, the question nevertheless remains: "How?" '

Process

How interventions fit within the process of participants' lives is important for future applications of the intervention. Research has shown that people often experiment with different types of complementary treatments and use 'trial and error' in making their disease management decisions. (Verhoef et al, 1998). This practice results in frequent changes in treatment. How patients integrate symptoms and management of symptoms with the practicalities of their lives is an important area of exploration.

The process of the intervention itself is important as well. Qualitative research could also provide profound insight in what flexibility and adjustment within an intervention involve. Last, implementation of an intervention is often very different from the way it was planned (Rabeneck et al, 1992). In such cases, qualitative methods can be used to assess how the intervention is actually enacted as well as the actors' responses to it (Sandelowski, 1996).

Multiple realities

Yerxa (1991) has contended that the experimental method does not represent the patient's reality because it excludes the patient's subjective experience and natural environment. While researchers, and to a lesser degree practitioners, find scientific evidence crucial, many patients tend to believe that CAM is natural, and thus, safe, and find scientific evidence of less importance than personal evidence. Patients' beliefs are closely related to their expectations and may have a major impact on trial results. Exploring how such expectations are related to the process of the intervention is of great importance.

DISCUSSION

RCTs are important in assessing the efficacy of CAM. Many adjustments to RCTs have been suggested that facilitate their conduct with respect to CAM. However, RCTs address only one, limited, question, namely whether the intervention has – statistically – an effect. They do not address why the intervention works, how participants are experiencing the intervention and/or how they give meaning to these experiences. These are different questions, that require a different design, so it would be wrong to fault RCTs for not being able to address these questions, just as it would be wrong to fault qualitative research for its lack of 'statistical significance.' We argue that both are needed to evaluate fully the usefulness of CAM interventions provided that both are conducted rigorously, meticulously, and with great attention to validity and interpretation of the data. When such methods are combined, the potential for increased validity of the results is enhanced by numerical as well as conceptual generalizability.

Qualitative methods may be used before starting an RCT, to assist in the development of appropriate outcome measures or they may be embedded in the trial to assist in understanding the measuring context and process of the intervention. Third, qualitative methods can be used after the trial is completed to explain the trial results.

The discussion of the use of combined methods is directly relevant to the tension between patient-centered care and the use of evidence in clinical practice. As Holman (1993) states, 'the practice of medicine, with its focus on the individual, lives an unrelieved tension between knowledge of the average effects of a disease or treatment upon a group and the individual effects upon a single patient.' Practitioners are interested in improving individual patient outcomes in specific situations, and, therefore, in understanding as much as they can about the application, operation, and outcomes of an intervention in particular cases. Accordingly, emphasizing individual variation as idiosyncrasies in responses to interventions over time may be more clinically relevant than group means per se, from which individuals will often deviate in subtle, but clinically important ways.

We argue that the best way to assess the advantages of combined methods research is to conduct such studies and to demonstrate the potential to contribute to improved health care delivery and ultimately health status.

REFERENCES

Alraek T, Baerheim A. Subjective experiences following acupuncture treatment – Expected or not? [abstract]. *FACT* 2001;6:69–100.

Becker M, Witt C, Bandelin K, Willich SN. Qigong for school children [abstract]. *Altern Ther Health Med* 2001;7:54.

Cohen SR, Mount BM. Quality of life in terminal illness: Defining and measuring subjective well-being in the dying. *J Palliat Care* 1992;8:40–45.

Di Blasi ZD, Harkness E, Ernst E, Georgiou A, Kleijnen J. Influence of context effects on health outcomes: A systematic review. *Lancet* 2001;357:757–762.

Green J, Britten N. Qualitative research and evidence based medicine. *BMJ* 1998;316:1230–1232.

Holman HR. Qualitative inquiry in medical research. *J Clin Epidemiol* 1993;46:29–36.

Jobst KA. Rigor and compassion: The paradoxical challenge of peer review. *J Altern Complement Med* 2001;7:1–3.

Levin JS, Glass TA, Kushi LH, Schuck JR, Steele L, Jonas WB. Quantitative methods in research on complementary and alternative medicine: A methodological manifesto. *Med Care* 1997;35:1079–1094.

Maxwell JA. *Qualitative Research Design: An Interactive Approach*. Thousand Oaks, CA: Sage Publications, 1996.

Mays N, Pope C. Rigour and qualitative research. *BMJ* 1995;311:109–112.

Nahin RL, Straus SE. Research into complementary and alternative medicine: Problems and potential. *BMJ* 2001;322:161–164.

Pope C, Mays N. Reaching the parts other methods cannot reach: An introduction to qualitative methods in health and health services research. *BMJ* 1995;311:42–45.

Rabeneck L, Viscoli CM, Horwitz RI. Problems in the conduct and analysis of randomized clinical trials: Are we getting the right answers to the wrong questions? *Arch Intern Med* 1992;152:507–512.

Sandelowski M. Focus on qualitative methods: Using qualitative methods in intervention studies. *Res Nurs Health* 1996;19:359–364.

Stewart BJ, Archbold PG. Focus on psychometrics: Nursing intervention studies require outcome measures that are sensitive to change: Part One. *Res Nurs Health* 1992;15:477–481.

Stewart BJ, Archbold PG. Focus on psychometrics: Nursing intervention studies require outcome measures that are sensitive to change: Part Two. *Res Nurs Health* 1993;16:77–81.

van Weel C. Examination of context of medicine [letter], *Lancet* 2001;357;733–734.

Verhoef MJ, Pope A, Hilsden RJ. Combining randomized controlled trials and qualitative methods to assess the efficacy of complementary medicine [poster]. Art & Science of Healing II: Integration of Conventional & Complementary Medicine Conference, Vancouver, Canada, November 2001.

Verhoef MJ, Scott CM, Hilsden RJ. A multimethod research study on the use of complementary therapies among patients with inflammatory bowel disease. *Altern Ther Health Med* 1998;4:68–71.

Vickers A, Cassileth B, Ernst E, Fisher P, Goldman P, Jonas W, Kang SK, Lewith G, Schultz K, Silagy C. How should we research unconventional therapies? *Int J Technol Assess Health Care* 1997;13:111–121.

Walach H, Jonas WB, Lewith G. The role of outcomes research in evaluating complementary and alternative medicine. In: Lewith G, Jonas WB, Walach H, eds. *Clinical Research in Complementary Therapies. Principles, Problems and Solutions*. Toronto: Harcourt Publishers Limited, 2002:29–45.

Yerxa EJ. Nationally speaking – Seeking a relevant, ethical, and realistic way of knowing for occupational therapy. *Am J Occup Ther* 1991;45:199–204.

CHAPTER 32

EVIDENCE-BASED COMPLEMENTARY MEDICINE: RIGOUR, RELEVANCE, AND THE SWAMPY LOWLANDS

Janet Richardson

The argument in support of evidence-based medicine is well-rehearsed and the extension of an evidence-based approach to complementary medicine seems to be a logical move that should be welcomed. Edward Mills and his colleagues have put together a comprehensive guide that should be of interest to researchers, educators, and practitioners (Mills et al, 2002). Access to published and unpublished research is fundamental for the development of evidence-based complementary medicine as is the ability to interpret the evidence in a way that is appropriate and relevant to clinical practice. This requires a community of 'research aware' practitioners who are skilled in critical appraisal techniques and who are able to assess the different forms of evidence the research might present.

Finding evidence for the effectiveness of complementary medicine, however, is problematic. There are two reasons for this. First, the evidence base is limited because insufficient research studies of high quality have been carried out. Second, finding the available evidence is not a straightforward process.

A number of important electronic databases exist that specialize in, or include, citations of research in complementary medicine (Richardson et al, 2001). However, searches using these databases will require different

Edited from an article in *Journal of Alternative and Complementary Medicine* 2002;8(3):221–3.

search strategies and are likely to produce different results. This is because the databases cover different journals and the index terms or keywords that are used vary from database to database. For example, reflexology is not a recognized 'index' term on MEDLINE® and articles on reflexology are indexed using the more general term 'massage.' Index terms, known as MeSH terms on MEDLINE, are the terms assigned by an indexer to reflect the overall concepts covered in papers.

Recent developments, such as the construction of a specialist complementary therapy thesaurus for the Research Council for Complementary Medicine (RCCM) Centralised Information Service in Complementary Medicine (CISCOM; see www.rccm.org.uk) database, and plans to develop Web technology for crossdatabase searching (Kronenberg et al, 2001) will go a long way toward addressing these problems. Training in the use of databases and search strategies will be essential if practitioners are going to be able to access and use relevant evidence-based literature to develop their practices.

Mills et al (2002) suggest that an evidence-based medicine (EBM) approach uses the 'best available evidence.' However, in practice, the pressure to adopt the 'gold standard' (high-level evidence) of randomized controlled trials (RCTs) and systematic reviews is overwhelming. The Cochrane Collaboration criteria for systematic reviews are very specific and tend to eliminate studies that do not adopt an RCT approach. This is understandable, being that, arguably, studies other than RCTs are limited when it comes to establishing cause and effect and treatment *effectiveness*. Although high-level evidence may be ruled out by clinicians because it is not relevant to their patients (Mills et al, 2002), in reality, the decision may be taken out of the clinicians' hands because decisions about health care are often made at the level of policymakers and commissioners. In the United Kingdom, the National Institute of Clinical Excellence (NICE) has been established to consider the research evidence for the effectiveness of particular treatments for specific conditions and to produce guidelines that are ultimately translated into commission decisions. It is naive to assume that bodies, such as NICE, and health care commissioners will base their decisions on evidence other than RCTs when making decisions about which kinds of health care to recommend or fund, particularly when resources are limited.

I fully support the development of evidence-based practice in health care and see how EBM may have direct benefits on patient care. However, my years of experience in clinical practice have demonstrated to me that delivering health care cannot always be subdivided into evidence-based components.

I have two concerns about evidence-based complementary medicine. The first is the possible tension between 'rigor and relevance' (Schon, 1983). In order to achieve rigour in complementary medicine research, 'holistic' approaches may be divided into separate components to examine their effectiveness. This may result in interesting research and could lead to new knowledge about, for example, the role of 'placebo' effects and specific aspects of therapeutic interventions. However, this approach may not be relevant to what actually happens in clinical practice, a fact that also applies to much of conventional health care. Although RCTs have a place in complementary medicine evaluation, the limitation of this approach has been the subject of many debates (Richardson, 2000a; Verhoef et al, 2002), and attempts have been made to develop pragmatic research designs that capitalize on 'packages' of care (Richardson, 2001). Adopting an evidence-based approach to complementary medicine will clearly require a balance between rigour and relevance.

My second concern relates to the nature of knowledge and the values a society invests in different ways of knowing. The 'evidence-based high ground' is rooted in a positivist epistemology in which practitioners can make use of research-based theory and technique (Schon, 1983). However, there is 'a swampy lowland where situations are confusing "messes" incapable of technical solutions' (Schon, 1983; see page 42). Much of what takes place within the therapeutic relationship lies within these swampy lowlands, and much of complementary (and conventional) medicine cannot be reduced to narrow, technical practice. Verhoef and colleagues (Verhoef, 2002) are prepared to immerse themselves in the swampy lowlands via the use of rigourous qualitative research techniques that facilitate an exploration of different dimensions of patient experience. Verhoef et al demonstrate how a narrow RCT approach that fails to include qualitative measures can miss important data about the impact of treatment on patients. The examples used in Verhoef et al's paper suggest that patients look for meaning in their illnesses and that some approaches, such as complementary medicine, might lead to positive outcomes that are more related to 'personal development' than measures of disease.

The multiple realities that cannot be captured via quantitative research need to be considered in the context of an evidence-based culture. Patients sometimes use illness to reassess their lives and find meaning (Jobst et al, 1999). These patients present their illness experiences as stories, and it is often via the telling of the story that a patient moves to some resolution (Richardson, 2000b). Our Western culture is science-driven and places little value on oral traditions and storytelling. Stories of patient recovery are dismissed as 'anecdotal evidence,' yet we define who we are by way of our own narratives. Mills et al (2002) suggest that complementary medicine practitioners' beliefs about scientific evidence and the philosophical underpinnings of complementary approaches contribute to the reticence of these practitioners to adopt an evidence-based approach. I think that this is a very important point that requires further exploration and deeper understanding. I suspect strongly that it relates to the nature of knowledge and the different ways of knowing inherent to complementary practitioners and the traditions from which the therapies arise.

Complementary practitioners often work with different narratives of health and illness that are difficult to reduce to a positivist epistemology.

Some time ago, Schon (1983) developed the concept of the 'reflective practitioner.' Structured reflection enables practitioners to access, make sense of, and learn from their experiences in practice (Johns, 1994). Many practitioners (conventional and complementary) are locked into a view of themselves as technical experts for which uncertainty is a threat (Schon, 1983). However, the development of a reflective 'mindful' approach to practice and research (Bentz and Shapiro, 1998; Johns, 2000; Schon, 1983) promotes an awareness of different kinds of knowledge as well as an understanding of self in relation to practice and context. Integration of reflective practice and research into complementary medicine will provide an opportunity to consider how the most relevant and appropriate knowledge can support the evidence base for complementary medicine.

So how can we develop evidence-based complementary medicine in the context of multiple realities and diverse narratives? Investment in high-quality primary studies that are relevant to practice and combine both quantitative and qualitative methodologies is essential. This must be supported by access to research information by way of specialist databases. Teaching practitioners how to use the available evidence via developing critical appraisal skills and an awareness of research methods will be an important part of the process. The ability to discriminate between different ways of knowing – and the relevance of different types of knowledge to the patient, the context, and the culture – will enable practitioners to assess and use the available evidence appropriately. Finally, we should not be afraid to admit that the pursuit of the Evidence-Based Holy Grail will only take us so far and that, ultimately, we may only come to a deeper understanding of the patient experience of care by engaging with each patient in the murky depths of the consultation.

REFERENCES

Bentz VM, Shapiro JJ. *Mindful Inquiry in Social Research*. Thousand Oaks, CA: Sage, 1998.

Jobst KA, Shotstack D, Whitehouse PJ. Diseases of meaning, manifestations of health and metaphor. *J Altern Complement Med* 1999;5(6):495–502.

Johns C. *Becoming a Reflective Practitioner*. Oxford, UK: Blackwell Science, 2000.

Johns C. Nuances of reflection. *J Clin Nurs* 1994;3:71–75.

Kronenberg F, Molholt P, Zeng ML, Eskinazi D. A comprehensive information resource on traditional, complementary, and alternative medicine: Toward an international collaboration. *J Altern Complement Med* 2001;7(6):723–729.

Mills EJ, Hollyer T, Guyatt G, Ross CP, Saranchuk R, Wilson K for the Evidence-Based Complementary and Alternative Medicine Working Group. Teaching evidence-based complementary and alternative medicine: 1. A learning structure to clinical decision changes. *J Altern Complement Med* 2002;8(2):207–214.

Richardson J. The use of randomized control trials in complementary therapy: Exploring the methodological issues. *J Adv Nurs* 2000a;32(2):398–406.

Richardson J. Clinical implications of an intersubjective science. In: Velmans M, ed. *Investigating Phenomenal Consciousness: New Methodologies and Maps*. Amsterdam: John Benjamins, 2000b.

Richardson J. Developing and evaluating complementary therapy services: Part 2. Examining the effect of treatment on health status. *J Altern Complement Med* 2001;7(4):315–328.

Richardson J., Jones C., Pilkington K. Complementary therapies: what is the evidence for their use? *Prof Nurs* 2001;17(2):96–99.

Schon D. *The Reflective Practitioner*. Guildford and Kings Lynn, UK: Biddles, 1983.

Verhoief MJ, Casebeer AL, Hilsden RJ. Assessing efficacy of complementary medicine: Adding qualitative research methods to the 'gold standard.' *J Altern Complement Med* 2002;8(3):275–281.

CHAPTER 33

THE EVIDENCE FOR OR AGAINST COMMON COMPLEMENTARY THERAPIES

Edzard Ernst

INTRODUCTION

An adequate definition of complementary/alternative medicine (CAM) is far from easy to provide. Often CAM is described by characteristics that exclude it from mainstream medicine, for example: it is not taught in most medical schools; it is not scientifically proven or plausible; it is not used in routine health care.

Such 'negative' definitions are neither totally correct nor remotely satisfactory. CAM can be positively defined as 'diagnosis, treatment and/or prevention which complements mainstream medicine by contributing to a common whole, by satisfying a demand not met by orthodoxy or by diversifying the conceptual frameworks of medicine' (Ernst et al, 1995). CAM encompasses a large variety of techniques which have little in common except that they are excluded from mainstream medicine, claim to offer help for a range of conditions, and pride themselves on a holistic approach to patient care (Table 33.1). Some relate to therapeutic modalities (e.g. herbalism), some to diagnostic techniques (e.g. iridology), and many include both diagnostic and therapeutic modalities (e.g. acupuncture).

There are considerable national differences in what is regarded as CAM or mainstream medicine. In Germany, for instance, massage therapy and herbalism are largely orthodox whereas in English-speaking countries they

This chapter has been commissioned by the editors for inclusion in this Reader.

are usually regarded as CAM. Acupuncture is CAM in the West, while in China it is a fully accepted therapy.

Since most of CAM is used as an adjunct to conventional treatments 'complementary' is a much more appropriate term than 'alternative'. When used as a true alternative (i.e. substitute for mainstream medicine) CAM almost invariably becomes a hazard to patients.

EPIDEMIOLOGY OF CAM

In the United States the prevalence of CAM increased from 33 to 42 per cent in the general population between 1990 and 1997, involving an annual expenditure exceeding US$20 billion (Eisenberg et al, 1998). In the United Kingdom, the current figures are around 20 per cent and £1.6 billion, respectively (Ernst and White, 2000).

In industrialised countries, typical users of CAM are middle-aged, female, well-educated and tend to belong to the higher socio-economic classes. Indications for CAM range from chronic benign conditions, for which mainstream medicine is usually unable to offer a cure (e.g. back pain), to life-threatening diseases like cancer and AIDS, for which patients tend to try anything that promises a cure. Most patients try CAM in parallel with conventional treatment, yet many do not tell their doctor. A comprehensive medical history should therefore include questions about CAM (Eisenberg, 1997).

Vis à vis the undisputed success of modern medicine, it may seem puzzling that so many patients try CAM. The following motivations may be important: to leave no option untried, to take control over one's own health, to accord one's health with one's (slightly alternative) world views, to be given time, understanding, and empathy by a practitioner, and to avoid the well-publicised adverse effects of conventional treatments.

EVALUATION OF THREE COMMONLY USED CAM METHODS

Because the CAM field is huge, this text must be confined to examples of only three popular modalities. For a more comprehensive overview of the evidence, see elsewhere (Ernst et al, 2001).

Acupuncture

According to the theories of Traditional Chinese Medicine, the life energy ('Qi') flows in particular channels (meridians) and governs the human body. 'Qi' is a balance of opposite characteristics; yin and yang. Illness is understood as an expression of an imbalance between yin and yang. One

Table 33.1 Examples of therapeutic and diagnostic methods used in CAM

Name	*Principle*	*Main indications*	*Efficacy*	*Safety*	*Risk-benefit balance**
Alexander technique	Training process of ideal body posture and movement; developed by FM Alexander	Musculoskeletal problems	Few clinical trials exist, no final verdict possible	No serious adverse effects	Uncertain
Applied kinesiology	Diagnostic technique using muscle strength as an indicator; developed by G Goodheart	Not applicable	Repeatedly shown to be not valid	Can delay reliable diagnoses, danger of false diagnoses	Negative
Aromatherapy	Application of essential oils usually through gentle massage techniques; developed by RM Gattefossé	Relaxation	Systematic review was inconclusive	Allergic reactions to oils	Uncertain
Autogenic training	Form of self-hypnosis for relaxation and stress reduction; developed by J Schultz	Stress management	Some evidence for effectiveness	No serious adverse effects	Positive
Chelation therapy	Intravenous infusion of EDTA used for 'deblocking' arteries from arteriosclerotic lesions	Circulatory disorders	Repeatedly shown in rigorous clinical trials to be ineffective	Serious adverse effects reported	Negative
Chiropractic	Popular manual therapy based on the assumption that most health problems are due to malalignments of the spine and treatable through spinal manipulation; developed by DD Palmer	Back pain	Conclusions of systematic reviews of chiropractic for back pain are not uniform. The methodologically best are not positive	Serious adverse effects have been reported, their exact incidence is not known	Negative
Colonic irrigation (or colon therapy)	Cleansing of the colon through water enemas, e.g. to 'free the system of toxins'	Various	No sound evidence for effectiveness	Serious adverse effects reported	Negative

Hypnotherapy	Induction of trance-like state to influence the unconscious mind	Various	Some evidence for effectiveness	Adverse effects probably infrequent	Positive
Iridology	Diagnostic technique using signs and impurities on the iris	Not applicable	Shown to be not valid	Can delay reliable diagnosis	Negative
Macrobiotic diet	Diet based on the yin/yang principle using whole grains and vegetables	Disease prevention	Positive effects on cardiovascular risk factors	Serious adverse effects reported	Negative
Massage	Various techniques of manual stimulation of cutaneous, subcutaneous, or muscular structures	Musculoskeletal problems	Some evidence for effectiveness in musculcskeletal and psychological problems	Few serious adverse effects	Positive
Osteopathy	Various techniques of spinal mobilisation; developed by T Still	Back pain	Systematic reviews of osteopathy for back pain are inconclusive	Adverse effects less than with chiropractic	Inconclusive
Reflexology	Internal organs correspond to areas on the soles of the feet and can be influenced through massaging these	Relaxation	Systematic review was inconclusive	No serious adverse effects	Inconclusive
Spiritual healing	Umbrella term for techniques of channelling of 'healing energy' through a healer into a patient	Re-establishing a wholesome balance	Clinical studies highly contradictory; the best recent studies are negative	No serious adverse effects	Negative
Yoga	Meditative, postural, and breathing techniques from ancient India	Various	Promising evidence for effectiveness in asthma, cardio-vascular risk factors and other conditions	No serious adverse effects	Positive

*for the most favourable indication

way of re-establishing the proper equilibrium is to insert needles in acupuncture points located along the meridians. Instead of needles one can also use other means of stimulating acupuncture points: pressure (acupressure), laser light (laser acupuncture), electrical currents (electroacupuncture), or heat (moxibustion). Neither the meridians nor the acupuncture points have a morphological basis, and the theory of yin and yang is, from a Western point of view, more a philosophy than a morphological or physiological reality.

How does acupuncture work?

Modern neurophysiological research has created two major theories for the mode of action of acupuncture: activation of brainstem nuclei and the release of neural transmitters and endorphins in the brain and descending inhibitory control systems.

Considerable differences exist between traditional Chinese and Western acupuncture. No conventional diagnoses are sought in traditional acupuncture, treatment is highly individualised according to each patient's particular yin/yang imbalance, and is often considered as a 'cure all'. The diagnostic techniques include pulse analysis and inspection of the tongue (Kaptchuk, 2000). Western acupuncturists tailor the treatment to the conventional diagnosis established beforehand and normally strive to identify those diagnoses for which acupuncture is helpful.

Evidence of efficacy?

Rigorous trials are possible but fraught with methodological problems, for example: What is an adequate sham procedure? How can the patient be blinded? How can the therapist be blinded? While some of these problems are difficult to solve, randomised clinical trials of acupuncture are clearly feasible, and about 200 such studies are available to date. Their results are often contradictory. Thus the most compelling evidence is generated through systematic reviews of this evidence.

Several systematic reviews and meta-analyses of clinical trials of acupuncture for defined conditions suggest that acupuncture is effective for the following conditions: back pain (Ernst and White, 1998), nausea and vomiting (Vickers, 1996), dental pain (Ernst and Pittler, 1998), migraine (Melchart and White, 2000), osteoarthritis of the knee (Ezzo et al, 2001). For all other conditions, the results of systematic reviews are inconclusive, negative or non-existent.

Evidence of safety?

The most serious complications of acupuncture include trauma (e.g. cardiac tamponade, pneumothorax) and infections (e.g. viral hepatitis).

These adverse events are extreme rarities as long as acupuncture is administered by an adequately trained professional. Mild adverse effects such as pain and minor bleeding occur with an incidence of around 7 per cent (White et al, 2001).

Herbal medicine

Medical herbalism is treatment with whole plants, parts of plants, or plant extracts. Treatment with single active constituents such as acetylsalicylic acid, originally from willow bark, is by definition no longer herbal medicine. Since all plants contain a multitude of chemicals, herbal medicine invariably involves treatment with a mixture of potentially active compounds. In many cases there is uncertainty about the active ingredients and their pharmacological actions (De Smet, 2002). Herbalists claim that the whole plant (extract) will yield more beneficial effects than any single isolated ingredient. In some instances this claim for synergy is supported by evidence but in most cases it is not.

All medical cultures have their version of traditional herbalism, e.g. Traditional Chinese Medicine, or its Japanese version Kampo. The Indian tradition has generated Ayurvedic medicine, which also relies heavily on plant-based remedies. Likewise, European herbalism has a tradition which is as old as European medicine itself. The scientific investigation of medicinal herbs (i.e. phytomedicine) is, however, a relatively recent innovation.

How does herbal medicine work?

Few differences exist in principle between pharmacotherapy and herbal therapy except that herbal remedies are multicomponent systems which render them pharmacologically more complex. The rules of pharmacokinetics and pharmacodynamics also apply to herbal medicine. For every plant-based medicine discernible modes of action can be identified. In some cases these have been elucidated; in many other cases they are still hypothetical (De Smet, 2002).

Evidence of efficacy?

Systematic reviews and meta-analyses of controlled clinical trials have found good if not compelling evidence for the efficacy of the following herbal remedies (Ernst et al, 2001; Ernst, 2001):

- garlic for hypercholesterolaemia
- ginger for nausea and vomiting
- *Ginkgo biloba* for intermittent claudication
- *Ginkgo biloba* to delay the clinical deterioration in dementias

Table 33.2 Possible interactions between some popular herbal remedies and synthetic drugs

*Herbal remedy**	*Usage or pharmacological effect***	*Possible interaction*
Aloe vera (*Aloe barbadensis*)	Various	With chronic use potentiation of cardiac glycosides or antiarrhythmic drugs due to loss of potassium
Arnica (*Arnica montana*)	Wound healing	Decreased effects of antihypertensives and anticoagulants
Black cohosh (*Cimicifuga racemosa*)	Oestrogenic	Increased effects of antihypertensives
Borage (*Borago officinalis*)	Anti-inflammatory	Interaction with anti-eplileptics, may increase risk of seizure
Broom (*Cytisus scoparius*)	Anti-arrhythmic, diuretic	Increased effects of antidepressants, β-blockers, and cardiac glycosides
Cascara (*Rhamnus purshiana*)	Laxative, cathartic	Loss of potassium with chronic use; potentiation of cardiac glycosides or antiarrhythmic drugs
Camomile (*M. chamomilla*)	Spasmolytic, anti-inflammatory	May potentiate effects of anticoagulants through its coumarin content
Cranberry (*Vaccinium macrocarpon*)	Urinary tract infections	May enhance elimination of drugs normally excreted in urine
Ephedra (*Ephedra sinica*)	CNS stimulant, sympathomimetic	Cardiac glycosides/halothane: arrhythmias; guanethidine: enhanced sympathomimetic effect; secale alkaloids/oxytocin: hypertension
Garlic (*Allium sativum*)	Hypocholesterolaemic	Increased effects of anticoagulants and antiplatelet drugs
Ginger (*Zingiber officinalis*)	Anti-emetic	Increased effects of anticoagulants
Ginkgo (*Ginkgo biloba*)	Circulatory diseases	Increased effects of anticoagulants
Ginseng (*Panax quinquefolium*)	Various	Interaction with MAO inhibitors; interaction with stimulants and phenelzine; increased effect of hypoglycaemics
Hawthorne (*Crataegus*)	Digitalis-like	Can increase hypotensive effects of nitrates, antihypotensives, cardiac glycosides, and CNS depressants
Hops (*Humulus lupulus*)	Hypnotic	Antagonism with antidepressants; can increase effects of CNS depressants and hypnotics; interference with hormonal drugs

Horse chestnut (*Aesculus hippocastanum*)	Anti-inflammatory	Increased effects of anticoagulants
Kava (*Piper methysticum*)	Anxiolytic	Potentiation with other anxiolytics; can increase Parkinson symptoms with levodopa
Kelp (*Laminaria digitata*)	Antitumour effects, antiobesity	Increased effects of anticoagulants and antihypertensives
Lavender (*Lavandula officinalis*)	Sedative	Increased effects of CNS depressants
Liquorice (*Glycyrrhiza glabra*)	Corticosteroid activity for gastric irritation	Potassium loss, e.g. with thiazide diuretics; water and sodium retention with corticosteroids; increased effects of digoxin; decreased effects of antihypertensives
Lily of the valley (*Convallaria majalis*)	Congestive heart failure	Increased (side-)effects of quinodine, calcium, saluretics, laxatives, glucosteroids, β-blockers, calcium channel blockers, and digitalis
Mistletoe (*Viscum album*)	Anticancer drug	Increased effects of CNS depressants, antihypertensives, and cardiac drugs
Nettle (*Urtica dioica*)	Diuretic	May potentiate effects of other diuretics
Pumpkin seed (*Curcubita*)	Anthelmintic, diuretic	Can increase effect of diuretics
Sage (*Salvia officinalis*)	Antispasmodic	Interaction with antiepileptics, may increase risk of seizure; decreased effect with antiglycaemics
St John's wort (*Hypericum perforatum*)	Antidepressant	Increased effects of digoxin MAO inhibitors or serotonin-uptake inhibitors; decreased effect of anticonvulsants, antidiabetic drugs and oral contraceptives; increased photosensitivity with other such drugs
Valerian (*Valeriana officinalis*)	Hypnotic	Increased effects of CNS depressants and hypnotics
Vitex (*Agnus castus*)	Hormonal effects	Increased effects of other hormonal drugs
Yew (*Taxus brevifolia*)	Antirheumatic, anticancer	Chemotherapeutic agents may potentiate its effects

* Latin name in brackets
** Not comprehensive
CNS central nervous system
MAO monamine oxidase

- hawthorn for congestive heart failure
- horse chestnut seed extract for primary venous insufficiency
- kava as an anxiolytic drug
- peppermint oil for irritable bowel syndrome
- saw palmetto for benign prostatic hyperplasia
- St John's wort for mild to moderate depression.

For many other popular medicinal herbs, efficacy has not yet been demonstrated through systematic reviews of clinical trials; too few clinical trials have been carried out, or the studies are methodologically flawed, or their results are contradictory. The efficacy of popular herbal remedies such as valerian, aloe vera and ginseng is thus undetermined (Ernst, 2001).

Evidence of safety?

Many medicinal herbs have been associated with serious adverse effects. For example, it has been shown that aconite and broom are cardiotoxic, aristolochia and chaparral are nephrotoxic, and comfrey, kava, pennyroyal and skullcap are all hepatotoxic (Ernst, 2000). Numerous other herbal remedies are associated with only mild adverse effects.

Some herbal remedies can also interact with other drugs (Table 33.2). In many countries (e.g. the United Kingdom and the United States) herbal medicines are marketed as food supplements with no stringent quality control. Therefore their quality can be less than optimal, and this can easily lead to safety problems (De Smet, 2002). Asian herbal medicines, for instance, have been repeatedly shown to be adulterated with synthetic drugs or contaminated with heavy metals (Ernst, 2002a).

Homoeopathy

Two hundred years ago, Samuel Hahnemann, a German Physician, developed the two major principles which form the basis of homoeopathy. The 'like cures like' principle postulates that, if a given drug induces symptoms (e.g. a headache) in healthy individuals, this very drug can be employed in patients who suffer from headaches. The second principle holds that 'potentising' (i.e. shaking and stepwise diluting) drugs makes them not less but more potent for the treatment of illness. Homoeopathic dilutions prepared thus are believed to be clinically more effective than placebo even if not a single molecule of the original medicine is contained in the potentised remedy (Kaptchuk, 2000). Scientists have always pointed out that these principles of homoeopathy fly in the face of science. Therefore, they argue, homoeopathy cannot possibly work beyond a placebo effect. Yet homoeopaths insist that homoeopathic remedies work via 'energy' transfer from the original substance to the diluent (the theory of a 'memory of water').

Homoeopaths do not treat diseases but claim to treat the whole individual. A homoeopath would take a detailed history at each patient's first visit. The aim is to match the totality of the symptoms and characteristics of that patient with a 'drug picture' according to the 'like cures like' principle (Kaptchuk, 2000). Many but by no means all homoeopathic remedies are based on botanical substances; in principle any material can be used, e.g. salts, animals, bodily fluids, synthetic drugs.

How does homoeopathy work?

Several hypotheses have been developed to explain the transfer of 'energy' from the original substance ('mother tincture') to the diluent (Kaptchuk, 2000). None have so far withstood the scrutiny of independent assessment. Neither has the 'energy' ever been defined in physical terms, nor are there rational explanations as to how this 'energy' (if it exists) might induce a healing process in a diseased body or organ. Therefore, homoeopathy remains among the least plausible forms of CAM.

Evidence of efficacy?

A meta-analysis of all 89 randomised or placebo-controlled clinical trials published by 1995 calculated an overall odds ratio of 2.45 in favour of homoeopathy (Linde et al, 1997). When only the 26 most rigorous studies were meta-analysed the odds ratio fell to 1.66 but remained statistically significant. This publication was celebrated by homoeopaths as the ultimate proof of efficacy. However, others criticised it for pooling data for all medical conditions and all homoeopathic remedies, for including trials that were not randomised and therefore biased, and for including studies of material (low dilution) remedies where efficacy is not disputed.

The results of further systematic reviews including a re-analysis of the original data by the original authors of the above-named article are summarised in Table 33.3 (Ernst, 2002b). Collectively these data seem to indicate that the clinical evidence for homoeopathy is not convincing.

Evidence of safety?

Highly diluted homoeopathic remedies must be safe in a toxicological sense. 'Homoeopathic aggravations' are claimed by homoeopaths to happen in about 20 per cent of all cases and are interpreted as a sign of having administered the optimal remedy. There is, however, no good evidence for the existence of this phenomenon (Grabia and Ernst, 2003). One 'indirect' safety problem deserves to be mentioned: homoeopaths who are not medically qualified sometimes tend to advise their clients against immunisation (Schmidt and Ernst, 2002). If this happens on a large scale, we are in danger of losing herd immunity against important infectious diseases.

Table 33.3 Systematic reviews of homoeopathy published after Linde's meta-analysis (1997)

Reference	*Included trials (number)*	*Total patient number*	*Results of meta-analysis*	*Overall conclusion*
Ernst* (1998)	All studies from Linde et al which received 90 (of 100) points in at least 1 of the 2 quality ratings, using highly dilute remedies, following the principles of 'classical'° homoeopathy (n = 5)	587	OR = 1.0 (no evidence in favour of homoeopathy)	Homoeopathic remedies are associated with the same clinical effects as placebo
Linde* (1998)	All studies from Linde et al which tested 'classical'° homoeopathic remedies against placebo, no treatment or another treatment (n = 32)	1778	19 placebo-controlled trials were submitted to meta-analysis; OR = 1.62; however, when this analysis was restricted to the methodologically best trials the effect was no longer significant	Individualised homoeopathy has an effect over placebo; the evidence, however, is not convincing
Linde* (1999)	All studies from Linde et al which could be submitted to meta-analysis (n = 89)	Ndp	The mean OR of the best studies was not in favour of homoeopathy	There was clear evidence that studies with better methodological quality tended to yield less positive results
Morrison* (2000)	26 trials classified by Linde et al as high quality (n = 26)	Ndp	No meta-analysis performed	No significant trend was seen when correlating security of randomisation and trial result
Ernst* (2000)	All studies from Linde et al which received quality ratings between 1 and 4 on the Jadad score (n = 77)	Ndp	No meta-analysis performed	There is a ...strong linear correlation between OR and Jadad score (r = 0.97, *P*<0.05); homoeopathic remedies are, in fact, placebos
Sterne* (2001)	89 trials of Linde et al review compared with 89 trials of allopathic medicines	Ndp	Strong evidence for publication bias causing a false positive result in favour of homoeopathy	When adjusting high quality trials [of homoeopathy] for publication bias, the OR changed from 0.52 to 1.19 but remained unchanged for allopathy
Barnes (1997)	All placebo controlled trials of homoeopathy for post-operative ileus (n = 6)	776	Weighted mean difference to time until first sign of peristalsis was in favour of homoeopathy (-7.4h)	Homoeopathic treatment can reduce the duration of postoperative ileus, however, several caveats preclude a definitive judgement

Ernst (1998)	All placebo controlled trials of homoeopathy for delayed onset muscle soreness (DOMS) (n = 8)	311	No meta analysis possible, all randomised trials were negative	The evidence does not support the hypothesis that homoeopathic remedies are more efficacious than placebo for DOMS
Ernst (1998)	All placebo-controlled trials of homoeopathic arnica (n = 8)	338	No meta-analysis possible, no clear trend in favour of homoeopathy	The claim that homoeopathic arnica is efficacious beyond a placebo effect is not supported by rigorous clinical trials
Ernst (1999)	All RCTs of homoeopathy for migraine prophylaxis (n = 4)	284	No meta-analysis possible, 3 of 4 trials were negative (including the methodologically best)	The trial data...do not suggest that homoeopathy is effective in the prophylaxis of migraine or headache beyond a placebo effect
Ernst (1999)	All controlled clinical trials of 'classical'° homoeopathy vs conventional treatments (n = 6)	605	No meta-analysis possible	No clear trend in favour of homoeopathy
Lüdtke (1999)	All controlled clinical trials of homoeopathic arnica (n = 37)	Ndp	No meta-analysis possible	No clear trend in favour of homoeopathic arnica was found
Cucherat (2000)	All RCTs of homoeopathy vs placebo with clinical or surrogate endpoints (n = 16)	2617	Combined 2–tailed *P* value was highly significant ($P = 0.000056$) in favour of homoeopathy	There is some evidence that homoeopathic treatments are more effective than placebo
Vickers (2000)	All RCTs of homoeopathic oscillococcinum vs placebo for influenza (n = 7)	3459	RR = 0.64 for influenza prevention RR = 0.28 for influenza prevention	Treatment reduced length of illness significantly by 0.28 days
Linde (2000)	All RCTs of homoeopathy vs placebo for chronic asthma (n = 3)	154	No meta-analysis possible	No clear trend in favour of homoeopathy
Jonas (2000)	All controlled clinical trials of homoeopathy for rheumatic conditions (n = 6)	392	Combined OR = 2.19	Homoeopathic remedies work better than placebo
Long (2001)	All RCTs of homoeopathy for osteoarthritis (n = 4)	406	No meta-analysis possible	No clear trend in favour of homoeopathy

* re-analysis of (part of) the data from Linde et al (1997)
RCT = randomised clinical trial
RR = relative risk
OR = odds ratio
Ndp = no details provided
° = classical homoeopathy = approach where remedies are individualised according to patient characteristics deemed important by homoeopaths

CONCLUSION

CAM is a very heterogeneous array of therapeutic and diagnostic techniques. Many of its modalities are hugely popular with patients. The three examples chosen here show that at least some treatments are effective. The safety issues in CAM are even less well-researched than efficacy. However, by and large, CAM is burdened with less risks than conventional medicines. As our research efforts continue and the evidence becomes more complete, we are likely to identify treatments which demonstrably generate more good than harm.

REFERENCES

De Smet PAGM. Herbal remedies. *New Engl J Med* 2002;347:2046–56.

Eisenberg DM. Advising patients who seek alternative medical therapies. *Ann Intern Med* 1997;127:61–9.

Eisenberg D, David RB, Ettner SL, Appel S, Wilkey S, Van Rompay M et al. Trends in alternative medicine use in the United States; 1990–1997. *JAMA* 1998;280:1569–75.

Ernst E. Risks associated with complementary therapies. In: Dukes MNG, Aronson JK (eds). *Meyler's Side Effects of Drugs*. 14th ed. Amsterdam: Elsevier 2000;1649–81.

Ernst E. Herbal medicinal products: an overview of systematic reviews and meta-analyses. *Perfusion* 2001;14:398–404.

Ernst E. Toxic heavy metals and undeclared drugs in Asian herbal medicines. *Trends Pharmacol Sci* 2002a;23:136–9.

Ernst E. A systematic review of systematic reviews of homeopathy. *Br J Clin Pharmacol* 2002b;54:577–82.

Ernst E, Pittler MH. The effectiveness of acupuncture in treating acute dental pain: a systematic review. *Br Dent J* 1998;184:443–7.

Ernst E, Pittler MH, Stevinson C, White AR. *The desktop guide to complementary and alternative medicine*. Edinburgh: Mosby, 2001.

Ernst E, Resch KL, Mills S, Hill R, Mitchell A, Willoughby M et al. Complementary medicine – a definition. *Br J Gen Pract* 1995;45:506.

Ernst E, White AR. Acupuncture for back pain. A meta-analysis of randomized controlled trials. *Arch Intern Med* 1998;158:2235–41.

Ernst E, White AR. The BBC survey of complementary medicine use in the UK. *Complement Ther Med* 2000;8:32–6.

Ezzo J, Hadhazy V, Birch S, Lao L, Kaplan G, Hochberg M et al. Acupuncture for osteoarthritis of the knee. *Arth & Rheum* 2001;44:849–55.

Grabia S, Ernst E. Homoeopathic aggravations: a systematic review of randomised, placebo-controlled clinical trials. *Homeopathy* 2003;92:92–8.

Kaptchuk TJ. *The web that has no weaver. Understanding Chinese medicine.* Chicago: NTC/Contemporary Publishing Group, Inc. 2000.

Linde K, Clausius N, Ramirez G, Melchart D, Eitel F, Hedges LV et al. Are the clinical effects of homoeopathy placebo effects? A meta-analysis of placebo-controlled trials. *Lancet* 1997;350:834–43.

Melchart D, White AR. Acupuncture for migraines. *The Cochrane Review* 2000.

Schmidt K, Ernst E. Aspects of MMR. *BMJ* 2002;325:597.

Vickers AJ. Can acupuncture have specific effects on health? A systematic review of acupuncture anti-emesis trials. *J Roy Soc Med* 1996;89:303–11.

White A, Hayhoe S, Hart A, Ernst E. Adverse events following acupuncture: prospective survey of 32000 consultations with doctors and physiotherapists. *BMJ* 2001;323:485–6.

CHAPTER 34

QUALITY, EFFICACY AND SAFETY OF COMPLEMENTARY MEDICINES: FASHIONS, FACTS AND THE FUTURE. EFFICACY AND SAFETY

Joanne Barnes

INTRODUCTION

There is a view that the criteria for efficacy and safety of complementary medicines should be the same as those for conventional drugs. Many complementary medicines, particularly herbal medicines, have a long history of traditional use. However, most are of unproven efficacy by today's standard, i.e. well-designed randomized controlled trials, and a history of traditional use does not comprise an adequate assessment of safety. The lack of evidence does not necessarily mean that complementary medicines lack efficacy or are unsafe, but that rigorous clinical investigation has not yet been undertaken and that extensive surveillance of the use of complementary medicines has not yet been carried out.

EFFICACY

Some products, such as certain, standardized herbal extracts, have undergone extensive clinical investigation, and clinical trials involving these

Edited from an article in *British Journal of Clinical Pharmacology* 2003;55:331–40.

herbal medicines have been subject to systematic review/meta-analysis, including Cochrane reviews. However, because the composition of products varies between manufacturers (Schulz et al, 2000), evidence of efficacy (and safety) should be considered to be extract specific. At most, evidence should be extrapolated only to preparations of the same herb with a very similar profile of constituents. For example, most clinical trials of ginkgo (*Ginkgo biloba*) have tested the standardized ginkgo leaf extracts EGb-761 and LI-1370 (Barnes et al, 2002; Schulz et al, 2000); it should not be assumed that the results of these studies apply to other ginkgo leaf extracts, which may have a different profile of constituents, or to other preparations of ginkgo leaf, such as tinctures and teas. However, many systematic reviews and meta-analyses of clinical trials of herbal medicines ignore important details of the products tested, such as the type of extract and the formulation.

It is questionable though whether products containing well-tested herbal extracts have been assessed to the extent required for a UK product licence (marketing authorization). With conventional drugs, a median (range) of 1120 (43–4906) patients has been involved in clinical trials before marketing (Rawlins and Jefferys, 1993). St John's wort has been tested in over 30 controlled trials involving around 3000 patients with depression, approximately half of whom will have received St John's wort. However, these studies tested different extracts of the herb and involved patients with different types of depression. Hence there may be insufficient evidence for the efficacy of one extract in a defined, licensable indication.

In the UK, one of the reasons for the lack of research with complementary medicines is the lack of available funding. Major funding sources for medical research in the UK include the NHS and medical research charities, although these organizations spend only a small proportion of their funds on research involving complementary medicines (Ernst, 1996; Ernst, 1999). Pharmaceutical companies are another major sponsor of medical research, but some manufacturers of complementary medicines lack the resources required to carry out or fund research involving their products. Furthermore, there is little incentive to conduct research because complementary medicines, as natural products, cannot be patented, thus manufacturers do not have a protected period in which they can recoup financial returns on investments in research and development. Also, at present, many complementary medicines can be marketed without undergoing the stringent testing procedures required to obtain a marketing authorization (product licence). Another reason for the lack of research is the lack of a research infrastructure; few research units have the remit to carry out research into complementary medicines, and few complementary medicine practitioners have the research skills necessary to develop, obtain funding, conduct and publish good-quality research (Vickers, 1999).

Herbal medicinal products

There is good evidence from systematic reviews/meta-analyses (including Cochrane reviews) of randomized controlled trials for the efficacy of certain standardized herbal extracts in particular clinical conditions, e.g. standardized St John's wort extracts in relieving symptoms of mild-to-moderate depression (Linde and Mulrow, 2003), saw palmetto extracts in treating symptoms of benign prostatic hyperplasia (BPH) (Wilt et al, 2003a) and standardized ginkgo leaf extracts in symptomatic relief of cognitive deficiency and dementia (Ernst and Pittler, 1999). A summary of these and several other systematic reviews (Pittler and Ernst, 2000; Pittler and Ernst, 2003; Stevinson et al, 2000; Wilt et al, 2003a) is provided in Table 34.1.

In some cases, further clinical trials have been carried out since these systematic reviews were published. For example, recent studies have generally confirmed that standardized St John's wort extracts are more effective than placebo in mild-to-moderate depression, and have provided some evidence that such extracts may be as effective as certain conventional antidepressant drugs, including imipramine, fluoxetine and sertraline, in relieving the symptoms of mild-to-moderate depression (Barnes et al, 2001). Some of these studies have been criticised for using doses of comparator conventional antidepressant drugs at the lower end of the therapeutic range. A randomized, double-blind, controlled trial, funded by the US National Institutes of Mental Health and the US National Center for Complementary and Alternative Medicine, reported recently that the St John's wort extract LI-160 was no more effective than placebo in patients with major depressive disorder according to DSM-IV criteria. However, the active control sertraline also failed to demonstrate a statistically significant effect over placebo for the two primary outcome measures (mean change in the Hamilton depression scale score and the incidence of full response at week 8) (Hypericum Depression Trial Study Group, 2002). Thus, the results of this study appear to be inconclusive. Furthermore, it is important to emphasize that St John's wort extracts are not recommended for use in patients with major depression.

For several other standardized herbal medicinal products, there is evidence of efficacy from at least one well-designed, randomized, placebo-controlled trial. For example, a randomized, double-blind trial involving 170 women with premenstrual syndrome (PMS) who received a casticin-standardized *Vitex agnus-castus* (chasteberry) fruit extract (ZE-440), or placebo, for three menstrual cycles found that at the end of the study, improvements in self-assessed PMS symptoms and clinical global impression scores for severity of condition, global improvement and overall benefit/risk were significantly greater in the agnus castus group ($P < 0.001$) (Schellenberg, 2001). In another randomized, double-blind trial, 143 patients with hyperlipoproteinaemia and baseline total cholesterol concentrations of >7.3 mmol l^{-1} received a standardized globe artichoke leaf

Table 34.1 Summary of selected systematic reviews of clinical trials involving herbal medicines.

First author (year of publication)	*Herbal product*	*Details of systematic review*	*Summary of results/ conclusion* *
Linde (2003; 1998 most recent substantive amendment)	Oral formulations of St John's wort (*Hypericum perforatum*) extracts†	27 RCTs involving 2291 patients with depression	St John's wort extracts significantly more effective than placebo for short-term treatment of mild to moderately severe depressive disorders
Wilt (2003a; 2002 most recent substantive amendment)	Oral formulations of saw palmetto (*Serenoa repens, S. serrulata, Sabal serrulata*) fruit extracts†	21 RCTs involving 3139 men with BPH	Saw palmetto extracts significantly more effective than placebo and similar to to finasteride in improving urinary symptom scores
Ernst (1999)	Oral formulations of standardized ginkgo (*Ginkgo biloba*) leaf extract*	Nine RCTs involving 891 patients with Alzheimer's and/or multiinfarct dementia	Ginkgo extracts were more effective than placebo in the symptomatic treatment of dementia, but further research required due to methodological limitations of several included studies
Pittler (2000)	Oral formulations of standardized ginkgo (*Ginkgo biloba*) leaf extract*	Eight RCTs involving 415 patients with intermittent claudication	Ginkgo extracts, compared with placebo, significantly improved pain-free walking distance, but effect size small and clinical relevance questionable
Stevinson (2000)	Oral formulations of garlic (*Allium sativum*) (oil/powder)	13 RCTs involving 796 patients with various disorders including CHD, hyperlipoproteinaemia, hypercholesterolaemia, hypertension	Garlic preparations significantly reduced total serum cholesterol concencrations compared with placebo, but effect size small and some studies had methodological limitations
Pittler (2003; 2001 most recent substantive amendment)	Oral formulations of horse chestnut (*Aesculus hippocastanum*) seed extract	14 RCTs involving 1146 patients with CVI	Horse chestnut seed extract significantly more effective than placebo in relieving symptoms of CVI, but additional studies required
Wilt (2003b; 1997 most recent substantive amendment)	Oral formulations of *Pygeum africanum* (African prune tree) extracts†	18 RCTs involving 1562 men with BPH	*Pygeum africanum* extracts significantly more effective than placebo in improving urological symptoms and flow measures, but additional placebo-controlled studies required

BPH, Benign prostatic hyperplasia; CHD, coronary heart disease; CVI, chronic venous insufficiency; RCTs, randomized clinical trials (controls were placebo or active treatments). *See full papers for quantitative results. †Studies of both mono- and combination herbal preparations were included.

extract (CY-450) 900 mg twice daily, or placebo, for 6 weeks (Englisch et al, 2000). At the end of the study, mean total cholesterol concentrations had decreased by 18.5% to 6.31 mmol l^{-1} and by 8.6% to 7.03 mmol l^{-1} in the globe artichoke and placebo groups, respectively ($P<0.0001$). However, further rigorous randomized controlled trials are required to confirm these effects, and to test the efficacy of numerous other herbal medicines for which there is little or no clinical evidence.

Although rigorous clinical investigations are lacking at present for many herbs, there is a vast literature on the phytochemistry, and *in vitro* and *in vivo* pharmacological effects of medicinal plants (Barnes et al, 2002; Bisset, 1994; Evans, 2002; Mills and Bone, 2000; Schulz et al, 2000; Wren, 1988). This information affords a rationale for further investigation of such plants and provides supporting data where clinical evidence exists.

SAFETY

The risks of a medical intervention for a particular patient, as well as its benefits, should be considered before use. However, benefit–risk assessments for complementary medicines are difficult as information is lacking in several areas relevant to safety. This section will focus on herbal medicines, as these are among the most widely used 'complementary medicines' in the UK and, from a biomedical perspective, are likely to have the greatest potential in terms of risk.

In the case of herbal medicines, generally, data are lacking on:

- active constituents; metabolites
- pharmacokinetics
- pharmacology
- toxicology
- adverse effects and their frequencies; effects of long-term use
- drug–herb interactions; interactions with food, alcohol
- use in specific patient groups: children, elderly, individuals with renal or hepatic disease, gender effects, individuals with a different genetic profile
- contraindications and warnings; use in pregnancy and lactation.

This lack of information also makes it difficult to compare the benefit–risk profile of certain herbal medicines with that of conventional drugs, where similar effectiveness has been shown. On the basis of clinical trial data, some herbal medicines have been shown to have a more favourable safety profile than conventional drugs of similar effectiveness. For example, in randomized controlled trials involving patients with depression, the frequency of adverse effects with extracts of St John's wort is significantly lower than that for conventional antidepressants (Linde and Mulrow, 2003). Findings in a similar direction have been reported for extracts of saw palmetto, compared with finasteride, in randomized controlled trials in men with BPH (Wilt et al, 2003). However, it cannot be assumed that this will apply to all comparisons of herbal medicines and conventional drugs: benefit–risk comparisons must be made for each case. Nor should it be assumed that a benefit–risk analysis is applicable to all preparations of a particular herb. As with evidence of efficacy, evidence of safety should be considered to be extract specific or, at most, extended only to preparations of the same herb with a very similar profile of constituents.

Generally though, little is known regarding adverse effects of herbal medicines and their frequencies. There is a common misconception that because herbs are natural, they are entirely 'safe'. Clearly, this is not the case (many plants are inherently poisonous), and plants used medicinally do, in some cases, cause adverse effects. Such effects are not limited to type A adverse drug reactions (ADRs), i.e. those that are common, dose-related, and pharmacologically predictable, nor are they always minor in nature. ADRs associated with herbal medicines include type B reactions (those that are uncommon, unpredictable, unrelated to dose and usually serious), as well as those that occur with chronic use, and delayed effects occurring remote from drug use in the user or offspring (e.g. carcino- and terato-genic reactions) (De Smet, 1995). Some important safety concerns that have arisen with particular herbal medicines are discussed below.

Kava

Kava (also known as kava-kava; *Piper methysticum*) root is used ceremonially in most Pacific Islands as an intoxicating beverage. In developed countries, standardized extracts of kava are used to help relieve anxiety and stress. Medical herbalists also use preparations of kava in their practice.

In 2001, 30 cases of hepatotoxicity associated with the use of kava extracts were reported from Germany and Switzerland, although some of these reports appeared to be duplicates. These cases range from abnormal liver function to liver failure; one case has been fatal, and four or five others have required liver transplants. It is difficult to assess causality in these cases as, with most, the evidence is complicated by other factors, e.g. concomitant drugs which have themselves been associated with liver toxicity. Nevertheless, the majority of the herbal sector in the UK voluntarily withdrew kava products from sale, pending a decision by the Committee on Safety of Medicines (CSM) and Medicines Control Agency (MCA). By July 2002, the MCA had received 68 case reports of hepatotoxicity worldwide, including the UK (Medicines Control Agency, 2002).

The CSM's advice was that the benefit–risk profile of kava appears to be negative and on 13 January 2003 a statutory order came into effect in the UK prohibiting the sale, supply and import of unlicensed medicines containing kava (The Medicines for Human Use (Kava-Kava) (Prohibition) Order, 2002).

Interactions with conventional drugs

Where herbal medicines or dietary supplements are used concomitantly with conventional drugs, there may be a potential for drug–herb or drug–supplement interactions to occur. Also, herb–herb or supplement–supplement interactions may occur where several products are used concurrently. It should come as no surprise that these groups of pharmacologically active substances may interact with conventional drugs.

However, for the most part, knowledge of drug–herb, drug–supplement, herb–herb and other such interactions is lacking. Information is limited mainly to isolated case reports (Stockley, 2002) and to lists of theoretical or potential drug–herb or drug–supplement interactions, predicted on the basis of what is known about the pharmacological effects of supplements and of the chemical constituents of herbal medicines (Barnes et al, 2002). While these lists provide useful guidance, they are no substitute for formal studies. However, research in the area of drug–herb/ supplement interactions is almost entirely lacking.

Most documented information on drug–herb interactions relates to preparations of St John's wort. In 1999, evidence emerged of pharmacokinetic interactions between St John's wort products and certain conventional drugs (warfarin, digoxin, theophylline, cyclosporin, HIV protease inhibitors, anticonvulsants and oral contraceptives) (Barnes et al, 2001). St John's wort products appear to induce certain cytochrome P450 (CYP) drug-metabolizing enzymes, including CYP3A4, CYP1A2 and CYP2C9 (thus leading to a loss of or reduction in the therapeutic activity of drugs metabolized by these enzymes), and to affect P-glycoprotein (a transport protein). There is also the potential for pharmacodynamic interactions to occur between St John's wort products and, for example, selective serotonin reuptake inhibitors (e.g. fluoxetine) and triptans (e.g. sumatriptan) (Barnes et al, 2001).

Identifying ADRs associated with herbal medicines

At present, the main system for generating signals of potential safety concerns associated with herbal medicines is the MCA's yellow card scheme for ADR reporting. The scheme has always applied to licensed products, including licensed herbal medicines and licensed dietary supplements (e.g. certain vitamin and mineral preparations), and was extended to include reporting on unlicensed herbal products in October 1996 by professions included in the yellow card scheme (Anonymous, 1996). While the MCA does not formally request reports of suspected ADRs associated with other types of unlicensed products, it is unlikely that the MCA would ignore a genuine report of a serious suspected ADR associated with a nonherbal unlicensed product.

The extension of the yellow card scheme to unlicensed herbal products followed the findings of a study of traditional remedies and food supplements carried out by a UK Medical Toxicology Unit. Over a 5-year period, almost 1300 enquiries were received from healthcare professionals regarding suspected ADRs associated with these types of products (Shaw et al, 1997). In 12 cases, the relationship between the product and the ADR was confirmed, in 35 cases it was deemed 'probable' and in 735 cases 'possible'. Several reports of suspected ADRs associated with homoeopathic remedies were also received, although homoeopathic products were not included in the study (Shaw et al, 1997).

In November 1999, the yellow card scheme was further extended to include reporting by all community pharmacists (hospital pharmacists were granted reporter status in April 1997); community pharmacists were asked by the MCA to concentrate on areas of limited reporting by doctors, namely conventional OTC medicines and herbal products (Anonymous, 1997).

There is no mandatory manufacturer reporting of suspected ADRs associated with complementary medicines, except for licensed products. However, the British Herbal Medicine Association (BHMA), whose members include many manufacturers of herbal products, has a voluntary code of practice for members which requires that manufacturers send reports of suspected ADRs associated with unlicensed herbal products to the BHMA which may, at its discretion, forward such reports to the MCA.

In the year 2000, the MCA received almost 140 reports of suspected ADRs associated with herbal products. For the period 1996 (when the yellow card scheme was extended to unlicensed herbal products) to 2000, around 320 such reports were received. Of these 320, over a quarter describe suspected ADRs associated with St John's wort, and many of these relate to reports of interactions between St John's wort and conventional drugs (see Interactions with conventional drugs).

Pharmacovigilance of complementary medicines

Pharmacovigilance for complementary medicines is in its infancy. Generally, there is a lack of clinical trial data for complementary medicines and, in any case, controlled clinical trials have the power only to detect common, acute adverse effects. Post-marketing surveillance studies with certain herbal medicines have been conducted by some manufacturers (usually those based in Germany), but this is the exception. Other tools used in pharmacovigilance of conventional drugs, such as prescription event monitoring (PEM) methodology ('green cards') and the General Practice Research Database (GPRD), now managed by MCA, are of little use, as general practitioners (who provide the data collected by both these tools) may be unaware of their patients' use of complementary medicines and, even if they are, are unlikely to record this.

In addition, there are several factors which make pharmacovigilance for complementary medicines more difficult than for conventional medicines. The yellow card scheme for ADR reporting, the principal tool used in complementary medicines pharmacovigilance at present, has recognized limitations, including the poor quality of some reports, and the difficulty in establishing causality. An important limitation is underreporting and, for several reasons, this is likely to be greater for complementary medicines than for conventional drugs. Because of the belief that complementary medicines are natural and safe, consumers may not associate ADRs with their use (De Smet, 1997). Furthermore, users of herbal medicines may be reluctant to report ADRs associated with these products to their GP or pharmacist (Barnes et al, 1998), and some healthcare professionals may be unaware that the yellow card scheme accepts reports for herbal products (Barnes, 2001).

Another issue relates to the reporting of ADRs which may first be identified outside the formal system. Complementary-medicine practitioners, including medical herbalists, are not formally included in the MCA's yellow-card scheme. The National Institute of Medical Herbalists (NIMH), the major organization for herbal practitioners in the UK, does have its own 'yellow card' scheme, based on the MCA scheme, which sends a summary report annually to the MCA. For the period January 1994 to November 2001, 23 'yellow card' reports were received by the NIMH (Broughton, 2001). Underreporting may be a problem with this scheme, as with other spontaneous reporting schemes. Also, health-food stores are a major outlet for complementary medicines, but it is not known if staff in such outlets receive reports of suspected ADRs associated with such products, or what action they take if they do.

Tools for investigating the safety of complementary medicines need to be developed. To this end, a feasibility study is planned to determine whether modified PEM methodology (involving provision of data by medical herbalists in addition to GPs) can be applied to herbal products as prescribed by medical herbalists (Personal communication, 2002). In the longer term, consideration could be given to the development of a Pharmacy Practice Research Database – similar to GPRD – where community pharmacists monitor patients registered with their practice and enter relevant data on use of prescription and OTC medicines, including complementary medicines (Barnes, 2001).

THE FUTURE FOR COMPLEMENTARY MEDICINES

On the basis of current trends in market research data, it has been predicted that sales of complementary medicines will continue to increase (Mintel International Limited, 2001). Longitudinal data on the utilization of complementary therapists who use complementary medicines in their practice, such as medical herbalists, homoeopaths and aromatherapists, are not available for the UK, although increasing numbers of such practitioners may suggest increasing public demand for treatment with these therapies.

With the traditional herbal medicinal products directive, the future is set to bring improved quality standards for herbal medicinal products from around 2004/2005 – manufacturers will need to meet standards for Good Manufacturing Practice (GMP) or remove their products from the market. Initiatives involving ethnic medicines are also aimed at improving quality standards for these preparations, although as this sector is less developed in the UK, it is likely that improvements in the quality of ethnic medicines will be seen over a longer time period.

In addition to requiring compliance with quality standards, the proposed traditional herbal medicinal products directive will require manufacturers of products to be registered under the scheme, to provide evidence of the safety of their products, and to comply with standard regulatory provisions on pharmacovigilance. At the same time, the increasing use of herbal medicines, particularly by patients using conventional drugs and those with serious chronic illness, may result in the emergence of new safety concerns, such as signals of uncommon ADRs, those occurring with long-term use, and interactions with conventional medicines.

At present, most research involving herbal medicinal products concentrates on establishing efficacy. The proposed traditional herbal medicines directive may have the effect of shifting the emphasis of herbal medicines research from efficacy to safety. However, manufacturers who aim at obtaining full marketing authorizations (i.e. with licensed indications) via the conventional route will still have an incentive to carry out well-designed randomized controlled trials of their products.

Against a background of widespread and increasing use of complementary medicines, it is recognized that complementary-medicine practitioners need to be regulated, and that conventional healthcare professionals need to be knowledgeable about complementary medicines and therapies. The House of Lords Select Committee on Science and Technology's report on complementary/alternative medicine (CAM) recommended statutory regulation of certain types of complementary-medicine practitioner, including herbalists, and recommended that regulatory bodies of healthcare professionals develop guidelines on competence and training in CAM (including complementary medicines) (House of Lords Select Committee on Science and Technology, 2000). The government accepted the recommendations made in the House of Lords report. Thus, in the future, conventional healthcare professionals should have a basic knowledge of complementary medicines and therapies, and doctors, pharmacists, and so on, may have interactions with state-registered herbal practitioners.

In its response to the House of Lords report, the government stated that if a therapy gains a critical mass of evidence, the NHS and the medical profession should ensure that the public has access to that therapy (Department of Health, 2001). Thus, in addition to homoeopathic treatment, which is already available through the NHS, licensed herbal medicines and licensed dietary supplements with a sound evidence base may become more widely utilised within the NHS.

A recommendation that was welcomed related to funding for research in CAM. As well as recommending that manufacturers of complementary medicines should invest more heavily in research and development, the House of Lords report also recommended that the NHS research and development directorate and the Medical Research Council should pump-prime CAM research with dedicated funding (Department of Health, 2001). In 2002, the UK Department of Health Research and Development programme invited applications for post-doctoral research awards in CAM (Department of Health, 2002).

Overall, it is likely that the immediate future will bring most change for herbal medicines. The effect of regulation of herbal medicinal products and herbal-medicine practitioners, training in herbal medicine for conventional healthcare professionals, and the promise of NHS provision of herbal medicines where there is sound evidence of efficacy, may be to move herbal medicines more towards the mainstream.

In the long term, the future for 'complementary medicines', particularly herbal medicines, may lie with pharmacogenetics and pharmacogenomics. These relatively new fields of research are widely held to be central to the discovery of new drugs and to the future of therapeutics, yet optimizing treatment on the basis of a patient's genotype has not been discussed in the context of complementary medicines. It is reasonable to assume that individuals with a different genetic profile will have different responses to herbal medicines as well as to conventional drugs.

ACKNOWLEDGEMENTS

The author thanks Dr Linda Anderson and Professor J. David Phillipson for helpful discussions during the preparation of this chapter, and the referees for their comments. Competing interests: J. B. has received research funding and hospitality from Lichtwer Pharma UK Ltd, manufacturer of LI-1370 and LI-160, and held a Lichtwer Pharma Research Fellowship (August 1999 to July 2002). J. B. held a research fellowship (February 1996 to July 1999) funded by Boots, retailer of herbal medicines.

REFERENCES

Anonymous. Extension of the Yellow Card scheme to unlicensed herbal remedies. *Curr Prob Pharmacovigilance* 1996; 22: 10.

Anonymous. Extension of the Yellow Card scheme to pharmacists. *Curr Prob Pharmacovigilance* 1997; 23: 3.

Barnes J. An examination of the role of the pharmacist in the safe, effective and appropriate use of complementary medicines. PhD Thesis, University of London, 2001.

Barnes J, Anderson LA, Phillipson JD. St John's wort (*Hypericum perforatum* L.): a review of its chemistry, pharmacology and clinical properties. *J Pharm Pharmacol* 2001; 53: 583–600.

Barnes J, Anderson LA, Phillipson JD. *Herbal Medicines. A Guide for Healthcare Professionals*, Second Edition, London: Pharmaceutical Press, 2002.

Barnes J, Mills SY, Abbot NC, Willoughby M, Ernst E. Different standards for reporting ADRs to herbal remedies and conventional OTC medicines: face-to-face interviews with 515 users of herbal remedies. *Br J Clin Pharmacol* 1998; 45: 496–500.

Bisset NG, ed. *Herbal Drugs and Phytopharmaceuticals*, ed. (German edition), Wichtl M. Stuttgart: Medpharm, 1994.

Broughton A. Yellow card reporting scheme. *Eur J Herb Med* 2001; Dec: 3–6.

De Smet PAGM. Health risks of herbal remedies. *Drug Safety* 1995; 13: 81–93.

De Smet PAGM, Keller K, Hänsel R, Chandler RF, eds. *Adverse Effects of Herbal Drugs*, Vol. 3. Berlin: Springer-Verlag, 1997.

Department of Health. *Government Response to the House of Lords Select Committee on Science and Technology's Report on Complementary and Alternative Medicine*. London: The Stationery Office, 2001.

Department of Health. *Department of Health Research and Development Programme. Guidance notes for Department of Health Complementary and Alternative Medicine Post-Doctoral Awards 2002*. http://www.doh.gov.uk/research/rdi/camresearch.htm [accessed 4 November 2002].

Englisch W, Beckers C, Unkauf M, Ruepp M, Zinserling V. Efficacy of artichoke dry extract in patients with hyperlipoproteinaemia. *Arzneimittelforschung* 2000; 50: 260–265.

Ernst E. Only 0.08% of funding for research in NHS goes to complementary medicine. *Br Med J* 1996; 313: 882.

Ernst E. Funding research into complementary medicine: the situation in Britain. *Complement Ther Med* 1999; 7: 250–253.

Ernst E, Pittler MH. *Ginkgo biloba* for dementia. A systematic review of double-blind, placebo-controlled trials, *Clin Drug Invest* 1999; 17: 301–308.

Evans WC. *Trease and Evans Pharmacognosy*, Fifteenth Edition, Edinburgh: W.B. Saunders, 2002.

House of Lords Select Committee on Science and Technology. *Complementary and Alternative Medicine*, Session 1999–2000 6th report. London: The Stationery Office, 2000.

Hypericum Depression Trial Study Group. Effect of *Hypericum perforatum* (St John's Wort) in major depressive disorder. A randomized controlled trial. *JAMA* 2002; 287: 1807–1814.

Linde K, Mulrow CD. St John's wort for depression (Cochrane Review). In *The Cochrane Library*, Issue 1, Oxford: Update Software, 2003.

Medicines Control Agency. Voluntary suspension of kava-kava sales by herbal sector following safety concerns. Http://www.mca.gov.uk [accessed 28 February 2002].

Mills S, Bone K. *Principles and Practice of Phytotherapy*. Edinburgh: Churchill Livingstone, 2000.

Mintel International Limited. *Complementary Medicines. Market Intelligence.* London: Mintel International Ltd, 2001.

Personal communication. Southampton: Drug Safety Research Unit, February 25, 2002.

Pittler MH, Ernst E. *Ginkgo biloba* extract for the treatment of intermittent claudication: a meta-analysis of randomized trials. *Am J Med* 2000; 108: 276–281.

Pittler MH, Ernst E. Horse-chestnut seed extract for chronic venous insufficiency (Cochrane Review). In *The Cochrane Library*, Issue 1. Oxford: Update Software, 2003.

Rawlins MD, Jefferys DB. United Kingdom product licence applications involving new active substances, 1987–1989: their fate after appeals. *Br J Clin Pharmacol* 1993; 35: 599–602.

Schellenberg R. Treatment for the pre-menstrual syndrome with agnus castus fruit extract: prospective, randomised, placebo-controlled study. *Br Med J* 2001; 322: 134–137.

Schulz V, Hänsel R, Tyler VE. *Rational Phytotherapy. A Physicians' Guide to Herbal Medicine*, Fourth Edition, Berlin: Springer, 2000.

Shaw D, Leon C, Kolev S, Murray V. Traditional remedies and food supplements. A 5-year toxicological study (1991–1995). *Drug Safety* 1997; 17: 342–356.

Stevinson C, Pittler MH, Ernst E. Garlic for treating hypercholesterolaemia. A meta-analysis of randomized clinical trials. *Ann Intern Med* 2000; 133: 420–429.

Stockley I. *Drug Interactions*, Sixth edition, London: Pharmaceutical Press, 2002.

The Medicines for Human Use (Kava-Kava) (Prohibition) Order 2002 (SI 2002/3170). London: The Stationery Office.

Vickers AJ. Reflections on complementary medicine research in the UK. *Complement Ther Med* 1999; 7: 199–200.

Wilt T, Ishani A, Stark G et al, Serenoa repens for benign prostatic hyperplasia (Cochrane review). In *The Cochrane Library*, Issue 1, Oxford; Update Software, 2003a.

Wilt T, Ishani A, MacDonald R, Rutks I, Stark G. Pygeum africanum for benign prostatic hyperplasia (Cochrane review). In *The Cochrane Library*, Issue 1, Oxford: Update Software, 2003b.

Wren RC. *Potter's New Cyclopedia of Botanical Drugs and Preparations* (Revised Williamson EM, Evans FJ). Saffron Walden: Daniel, 1988.

CHAPTER 35

THE CRACK IN THE BIOMEDICAL BOX: THE PLACEBO EFFECT

Zelda Di Blasi

Crocodile dung, lozenges of dried vipers, blisters and bloodletting. Until this century most medications were pharmacologically inert, if not harmful. Since the age of the scientific revolution the realms of magic, spirituality and superstition have been pushed aside by the rational, objective and scientific biomedical model. The discovery of penicillin, aspirin and cortisone are only a few examples of the triumph of science and rationality in the conquest of illness and the combat of quackery and charlatanism.

But, interestingly, remarkable medical achievements and scientific proof have often been obtained by using the very thing that was associated with trickery and deceit – the placebo.

THE PLACEBO AS DESIGN AND EFFECT

In his classic meta-analysis of placebo-controlled trials, Beecher found that a third of patients responded positively to placebos (Beecher and Boston, 1955). This discovery prompted researchers to carry out studies on university students and in clinical populations suffering from a variety of conditions. Many undergraduates took part in drug experiments and were found to display various drug-related behaviours (e.g. alcohol-induced sexual arousal: Hull and Bond, 1986), even though the substance taken

Edited from an article in *The Psychologist* 2003;16(2):72–5.

was totally drug-free. In asthma patients, airways could be dilated simply by telling people they were inhaling a bronchodilator, even when they weren't (Luparello et al, 1970; Neild and Cameron, 1987).

Over the past 20 years therapies have been compared using an experimental design known as the randomised controlled trial or RCT (Lilienfeld, 1982). To evaluate the specific effectiveness of a new 'active' treatment, patients are randomly allocated either to the experimental treatment or to a sham or 'inert' placebo treatment (Armitage, 1982).

Placebos were designed to simulate the treatments being investigated but had no specific therapeutic properties. For example, in pharmacology a fake drug would usually be a white sugar pill or a saline injection. In physiotherapy the ultrasound machine would be turned off for the placebo group (Hashish et al, 1988). In surgery, sham operations merely involve making a skin incision – this has been found to have an especially powerful placebo effect (Cobb et al, 1959; Dimond, 1960). In acupuncture, patients would get their needles in the 'wrong' pressure points (Berk et al, 1977). A more recent study of placebo surgery published in the *New England Journal of Medicine* found no difference between patients randomised to surgery for the knee and placebo surgery (Moseley et al, 2002).

To study the direct effects of treatment on health, clinical researchers controlled for any possible experimenter bias by following very strict guidelines in the conduct of RCTs, such as double-blind designs, randomisation and power calculations (Pocock, 1983). In controlling for potential biases, researchers created a 'biomedical box' that allowed them to get rid of any possible variable that might 'threaten the fastidious detection of a predictable cause and effect outcome' (Kaptchuk, 1998, p.1723). Among these variables were placebo effects. Seen as 'noise' in the machine to be filtered out of the scientific data, placebo effects were 'boxed'.

The challenge for biomedical scientists was to prove that the therapeutic intervention was better than a placebo, because if clinical trial findings showed little or no difference between the two treatments, the therapy would have to be abandoned. But despite rigorous and systematic adherence to strict clinical guidelines, placebo effects would still appear – unpredictably and uncontrollably (Hrobjartsson, 1996). This was a nuisance for scientists who had devoted time and energy to carefully developing the therapy, for healthcare practitioners who needed effective treatments, and most importantly for patients desperately seeking a relief to their symptoms.

If the treatment consisted of a placebo, there were problems even when patients *did* get better, as the medical condition of patients who responded to placebos would often be thought of as 'psychosomatic' or 'all in their head'. Furthermore, discovering that they had improved thanks to a fake therapy threatened the doctor–patient relationship, as patients might feel they had been tricked. It also risked cutting short the healing response. It is perhaps because of this that people who *do* respond to placebo treatment are often not told what they got when the study closes (Di Blasi et al, 2002).

Scientists, physicians and practitioners are not the only ones to be frustrated and mystified by the placebo effect. The phenomenon has been an attack on the whole scientific paradigm, clearly shaking the solid foundations of the biomedical model. Harvard historian Anne Harrington described placebos as 'ghosts that haunt our house of biomedical objectivity ... and expose the paradoxes and fissures in our own self-created definitions of the real and active factors in treatment' (Harrington, 1997, p.1).

THE DEBATE HOTS UP

Puzzled by the thought that a harmless white pill could have such overwhelming effects on the physical state of patients, biomedical researchers pulled up their Sleeves to take a good look at what might be happening. In Beecher's meta-analysis no systematic strategy had been used to identify the studies. While these were selected 'at random', seven of the 15 trials had been conducted by the author himself. The trials had not been conducted prospectively to investigate placebo effects, and while some of these had both placebo and no treatment arms, the difference between these groups was not discussed. Having noted various such flaws in the evidence for placebo effects, a group of reviewers from Germany explained the effect, not as a powerful therapeutic tool, but as merely an 'illusion' created by a scientific artefact (Kienle and Kiene, 1998, 2001).

Kienle and Kiene (2001) listed a number of factors 'that cause a false impression of a placebo effect', such as natural course of disease (e.g. spontaneous improvement, fluctuation of symptoms), additional treatment, observer bias (e.g. scaling bias, conditional switching of treatment), no placebo given at all, and patient bias (e.g. polite answers, neurotic or psychotic misjudgement).

The debate became a hot topic in the media and internet discussion lists when the views of Kienle and Kiene were supported by the findings of two Danish researchers, published in the *New England Journal of Medicine*. Asbjorn Hrobjartsson and Peter Gøtzsche felt that a 'true' placebo effect should be examined by comparing the difference not between 'active treatment' and 'placebo' but between 'placebo' and 'no treatment' groups. This is because it is normal for placebo effects to be observed in randomised controlled trials when comparing an active drug with a placebo control; a waiting-list group would control for the effects of natural progression of the disease. They identified 114 such trials and found 'little evidence in general that placebos had powerful clinical effects'

(Hrobjartsson and Gøtzsche, 2001). This finding delighted placebo sceptics and reinforced the view of placebos as fictitious, powerless phenomena when compared with biology and medicine. Was the biomedical box safely shut once more?

A new challenge to its solid structure came when a group of psychiatrists from Los Angeles identified brain changes in patients randomised to placebos (Leuchter et al, 2002). Perhaps placebo effects *were* real, and even more powerful than previously thought. Once the LA study was over and placebo responders were told about their treatment allocation, most of them relapsed and had to be put on 'active' treatment. According to a Reuters report, 'placebo responders, when told they were on a placebo, had a deterioration of their mood. Within a month, most of the placebo responders had enough depressive symptoms that they actually ended up on medications' (Fox, 2002).

Yet not all placebo responders are upset to find that their medicine was a sham. In a study conducted in collaboration with John Weinman from University College London, I interviewed a man whose heel pain had vanished following a placebo injection. When told about his treatment allocation he excitingly replied: 'This is fantastic, this is a real discovery ... Human chemistry is the most important of them all ... It is the faith, the trust we put in people!'

DIGGING FOR PLACEBO GOLD

Social psychologist W.J. McGuire describes 'three stages in the life of an artefact: first it is ignored; then it is controlled for its presumed contaminating effects; and finally, it is studied as an important phenomenon in its own right' (quoted in Harrington, 1997, p.2). This has been the case with the placebo effect: rather than attempting to repair the cracks of the biomedical box, some researchers have been curious to see what lay inside. And indeed, something appeared to glitter.

The possibility of striking gold moved researchers towards digging to explore what they increasingly felt was the most magical, mysterious and most widely misunderstood phenomenon in medicine. The 'gold rush' grew in the year 2000 when the National Institutes of Health (NIH) in America organised a placebo effect conference, putting forward major grants to study placebo effects (see weblinks).

Interestingly, the pharmaceutical industry has indirectly exploited the placebo effect in the form of marketing and advertising. We only need to think of the diamond-shaped sex pill Viagra to get excited! Drugs are promoted in ways that attempt to maximise their effect with allusive names such as 'Regaine' for male baldness, 'Welldorm' for insomnia, 'Marvelon' as a marvellous contraceptive (Holm and Evans, 1996). The colour of a drug has also been shown to affect its perceived effects, with red, yellow and orange pills perceived as stimulants and blue and green as tranquillising or sedative drugs (de Craen et al, 1996).

Despite the fact that placebo effects are basically psychological processes, psychologists were the last discipline to join the placebo gold rush (Shapiro and Shapiro, 1997). Perhaps we felt that researching placebo effects threatened the scientific soundness of the discipline, or that it risked reawakening ghosts like Freud. Rather than advancing our understanding of the mechanisms of this phenomenon, we have generally tended to adopt placebo controls in our trials to evaluate the efficacy of specific psychological therapies.

Enthusiasm in researching placebo effects dwindled when studies failed to identify a placebo-responding personality (e.g. Shapiro and Shapiro, 1997), but was reawakened yet again in the 1980s and 1990s with the boom in complementary and alternative medicine (Eisenberg et al, 1993; Fulder and Munro, 1983). Sceptical of the growing popularity of 'CAM', clinical researchers challenged its real worth by assigning any effectiveness to placebo effects alone (Lynoe, 1990). This left alternative practitioners with the challenge to prove that their therapy is actually more effective than a sugar pill. Interestingly, CAM practitioners are among the few health professionals to recognise that it is not their treatment alone (homeopathy, acupuncture, etc.) but also the way this is delivered (e.g. empathically, reassuringly) that is therapeutic. It is for this reason that some of the major placebo effect experts have a background in CAM research.

It is with the guidance of some of these experts that I began to examine whether the way treatment was delivered by healthcare professionals could actually affect the healing process. We conducted a systematic review of all relevant placebo-controlled randomised controlled trials conducted in patients with a physical illness. Complex psychological and psychotherapeutic interventions (e.g. training health professionals in patient-centred care or in preparing patients for stressful interventions) were excluded to focus on situational or context factors (e.g. the manipulation of treatment expectations).

We used Leventhal's self-regulatory theory (Leventhal et al, 1980) to guide this work. Leventhal's theory was chosen because it takes account of the dynamic nature of psychological processes, and in predicting how patients cope in reaction to a health threat it takes account of both cognitive and emotional responses. It appears to embrace various theoretical approaches commonly used to understand the mechanisms and determinants of the placebo effect, such as expectancy, anxiety, appraisal and conditioning.

Our aim was to see if healing could be 'triggered' by influencing the way patients thought ('cognitive care') and felt ('emotional care') about their illness and their treatment. For example, by giving a positive vs. a negative/neutral diagnosis or prognosis, or by increasing or decreasing expectations (e.g. 'This is a new, fast-acting drug, very effective in reducing pain' vs. 'This is a new drug which I have not found to be very effective in reducing pain').

We searched 11 electronic databases, including PsycLIT. Our search strategy for Medline alone included 183 search terms. Our findings, published in *The Lancet* (Di Blasi et al, 2001), showed that out of a total of 25 trials that met our inclusion criteria, approximately half of these studies found significant effects on patients' health status. No clear patterns emerged when clinical conditions were analysed separately. However, there were some interesting findings, though not always consistent. Systolic blood pressure was found to be higher in hypertensive patients who were told to expect this to be higher in a second assessment, than in patients who were informed that it would be low or that there would be no change. We also found that physicians who adopted a warm, friendly and reassuring manner while increasing expectations were more effective than those whose consultations were formal and did not offer reassurance.

You will probably wonder how some of these variables (such as 'warmth' and 'friendliness') were operationalised. Unfortunately, these studies do not go beyond giving a simple description of the intervention; for example, 'warm, a lot of verbal interaction' vs. 'neutral, minimal interaction' (Freund et al, 1972). Furthermore, even though 'expectancy' was the main variable being manipulated (i.e. 'high' vs. 'low') in 19 of the 25 studies, only five studies actually measured whether expectations had indeed been influenced by the intervention. When expectations were assessed, measures tended to be crude, single-item scales and administered at one point in time.

Furthermore, while the RCT is perceived to be the 'gold standard' research method in health sciences, it is limited in its application. For example, by focusing on outcomes it tends to overlook processes such as healthcare interactions, making it difficult to extrapolate on the findings. It is also important to bear in mind that human interactions are often spontaneous, creative and unpredictable. For this reason, video or tape recordings of interactions could help advance our understanding of the types of therapeutic processes that are influencing the effects of therapies and placebos.

CONCLUSION

In the 17th century Descartes, one of the great fathers of the Age of Science, wrote: 'there is nothing included in the concept of the body that belongs to the mind; and nothing in that of mind that belongs to the body' (quoted in Sommers, 1978). Our current system of care is founded upon this assertion. It is no wonder that four hundred years later we are finding so many cracks in our system. This artificial split cannot be sustained much longer.

With growing evidence on mind–body interactions in healing and with our current crisis in health care, a revolutionary paradigm shift needs to occur. Rather than fixing the cracks of the biomedical model, we need to break the box, remove the gap between medicine and psychology and welcome back the discredited sister of scientific medicine.

REFERENCES

Armitage P. The role of randomization in clinical trials. *Statistics in Medicine*, 1982;1:345–52.

Beecher HK, Boston MD. The powerful placebo. *Journal of the American Medical Association*, 1955;1602–6.

Berk SN, Moore ME, Resnick JH. Psychosocial factors as mediators of acupuncture therapy. *Journal of Consulting and Clinical Psychology*, 1977;45:611–19.

Cobb L, Thomas GI, Dillard DH et al. An evaluation of internal-mammary-artery ligation by a double-blind technic. *New England Journal of Medicine*, 1959;260(22):1115–18.

de Craen AJM, Roos PJ, de Vries AL, Kleijnen J. Effect of colour of drugs: Systematic review of perceived effect of drugs and of their effectiveness. *British Medical Journal*, 1996;313:1624–6.

Di Blasi Z, Harkness E, Ernst E et al. Influence of context effects on health outcomes: A systematic review. *The Lancet*, 2001;357:757–62.

Di Blasi Z. Kaptchuk TJ, Weinman J, Kleijnen J. Informing participants of allocation to placebo at trial closure: Postal survey. *British Medical Journal*, 2002;325:1329–31.

Dimond EG, Kittle CF, Crockett JE. Comparison of internal mammary artery ligation and sham operation for angina pectoris. *American Journal of Cardiology*, 1960;5:483–6.

Eisenberg D, Kessler RC, Foster C et al. Unconventional medicine in the United States. *New England Journal of Medicine*, 1993;328:246–52.

Fox M. *Brain scan study shows how placebo aids depression.* Reuters. Retrieved 8 February 2002 from www.forbes.com/newswire/2002/01/01/rtr467478.html

Freund J, Krupp G, Goodenough D, Preston LW. The doctor–patient relationship and drug effect. *Clinical Pharmacology and Therapeutics*, 1972;13(2):172–80.

Fulder SJ, Munro RE. Complementary medicine in the United Kingdom: Patients, practitioners, and consultations. *The Lancet*, 1983;2(8454):542–5.

Harrington A. *The placebo effect: An interdisciplinary approach.* Cambridge, MA: Harvard University Press, 1997.

Hashish I, Hai HK, Harvey W et al. Reduction of postoperative pain and swelling by ultrasound treatment: A placebo effect. *Pain*, 1988;33:303–11.

Holm S, Evans M. Product names, proper claims. More ethical issues in the marketing of drugs. *British Medical Journal*, 1996;313:1627–9.

Hrobjartsson A. The uncontrollable placebo-effect. *European Journal of Clinical Pharmacology*, 1996;50(5):345–8.

Hrobjartsson A, Gøtzsche PC. Is the placebo powerless? An analysis of clinical trials comparing placebo with no treatment. *New England Journal of Medicine*, 2001;344:1594–602.

Hull JG, Bond CF. Social and behavioural consequences of alcohol consumption and expectancy: A meta-analysis. *Psychological Bulletin*, 1986;99:347–60.

Kaptchuk TJ. Powerful placebo: The dark side of the randomised controlled trial. *The Lancet*, 1998;351:1722–5.

Kienle GS, Kiene H. The placebo effect: A scientific critique. *Complementary Therapies in Medicine*, 1998;6:14–24.

Kienle GS, Kiene H. A critical reanalysis of the concept, magnitude and existence of placebo. In: *Understanding the placebo effect in complementary medicine: Theory, practice and research*, Peters D (ed). London: Churchill Livingstone, 2001; 31–50.

Leuchter AF, Cook IA, Witte EA, Morgan M, Abrams M. Changes in brain function of depressed subjects during treatment with placebo. *American Journal of Psychiatry*, 2002;159(1):122–9.

Leventhal H, Nerenz D, Straus A. Self-regulation and the mechanisms for symptom appraisal. In: *Symptoms, illness behavior and help-seeking*, Mechanic D (ed). New York: Neale Watson Academic, 1980; 55–86.

Lilienfeld AM. Ceteris paribus: The evolution of the clinical trial. *Bulletin of the History of Medicine*, 1982;56:1–18.

Luparello T, Leist N, Lourie CH, Sweet P. The interaction of psychologic stimuli and pharmacologic agents on airway reactivity in asthmatic subjects. *Psychosomatic Medicine*, 1970;32:509–13.

Lynoe N. Is the effect of alternative medical treatment only a placebo effect? *Scandinavian Journal of Social Medicine*, 1990;18(2):149–53.

Moseley JB, O'Malley K, Petersen NJ et al. A controlled trial of arthroscopic surgery for osteoarthritis of the knee. *New England Journal of Medicine*, 2002;2:81–8.

Neild JE, Cameron IR. Bronchoconstriction in response to suggestion: Its prevention by an inhaled anticholinergic agent. *British Medical Journal*, 1987;290:674.

Pocock SJ. *Clinical trials: A practical approach*. Chichester: Wiley, 1983.

Shapiro AK, Shapiro E. *The powerful placebo: From ancient priest to modern physician*. Baltimore, MD: Johns Hopkins University Press, 1997.

Sommers F. *Dualism in Descartes: The logical ground*. In: *Descartes*, Hooker M (ed). Baltimore, MD: Johns Hopkins University Press, 1978.

SECTION 6

CAM IN PRACTICE: DIVERSITY, INTEGRATIONS AND DEVELOPMENT

INTRODUCTION

Geraldine Lee-Treweek

This section brings together the key themes of the collection. It does this by focusing upon CAM in practice, the various and diverse settings in which CAM are currently being used and the diverse experiences that using CAM can bring. The readings stretch the reader's imagination to think about the possibilities that come with integrating CAMs; in palliative and terminal care, in obstetrics and midwifery, in the care of people with dementia, in nursing and in general practice. CAM is often used with types of illness that do not respond well to traditional orthodox care, such as chronic pain, migraine, stress and mental distress and this section illustrates the ways in which CAMs may approach these conditions. Finally, the section explores the personal journeys of some people who have chosen to become practitioners of CAM.

Jan Wallcraft's reading explores the issue of the use of CAM with people with various forms of mental distress, raising the important issue of evidence. She shows that the user's subjective experience of massage and aromatherapy is important to assessing its value. Likewise, Alison Faulkner and Sarah Layzell highlight the experience of people who use CAM to help them when they are going through a period of mental distress. Together these readings show how alternatives are being used to bring relief to traditionally 'hard to treat' conditions. Maintaining the same theme, Ann Wiles and Dawn Booker's reading discusses how CAM is being used to help people with dementia. This includes the examination of the use of sensory stimulation (through aromatherapy for instance) and massage to help reconnect and maintain connections to the present and to the past in people with this disease.

Marion Garnett's reading focuses on the empowering qualities of using CAMs in palliative care settings. Using social theories about the effect of living in an anxious and risky society in general, she transposes these ideas into a discussion of the care of people facing life threatening illness. Garnett argues that use of CAM empowers people and supports and cushions them emotionally in situations in which, often, curative care has ended. Her touching account is followed by Leslie Nield-Anderson and Ann Ameling who discuss the use of Reiki healing in a nursing context. The reading has been edited to focus upon a case study of how Reiki was used to aid the care of a person who was dying. Again the focus is upon empowerment and the way CAM can often provide a form of care and support that orthodox nursing cannot. Lorraine Williams' work examines the way that the integration of CAM into orthodox maternity care is providing choices for women during pregnancy and childbirth. She reviews the ways in which CAM is being integrated and discusses models of best practice that are arising out of the growing midwifery and obstetric interest in integrating a range of techniques.

Finally, Sheelagh Donelly and Sue Spurr discuss their journeys to become practitioners in CAM and their personal experience of the use of CAM. Donnelly's reading describes how as a general practitioner she became aware that there were other ways of treating illness and helping people towards regaining health than those offered by orthodox treatment. She outlines how making this discovery affected how she saw her role and encouraged her towards integrating spiritual healing into the range of skills she offered. Sue Spurr's reading focuses on her personal journey from CAM user to training to become a Shiatsu practitioner. Both pieces conclude the selection of readings by bringing focus to the diverse subjective experiences people have with CAM, as both users and practitioners.

CHAPTER 36

HEALING MINDS: WHAT EVIDENCE IS THERE THAT MASSAGE OR AROMATHERAPY HELPS PEOPLE IN MENTAL DISTRESS?

Jan Wallcraft

There are a number of forms of complementary therapy that are currently being used with people who are going through a period of mental distress in their lives. This chapter selects massage and aromatherapy and examines the claims for efficacy made by practitioners of these therapies.

MASSAGE

Massage is the use of physical manipulation, pressure, friction, stretching and kneading of the body for therapeutic purposes.

What claims are made for its use in mental health?

Massage is claimed to reduce stress and anxiety, insomnia and tension, and aid relaxation, by a 'combination of mechanical, neural, chemical and psychological factors' (Cochran-Fritz, 1993).

Edited from Wallcraft J. *Healing Minds; a report on current research, policy and practice concerning the use of complementary and alternative therapies for a whole range of mental health problems.* London: Mental Health Foundation, 1998.

Whatson (1993), who worked as a volunteer giving massage in a psychiatric hospital for 11 months, says that many psychiatric patients may not have felt relaxed for a long time; if massage can enable them to feel relaxed, they may learn to recognise tension in its early stages and get treatment before it gets out of hand. She says that patients appreciate the experience of a 'little warmth, comfort and respite' from depression and anxiety.

Davey (1993) suggests that massage is:

> ... a gentler way of changing mood which in acute crisis would usually be in the direction of calming people.

However, he cautions that the touch involved may be too emotionally explosive where a patient is seriously disturbed and suggests that reflexology may be the least threatening form of touch at these times.

Stevensen (1992) trained in iridology, massage, aromatherapy and shiatsu, and has since helped to train several hundred other nurses in the rudiments of massage and the concepts and safety factors in complementary therapies. Friends or relatives of the patient, she points out, can also be taught simple massage, making them feel less isolated from their loved ones and more able to contribute to their care. However, it is often hard for nurses to find the time and energy amid a busy ward schedule to practice hands-on care.

Is there any evidence to support these claims?

Accounts of personal experience

A client of the Complementary Therapy Service in Leeds (Leeds Social Services, 1997) wrote to say the following:

> I have benefited enormously from the treatments; initially I found the relaxation was most important, both physically and emotionally. After a while, in addition to relaxation, I began to feel a change in my attitude to my body – I valued myself more and felt enabled and encouraged to tackle my physical and emotional problems in a different way ...
>
> (Leeds Social Services, 1997, pp. 25–6)

James (1993) recounts her own experience of recovery from mental illness which she attributes to massage. She was hospitalised twice and diagnosed as suffering from manic depression. In hospital she was given a couple of massage sessions which, in hindsight, she considered to be a turning point in her recovery from depression at that time:

> In the cold, clinical, efficient atmosphere of a hospital this massage therapy had had a great impact on me. It felt wonderful to be touched, cared for and to feel valued, and led me to take an active interest in myself again. The seed of recovery has been sown for me only to come to light much later in my life.

Gradually she learned 'to trust myself, listening to my own body and having support from aromatherapy and complementary therapies, I walked away from clinical drug dependence to a healthier future'. James eventually trained as a massage therapist herself.

> A little tender loving care was what I needed. I believe that massage can help a person get in touch with all aspects of themselves. It stimulates the soft body tissues, releasing tensions and unblocking the energy paths thus allowing the mind to meditate and letting ideas, talents and the true latent potential of the person come to the fore.
>
> (Hilliard, 1995, p. 30)

Evaluated projects

Brassington (1996) carried out a small study with Bromley Users' Group (a group for mental health service users), with the aim of introducing massage to the group and finding out their views and experiences on massage. She demonstrated massage to the group and encouraged them to try out massage techniques on each other.

Comments included:

> I generally have a back massage once a month ... Most times I come out of these sessions feeling very balanced.
>
> When my friend was taking her qualifications in massage and aromatherapy she used me as her subject. I found that afterwards I was able to sleep well and usually better than usual.
>
> (Brassington, 1996, p. 4)

The Mental Integration Project in Lewisham provided a series of courses for people experiencing mental health difficulties, including a course on therapeutic touch and massage. The courses were developed in partnership with Lewisham Mental Health Service Users. Students are offered massage, taught basic massage techniques, and explore issues around touch and emotion and physical well-being. Jones (1997), who developed the course and teaches on it, provided information on students' views of the classes, including the following comments:

> What you [Hearing Voices Project] have done for me is amazing. I'm transformed, I change my shirts now and want to look as good as I feel.
>
> Since joining the classes I've been able to identify more when I get stressed and do something about it.

Clinical trials

Field et al. (1993) carried out a study of 52 hospitalised, depressed and adjustment disorder children and adolescents, who were given daily back massage for five days, compared to a matched control group of 20 who viewed relaxing videotapes. Improvement was measured by a series of mood-state rating scales, and physiological tests. Clear differences were recorded between the two groups, with massage patients reporting lower depression levels than the control group at the end of the five-day period. They were observed by the nurses to be more co-operative and less anxious and fidgety.

The staff were concerned about a number of issues regarding the children being massaged. There were fears of accusations of sexual abuse (resolved by using same-sex masseurs and restricting areas to be massaged), and fears about how the children would respond to unaccustomed physical touch:

> Many of the children did not recall ever having been touched by their parents, and none of the children had ever received a massage.
>
> (Field et al, 1993, p. 27)

However, the study did not lead to any problems, and appeared to show that massage could have positive effects on child and adolescent psychiatric patients.

A trial of the effects of massage on anxiety, stress and depression was carried out in Florida (Field et al, 1996). A group of 26 adults was given a twice weekly massage for five weeks, while a control group of 24 adults was asked to relax in the massage chair for 15 minutes. All the participants were monitored by EEG on the first and last days of the study, and before, after and during the sessions, along with a range of depression, stress and anxiety scales. At the end of the sessions, both groups were more relaxed, but the massage group had lower anxiety and depression scores, while the control group had only lowered depression scores.

At the end of the five weeks, the massage group had lower job stress and depression scores and increased mental alertness, whereas the control group had improved only on depression scores. This trial appeared to show that massage relieves anxiety and improves mental alertness.

Research reviews

Brassington (1996) carried out a literature review on massage in mental health and found that only a very few scientific papers on massage related to any aspect of mental health out of 100–150 scientific papers on massage each year. Even fewer were directly concerned with the use of massage for people diagnosed as mentally ill.

Cochran-Fritz (1993) summarised a number of studies of the effects of massage on stress. However, she did not critically assess the trials cited. The studies link the stress-relieving effects of massage to its effect on the autonomic nervous system (the reflex nervous system which enables a person to tense and relax automatically in response to different stimuli) and the endocrine system (the system of glands which produce hormones which affect both body and mind). Massage is claimed in these studies to enable the body to dissipate stress hormones associated with the sympathetic nervous system, the 'fight or flight' mechanism; excessive stimulation of this system is related to a variety of stress-related diseases.

Cochran-Fritz concludes that therapeutic massage methods are a simple and effective means of affecting the nervous system, and could be used to replace pharmaceuticals for mild manifestations of symptoms, and as a supporting adjunct to drug therapy to reduce dosages and duration of treatment, thus reducing the risk of side-effects.

AROMATHERAPY

Aromatherapy is the use of essential oils from plants in treatment. They are generally used externally in massage.

What claims are made for its use in mental health?

Moate (1995) says that aromatic plants have been used as tranquillisers for centuries, but that it is only recently that systematic research has begun to look at how aromatherapy can affect depression and anxiety.

Aromatherapists claim that essential oils can reduce fear, stress, agitation, fatigue, anger and other negative emotions and relieve grief and trauma; aid sleep; and restore energy, harmony and balance (Davis, 1991; Mojay, 1996; Worwood, 1995). Specific essential oils are linked to symptom relief for a wide range of mental and emotional symptoms, for instance, lavender for relaxation and sleep, rose for grief, chamomile for anger, geranium for depression. Worwood (1995) recommends aromatherapy for people with schizophrenia or manic depression to help with controlling symptoms.

Aromatherapy massage uses essential oils with massage, and, according to Davey (1993), provides:

> ... a means to stress reduction, relaxation and the reduction of aroused states found in emotional crisis. An increase in self esteem and a reduction in depression may be possible.
>
> (Davey,1993, p. 2)

Moate (1995), who provided aromatherapy at a psychiatric day unit, said:

> I have found that aromatherapy is able to work alongside psychiatric medication – aromatherapy could also be used to counter some of the side-effects of chemical drug treatment such as achy limbs and nausea.
>
> (Moate, 1995, p. 21)

It is claimed that aromatherapy affects mood by altering the brain chemistry:

> Odour stimuli in the limbic system or olfactory brain release neurotransmitters – among them encephaline, endorphins, serotonin, and noradrenaline. Encephaline reduces pain, produces pleasant euphoric sensations, and creates a feeling of well-being. Endorphins also reduce pain – and produce a feeling of well-being. Serotonin helps relax and calm, and noradrenaline acts as a stimulant that helps keep you awake.
>
> (Lawless, 1994, p. 75)

Lawless (1994) claims that aromatherapy affects the nervous system and brain wave patterns as measured on EEG machines. She quotes research which claims to show that bergamot, lime, neroli, petitgrain, lavender, marjoram, violet leaf, rose, cypress and opopnax are effective anxiety relievers, while lemon, orange, verbena, jasmine, ylang ylang and sandalwood relieve depression.

Rankin-Box (1991) warns:

> There seems to be a popular misconception that essential oils are natural and therefore safe, however a few are extremely toxic. Essential oils are highly concentrated and so their use should occur only after competent and thorough training through validated bodies such as the International Federation of Aromatherapists ...

> Additionally, the physiological effects of certain oils imply pharmacological properties and their use upon already immunocompromised clients should be closely monitored and interactions with other drugs carefully recorded.
>
> (Rankin-Box, 1991, p. 14)

She argues that, if the oils are proven to have properties synonymous with those of herbs, as is claimed, they should be subject to scrutiny under the Medicines Act and the EEC directives.

Is there any evidence to support these claims?

Case study report

Sanderson and Ruddle (1992) describe the treatment of a retired carpenter suffering from depression, anxiety, hyperventilation when distressed, and sleep problems, as well as a range of physical problems. After six months of treatment with aromatherapy massage and therapeutic baths using essences he had reduced his medication by 50%, had no sleep problems, reduced anxiety and sadness, increased assertiveness, and reported less pain and physical problems.

Evaluated projects

A study by a service user (Alexander, 1993) of complementary therapies offered at a Nottingham psychiatric hospital combined personal experience of treatment with evaluation of aromatherapy by other service users in the Day Unit and the Acute Ward. Alexander's own experience was that lavender oil enabled her to regain a natural sleep pattern and to reduce withdrawal symptoms after she discontinued her lithium treatment.

Two users in the Day Unit commented that aromatherapy was beneficial in easing tension, helping them express problems in a relaxed atmosphere, and helping with anxiety problems. The touch aspect was valued because of a lack of hugs in childhood. Users on the Acute Ward who had received aromatherapy and reflexology commented that they 'felt less aggressive after aromatherapy', that it eased tension. Improved well-being, 'helped ease the stress of disturbed thoughts', 'side effects of drugs seemed to lessen', and they were 'able to talk more easily to a caring nurse' (Alexander, 1993, p. 4).

No side-effects were experienced by any of the users, and all considered they had had positive benefits from treatment.

Alexander concludes that mental health service users are concerned about the side-effects of medication, and would benefit from a more flexible approach to treatment, including aromatherapy and reflexology, which could ease the stress factor for both professionals and users, and aid patients in the transition from the acute unit back to the community, and back to work.

Of the seven completed assessments after 12 sessions at the Leeds Complementary Therapy Project (Leeds Social Services, 1997), three had improved energy, two improved mood and two improved sleep. However, five experienced no change with regard to stress, four no change in mood and three no change in energy. The overview showed that scores were highest during therapy, suggesting that benefits were immediate but not sustained. The immediate benefits may have increased expectations and led to lower scores at the end. Several clients expressed disappointment that they could not have more sessions.

Moate (1994) gave aromatherapy massage treatment to clients at a psychiatric day unit as part of a massage project. She worked with the consultant psychiatrist to eliminate possible contraindications regarding the use of essential oils for clients taking psychiatric medications. The psychiatrist contacted the Drug Information Unit at St Thomas' Hospital to see if there were any reported safety cautions in this area, but no information was found. The psychiatrist advised careful monitoring of clients taking monoamine oxidisase inhibitor (MAOI) antidepressants. Clients were reported to be very receptive to receiving aromatherapy massage treatments even though for most it was their first experience of any form of complementary therapy.

Evaluation of the day unit services showed a high attendance rate for aromatherapy. Informal feedback from clients about sessions with Moate (1994) included:

> The best therapy being offered because it was physical. (p. 16)
>
> Felt relaxed and lighter. (p. 17)
>
> Not over-thinking as much. (p. 23)
>
> Felt as if everything was flushing out, leaving a cleansed feeling, (p. 32)

Three nurse colleagues at the Wirral Hospital Trust (Scott, 1995) gave treatment to 900 staff of the service over 12 months. An evaluation was carried out on 50 people who used the service during a two-month period, with self-rating anxiety scales filled in before and after two sessions. The results indicated that both new and existing clients experienced a 'feel good' factor and symptom relief following treatment. They also suggest that the fact that, of the 900 staff clients during the first year, 97% returned for more, indicated that most people perceived the treatment as beneficial.

Clinical trials

A small study (not double-blind or controlled) of four older people with mental distress (Hardy et al, 1995) measured the length of time asleep using the normal amount of medication, then withdrew medication for two weeks, and finally replaced medication with lavender oil for another two weeks. The findings showed that sleep was reduced without medication, but with the use of lavender oil, sleep returned to the previous level, and patients were less restless during sleep. The study suggested that lavender oil might be used as a temporary relief from continued medication for insomnia, thus reducing side-effects. The authors suggest that it might be worthwhile to investigate this effected under controlled conditions.

A study (not blind) of the use of citrus fragrance on the immune function and depressive states was carried out in Japan (Komori et al, 1995). In this study, 12 male patients suffering major depressive disorders were treated with citrus fragrance (a mixture of lemon, orange, bergamot and other oils) which was added to the airflow in their room, day and night. Simultaneously with the fragrance, anti-depressant doses were reduced by half, and thereafter by as much as the patients agreed each week. A control group of eight male patients with similar symptoms received their normal anti-depressant treatment. Depression scores were measured on the Hamilton rating scale and SDS self-rating scales. By the third week of the treatment, nine of the fragrance group had stopped taking anti-depressants, while the control group still needed the usual doses of anti-depressants.

A double blind RCT (Buckle, 1993) was carried out on the value of lavender oil in stress reduction, testing the value of two different types of lavender oil used on patients in an intensive care unit. Twenty-eight patients were given massage several days after their operations, on two consecutive days. All treatments were carried out by the researcher, with oils marked by the supplier as A and B. Neither the researcher nor the patients knew which oil was which. Treatments were standardised in terms of length and areas of the body massaged. The results were evaluated by using physiological measures and a semi-structure questionnaire asking about anxiety, mood and coping before and after treatment. The results showed a clear difference between the two oils in relation to anxiety, one showing twice as much anxiety relief as the other, though both achieved similar positive effects on mood and coping.

This study appeared to show that the therapeutic effect of aromatherapy massage was not due entirely to the massage, touch or placebo effect, and that different types of lavender had different therapeutic benefits. The results were unexpected, as the hybrid lavender (*lavandula burnatii*) scored better than the naturally occurring lavender (*lavandula angustifolia*), which according to the literature is reputed to be more therapeutic.

Buckle points out that the study was small and that the methods for measuring improvement (questionnaire) were not very sophisticated. She suggests that the accuracy of measurement of stress and anxiety could be improved by testing the blood for adrenocorticosteroids, but argues that, if anxiety levels can be significantly altered, from 'very tense' to 'very relaxed' with a 20-minute massage, as was the case in six of the 12 patients treated with the hybrid lavender, then this may be considered an alternative to orthodox drugs.

REFERENCES

Alexander B. The Place of Complementary Therapies in Mental health, unpublished report, Nottingham Advocacy group, 1993.

Brassington J. C. E. Massage and Mental health, unpublished project for ITEC Diploma, 1996.

Buckle J. Does it matter which lavender essential oil is used?, *Nursing Times* 1993;89(20):32–5.

Cochran-Fritz S. Physiologiucal effects of therapeutic massage on the nervous system, *Int J Altern Complement Med* 1993;September:21–5.

Davey B. The place of complementary therapy in mental health, Nottingham Advocacy group, unpublished paper, 1993.

Davis P. *Subtle Aromatherapy*. Saffron Walden: C. W. Daniel Company, 1991.

Field T., Morrow C., valdeon C., Larson S., Kuhn C., Schanberg S. Massage reduces anxiety in child and adolescent psychiatric patients, *Int J Altern Complement Med* 1993;July:22–7.

Field T., Ironson D., Scafidi F., Nawrocki T., Goncalves A., Burman I., Pickens J., Fox N., Schanberg S., Kuhn C. Massage therapy reduces anxiety and enhances EEG pattern of alertness and math computations, *Int J Neurosci* 1996;86(3–4):197–205.

Hardy M., Kirk-Smith M. D., Stretch D. D. Replacement of drug treatment for insomnia by ambient odour, *The Lancet* 1995;356:701.

Hilliard D. Massage for the seriously mentally ill, *J Psychosoc Nurs Mental Hlth* 1995;33(7):29–30.

James E. Mind and matter: massage for mental health, *Massage* 1993;Summer:11–12.

Jones A. Personal communication, 1997.

Komori T et al. Effects of citrus fragrance on immune function and depressive states, *Neuroimmunomodulation* 1995;2:174–80.

Lawless J. *Aromatherapy and the Mind*. London: Thorsons, 1994.

Leeds Social Services. Report on the complementary therapy project based at Roundhay Road Day Centre, August, unpublished report, 1997.

Moate S. Anxiety and depression, *Int J Aromather* 1995;7(1):18–21.

Mojay G. *Aromatherapy for Healing the Spirit*. London: Gaia Books, 1996.

Rankin-Box D. Complementary therapies in nursing, *Nursing* 1991;4(46):12–14.

Sanderson H., Ruddle J. Aromatherapy and occupational therapy, *Br J Occupational Ther* 1992;55(8):310–14.

Scott E. Body and soul, *Nurs Stand* 1995;9(37):22–3.

Stevensen C. Holistic power, *Nursing Times* 1992;88(38):68–70.

Watson J. Homoeopathy for emotional and mental health problems. Workshop handout for Pavilion Conference on Complementary therapies in Mental Health Services, 26 February 1998.

Worwood V. *The Fragrant Mind – Aromatherapy for Personality, Mind, Mood and Emotion*. London: Doubleday, 1995.

CHAPTER 37

COMPLEMENTARY THERAPIES AND MENTAL HEALTH

Alison Faulkner and Sarah Layzell

INTRODUCTION

This section covers the range of complementary therapies experienced by the people we interviewed, and explores the ways in which they were found to be helpful. Some approaches, like relaxation techniques, are not always thought of as therapies, but as they were used therapeutically by some people, classifying them as complementary therapies is a useful collective shorthand.

Complementary therapies have become increasingly popular in recent years, and studies have shown that they are beginning to become more easily available on the NHS – predominantly in the treatments of drug and alcohol abuse, HIV and Aids, and some other physical conditions. They are more rarely given or considered in relation to mental health services, although this too is beginning to change; due to the increased interest in this area, the Mental Health Foundation published a comprehensive review of research into complementary therapies in mental health in 1998 (Wallcroft J, 1988). In *Knowing our own Minds* (Faulkner A, 1997: ch. 3), complementary therapies constituted one of the main themes under investigation, alongside other alternative approaches. We categorised them under headings of: art/creative therapies, physical (touch) therapies, exercise/postural therapies, and dietary/herbal therapies. The most commonly experienced of these were the art and creative therapies, perhaps more often provided through statutory and voluntary sector day

Edited from Faulkner A, Layzell S. *Strategies for Living*. London: Mental Health Foundation, 2000.

Table 37.1 Complementary therapies used

- Reflexology
- Healing and Reiki
- Relaxation
- Meditation
- Yoga
- Tai Chi
- Homeopathy
- Herbal remedies
- Acupuncture
- Aromatherapy and massage
- Aromatherapy oils at home (bath or burner)

services than others. However, all of the complementary therapies were very popular, and many people in the survey expressed the wish to gain access to more of them.

In this study, although relatively few people had used complementary therapies, we were able to explore in more depth the ways in which they had found them helpful or therapeutic. Table 37.1 lists the different therapies people had tried. There were no particular groups within our sample, whether by personal characteristics or experience or by geographical area, who had particular experience of using complementary therapies. Rather, the dominant factor appeared to be easy access to therapies through local services or contacts.

WHY DID PEOPLE USE COMPLEMENTARY THERAPIES?

Overall, people's comments suggest that they saw complementary therapies as distinctly complementary to conventional approaches rather than as a substitute. In this sense they were truly complementary rather than alternative therapies. Indeed, some mental health professionals recommended that people try these approaches in addition to medication or talking therapies. This woman, who was going to see a herbalist, is typical:

> 'I am hoping she will give me something, she won't be able to substitute my medication, although it would be great if she could, but something that works alongside the medication and improves my life a bit more, then I am willing to do it.'

Very many people hoped complementary therapies would help them relax, recognising that relaxation was good for their mental health. Obviously this was the reason people tried relaxation classes, but also why they had massage or reflexology and tried more active therapies like yoga and Tai Chi. The few people who saw a healer did not, apparently, expect to be 'cured', but rather to feel calmer and more at ease with themselves.

Some of the support groups and day centres that people attended offered relaxation classes and other therapies, such as massage or reflexology, free of charge, although often on a short term basis; it seemed that some people had tried them because of this ready accessibility. A few people paid for massage, aromatherapy or to see a herbalist; these people were convinced of the benefits of their chosen approach. A relatively small number of people had tried several different complementary therapies; it seemed that once someone had tried one, they were more likely to try another. Perhaps this suggests that there are some people who are generally open-minded about, or convinced of, the potential benefits of complementary therapies, whereas those who are more sceptical are less likely to try them in the first place.

CHOICE OF COMPLEMENTARY THERAPY

As suggested above, people were more likely to use complementary therapies because they wanted to, rather than because they had been prescribed to them; in other words, there was a more active choice involved (as long as money was not an issue). Determining which therapies were most beneficial depended on individual factors: therapies that some people found very helpful were described by others as not at all helpful and even potentially frightening. Most people had a prior idea about what they would find helpful and so hadn't tried things that they were sceptical about. However, some people had been surprised when a therapy they thought would be relaxing had brought uncomfortable issues to the fore. For instance, although the majority of people enjoyed massage, some women who had been sexually abused found the level of physical intimacy difficult:

> 'I did find that I just could never relax with, like aromatherapy, and I just couldn't. If I tried to mention my history, I'd get to a certain point and then it just all comes crashing back.'

People's attitude towards complementary therapy overall, or to particular therapies, influenced whether or not they found it helpful. One woman pointed out that sometimes it can be difficult to get into a frame of mind which would give a therapy a chance to work. She was talking here about relaxation:

'... one of the things that I have always found rather contradictory is that people with anxiety and depression are told to relax and listen to relaxation tapes and it is one of the most difficult things to try and make yourself do when you are actually tensed up. I found that I could do it sometimes, but it had to only be at a certain time and I was better actually trying not to relax, and doing something while I calmed down a bit, and then try and relax when I was on a more even keel, because to try and relax when you were... is just counter-productive to me, it made me worse.'

It might be that a different approach, such as massage, would have helped these people to unwind sufficiently to then be able to practice relaxation techniques themselves. One woman said that she was only able to benefit from relaxation classes once she was on medication which allowed her to start to unwind, again showing how the two approaches can complement each other:

'I went there for relaxation every week or every day I suppose for seven years... I found it really helpful once I was on the medication and my body was settling down and stayed down and my thoughts went elsewhere – I found that really helpful.'

However, one person found that medication interfered with her ability to use meditation as an aid to relaxation. These examples show how difficult it is to generalise about approaches which require active engagement on the part of the person trying them, yet most people felt that a positive attitude was necessary if they were to benefit from complementary therapies:

'I think you have got to have your mind in focus usually for complementary therapies. I don't think you can just go and say it will work for me, I think you have got to apply some thinking – like I am sure it is going to work.'

It follows that if it is necessary to feel positive or at least open-minded about complementary therapies, people should be able to choose which approach they want to try. The importance of matching the therapy or technique to the individual is further illustrated by the following:

'... the one thing the psychologist did for me that was helpful, was taught me how to do deep breathing. To relax... It really works as well... It takes away the tightness in the chest and all that. [Whereas]

I've been to meditation. I been there, didn't find that helpful. It really terrified me... Focusing on myself. I didn't want to do that.'

WHAT WAS HELPFUL ABOUT PARTICULAR THERAPIES?

In this section, we first look at what people had to say about individual groups of complementary therapies, and then draw out the common themes emerging across all of the therapies.

Massage, aromatherapy and reflexology

Many people found massage and reflexology very relaxing, either on their own or using aromatherapy oils. A very specific benefit was to help manage the side-effects of medication, by inducing physical relaxation:

> 'My medication stiffens up my muscles, and knots them all up, makes them all knotted and horrible, so the massage part of the aromatherapy treatment is absolutely wonderful to say the least. It just, you know, knocks about 20 years off me.'

Other people talked about the connection between physical and mental relaxation:

> '[Massage] helped me a lot. An awful lot. [I felt] more relaxed. Like, there was tension... taken... being taken away from you, from your muscles. And all the strain in your muscles, tensions being taken away from your muscles. And it's like, when you exercise your muscles, that's what it's like. It's stress being taken away. It's a nice feeling.'

Massage and reflexology differ from other approaches in that they involve physical contact. Whereas for some people, as mentioned earlier, touch could be experienced as quite threatening or invasive, there were others who found this aspect of physical therapies especially beneficial:

> 'I guess because I don't have physical relationships with guys and I am not married yet... I find the sensation of touch very, very comforting and very relaxing... and because it touches certain parts of your body, and sort of, um, is connected to certain other muscles and stuff, I just find it very relaxing.'

> 'I need a massage, or I need some kind of physical, you know, contact with another human being, is the only thing that's going cure it, it's not going to be, you know, drugs or what have you.'

This woman went on to say that physical touch was also helpful because it would release things that she could not let go of through talking alone. For this reason, the counsellor she had found most useful was a woman who had occasionally used touch:

> '... it released so much in my body, from what had happened in the past, and brought everything up to the surface, in a way that talking never had.'

Aromatherapy alone, without massage, could also be relaxing. Some people used aromatherapy oils at home, believing that their properties would be beneficial. They were used for relaxation or to influence mood; either by self-massage, burning the oils or putting them in the bath:

> 'I buy things that are for the nerves, you know, for my ailment... It wakes me up and makes me more alert, yes.'

Relaxation and meditation

Many people had been offered relaxation classes held at their support group or day centre. Some had used relaxation tapes at home, either on their own initiative or because they had been recommended by their keyworker or mental health care team. They described how relaxation techniques made them feel:

> 'Made me feel quite, um, I don't know a word for it, just relaxing really, and dreaming of stuff. I had some good dreams. If I can keep me eyes shut of course. Eh, that was quite good actually, I used to like relaxation.'

> 'I just felt rested and relaxed – thoughts were away somewhere else and you were able to get up from your relaxation and go to another group without having all these weird thoughts going round your head or really feeling anxious, you just went and did it, instead of before it would be 'oh no I am not going' – you would just sit and do nothing. I found it really helpful – relaxation.'

A few people found meditation helpful. One woman had begun meditating as a result of reading the Bible and found that it helped to clear her head; one man combined relaxation and meditation:

'... when I relax I just don't think about anything – I just give my mind a rest and give my back a rest at the same time, and usually while I am relaxing I drift into meditating and I am thinking about ways I can improve my situation, like when I started meditating about work and getting back to work, I was thinking of ways I can do that myself rather than depending on somebody else to do it for me.'

Yoga and Tai Chi

Yoga was another therapy that people found helped them to relax. One woman preferred it to relaxation classes:

'Yoga was good. I found that helpful. I don't like relaxation. I found if I lie on the floor and try to relax, I immediately tense up and that always makes me worse. [Yoga was] relaxing and calming... it helps your concentration.'

Yoga and Tai Chi use a series of movements and postures to focus awareness and develop physical and mental strength. These people were in no doubt that they were helpful:

'I had a breath problem as well, I couldn't breathe properly... He [doctor] sent me to yoga classes and that was good. Physically and mentally it's good. I'm OK now, I breathe now, I'm OK now. [It helped with] breathing, physical exercise and mentally relaxing.'

'... it was something relaxing, you could focus your mind and lose all the stresses and strains from wearing yourself out... You're exercising and you're relaxing at the same time... You're concentrating and relaxing on something and nothing. Whenever I concentrate on something I feel better.'

'[Tai Chi] was so – it was relaxing and somehow cleared your mind. You had to concentrate so much on learning the movements that whether it was the process of concentrating to learn the movements that took your mind off your problems, or whether it was the actual doing of the movements that made you feel better – but it really did have a positive effect.'

Most forms of Yoga and Tai Chi involve elements of meditation practice, or induce a similar state of mind:

> 'Meditation I've found useful... I find it helps me to be aware of the moment rather than, you know, worrying about what's going to happen next week or something... I think meditation's very useful. Tai Chi also, I've tried that... that's the same thing, I mean it's a bit like moving meditation really.'

Other therapies

A few people had seen a herbalist or used herbal remedies. One woman had been prescribed camomile tea from a herbalist, which helped her to sleep:

> 'I used to wake up a lot and have broken sleep and wake up a lot in the night, and walk around. Now it has sort of got me a little bit more rested, I do wake up but I don't walk about, I am a bit more relaxed and lie in bed until I fall asleep again.'

A small number of people had seen healers. One of these, an African-Caribbean man, spoke about his experiences at length. He had seen three different healers: two who practised forms of hands-on healing and one who did Reiki. He described how healing had helped overall:

> '[They] actually helped me work out a load of baggage, and get rid of a load of stuff that wasn't there, that, that was there, and shouldn't have been... I think it helped me at the time to, how can I say, um, it helped me to sort of, I think, be a freer person in my mind, um, I think it helped me to be, helped me to be more together with myself inside, but I think, um, it was beneficial, it was beneficial... I felt at one with myself, I felt peaceful with myself.'

He talked at length about what was helpful about seeing a particular healer, who was:

> 'A black, black guy, very nice person, understood where I was coming from, and understood what was happening in my mind... he was working with guides that had been... channelled through him. And this was, er, quite productive, very helpful... it seemed to reconnect me back to how I wanted to be with myself, and the person that I was trying to be before I saw all of these healers before. It seemed, he seemed to sort of like, clear out a lot of the crap that was going on in my mind. And, sort of like, help me to get back to being together with myself. Um, he was a very nice person and quite understanding, quite compassionate as well.'

He explained that he did not think it was because he was black that he had been more helpful than the other healers he had seen:

> 'I wasn't looking at it in terms of colour... I think it was just a different way of understanding, he was much more compassionate, and much more caring, and much more gentle... I think the most helpful thing that I've had is going to see this black healer. And that's been the most helpful.'

The black healer listened to his story without judging him and showed compassion, qualities we have seen emerge as valued within other relationships.

COMMON THEMES ACROSS THERAPIES

A number of strong common themes emerge from this exploration, which demonstrate that complementary therapies do tend to provide similar benefits to people but that individual factors about both person and therapy will affect the choice of therapy. Equally there were a small number of people who are more likely to try many different complementary therapies because they perceive the general approach to be a natural alternative for them.

Common themes

- Relaxation
- Concentration/focusing the mind
- Help with sleep
- Peace
- Taking control
- Compassion, caring
- Time to talk

Of these, by far the strongest theme was relaxation. As we have seen (above) many people spoke of the value of achieving a state of relaxation through sometimes different routes. This woman explains the value of relaxation:

> 'I only had neck massage and the hands. I found that really comforting and warm and I almost fell asleep with that as well, and I felt

really relaxed – having been all tensed up and frightened, it was like, 'oh, I feel great' and off I went.'

Another important theme to emerge was the role that complementary therapies could play in enabling someone to take some kind of action in alleviating their own symptoms or distress. This could be an important contribution towards beginning the process of taking control over distress or self-management:

> 'I'm pretty certain that there is something to do with, I don't know, a biochemical or pharmacological effect. But also, I do think there is an effect in like, actually taking, beginning to take action again. And actually taking control. I mean, I'm sure that there'd be some effect if I was given a Smartie and told it was a homeopathic remedy. Just taking it would have some effect. Because again, I'd feel like, yes, I've taken some action about it.'

The third major theme concerned the role of the therapists themselves, and as we have seen elsewhere, this could be vital in enabling the person to feel relaxed and accepted within the therapy. People valued the fact that complementary therapists were calm and non-judgmental and gave them sufficient time to express themselves and relax. Their experience of using complementary therapies often contrasted sharply with conventional medicine, which was characterised by a long wait for a hurried consultation. In other words, those aspects that were peripheral to the action of the therapy, itself, were therapeutic because they fostered people's self-esteem and potential for healing.

COMPLEMENTARY THERAPIES AS 'MOST HELPFUL' STRATEGY

Only two people named complementary therapies amongst the 'most helpful' strategies or supports they had encountered. One of these was the African-Caribbean man mentioned above, whose experience of the black healer was so compassionate and healing. The other was a man who combined homeopathy with counselling for his 'winning formula'. This man had lived in a town where all the doctors in the NHS general practice used homeopathy as well as conventional medication, and although he had now moved, he continued to see a homeopath as well as having counselling. He had subsequently come to accept it as an important part of his treatment, demonstrating the mediating influence of accessibility on the use of complementary therapies.

ACCESS AND CHOICE

Many of the people who took part in the study were able to get these therapies free of charge from the day centres/user groups they attended. However, some had to pay for them and this meant that they could not have treatments as often as they would have liked. As these women said:

> 'I really think it would be something brilliant to put on the NHS. If I could choose anything, I wouldn't choose any drug, I'd choose that.'

> 'I used to go to... a mental health users group and it was run by two females and they had lots of things going on – aromatherapy, reflexology – just different things... and I found the reflexology really wonderful and the massage, and that really helped a lot, you felt so relaxed, it was lovely. But there is not a lot of it going round, that is one problem, and obviously I think it would be great if they had it in doctors' surgeries, so that you could use it as a service on the National Health Service, because it did me a lot of good.'

As with talking therapies, access and choice affect people's ability to experience and to benefit from complementary therapies. From the interviews, it is clear that whilst many people had found complementary therapies very helpful, they had rarely continued with them for long periods, or had tended to drop in and out of them. Closer examination reveals that local services may have made certain therapies available to service users for periods of time, but were rarely able to do so on a long term basis. Consequently people's ability to use these therapies as a long term strategy is inevitably limited by cost and availability.

A number of people, including a couple of Asian women attending a voluntary sector project, had experience of receiving a combination of counselling and a physical therapy, such as aromatherapy massage or reflexology. They were very appreciative of the effects that this combination could achieve for them, feeling that the two approaches treated things in different ways and so increased the relative benefits:

> 'It was almost like having a lot of the stress massaged out of your body; so having released it orally and having expressed it, it was physically removed and it felt as though – I was just completely lighter all over, and very, very relaxed.'

REFERENCES

Faulkner, A. *Knowing our own Minds*. London: Mental Health Foundation, 1997, chapter 3

Wallcraft, J. *Healing Minds*. London: Mental Health Foundation, 1998.

CHAPTER 38

COMPLEMENTARY THERAPIES IN DEMENTIA CARE

Anne Wiles and Dawn Booker

The use of a range of complementary therapies with people with dementia appears to have increased in recent years. This may in part reflect the increasing use of complementary therapies by the general public as well as the shift in focus to a more holistic approach to the care of people with dementia. The aim of some of these therapies, particularly herbal remedies, has been to improve cognitive functioning. Other aims include more general improvements in well-being and quality of life, and a decrease in anxiety and distress.

AIMS OF THE STUDY

The aims of a study conducted in 2001 were to explore the extent to which complementary therapies were being used with people with dementia, and to ask whether they had been found to be effective. As there are a large number of such therapies, it was thought necessary to focus the study on those most frequently offered, and to ask about both the specific therapies and the therapists.

The information was collected in two ways

1. Review of the published literature and consultation with those engaged in relevant research;

Edited from an article in *Journal of Dementia Care* 2003;May/June:31–6.

2. Questionnaires to those persons known to be providing the selected complementary therapies to people with dementia.

The number of completed questionnaires returned from within the UK and Ireland was 85. It should be noted that this was a small self-selected group which may not be representative of those providing care. These findings are therefore only tentative.

WHAT WERE THEY DOING?

When asked to identify the therapy or therapies being offered to people with dementia, the replies were as shown below. Some therapists were offering more than one therapy, so the numbers in the table do not add up to 85.

Massage	51
Aromatherapy	49
Reflexology	31
Healing	14
Reiki	8
Herbal medicine	7

Aromatherapy and massage

The most popular therapies were massage and aromatherapy, but not necessarily offered together. 16 respondents provided massage but not aromatherapy, whilst 14 of the aromatherapists did not offer massage. Where aromatherapy was offered, the essential oil was usually applied to the skin, diluted in a carrier oil or cream. However, it was also being vapourised, added to baths, or sprinkled on tissues or cotton-wool, and left near the client.

The choice of essential oils was generally made according to the current need of clients; their mood, medical history, physical state and current medications were taken into account. A full assessment would usually be made and, in some cases, it was thought necessary to consult a medical practitioner before starting treatment. 40 of the aromatherapists said they were qualified to practice. 3 other practitioners, who were unqualified, said that the essential oils were prescribed on an individual basis by a qualified aromatherapist, but could be applied by others. It was unclear how the remaining six gained their knowledge.

It was often reported (11) that a particular essential oil may be chosen because its smell was liked or recognised by a client; lavender and rose most frequently fell into this category. Others were selected because it was believed they would have a particular therapeutic effect. Essential oils mentioned in connection with these effects included lavender or ylang ylang to calm and relax, and lemon, grapefruit, rosemary, basil or geranium for stimulation and 'clearing the mind'. Others such as frankincense, bergamot or neroli were thought to have a beneficial effect on depression. Perhaps surprisingly, given the literature (Ballard et al, 2002), the use of lemon balm was only mentioned once; but this may be due to the costliness of this oil. A reason for the selection of a particular oil was not always provided. Where the reason was given, the stated purpose could generally be justified, given the actions of individual essential oils suggested by Lawless (1995) and Price and Price (1999). However, it should be noted that the evidence for the claims made by these publications is unclear. This knowledge seems to be based on tradition and requires further research.

Where massage was offered, it was often of the hands, arms or feet. However, massage of the back and shoulders was also enjoyed by some. Shiatsu massage was offered by 4 respondents, who emphasised the gentle nature of the movements used.

Reflexology

More than a third of the respondents (28) offered reflexology, including 3 physiotherapists and 2 chiropodists who integrate the therapy into their practice. The usual practice of this therapy seemed to involve treating the whole body but giving extra attention to those areas of the feet which are believed to correspond to the head, brain, and spine, and to any other functions, such as elimination, which require specific treatment. It seems that there are also particular techniques which may be used to produce relaxation and calmness and to reduce agitation. The hands, as well as the feet, may be treated using similar therapy. However, no literature was identified which discusses the use of reflexology for the person with dementia.

Healing and Reiki

Descriptions of Reiki or healing included the 'laying-on of hands', distant healing or prayer; some practitioners also declared that they used prayer without defining themselves as healers. The various forms of healing have been used for calming, releasing tension, or for producing a sense of well-being. Healing was also described several times as a way of communicating with clients.

Herbal remedies

Only 7 respondents claimed to be using herbal remedies; all of them mentioned *Gingko biloba*. However 3 of the 7 held qualifications in herbal medicine and prescribed preparations according to the health needs of a particular client. These needs were said to change over time. Tinctures or capsules would be individually prepared for a client by the herbalist.

ARE THE THERAPIES THOUGHT TO BE EFFECTIVE?

Perhaps the most important question asked was whether the therapies were thought to be effective. No definition of effectiveness was provided; this interpretation was left to the respondents. The response was overwhelmingly positive, with only 4 respondents not being convinced of beneficial effect. Only one, a carer, felt that the therapy had not affected his wife's condition but he continued to support the treatment because he appreciated the close relationship which had developed between his wife and her therapist.

When asked how they knew that a therapy was effective, 61 of the respondents provided information. This ranged from a phrase or brief notes to a detailed description of behaviour with specific examples. These responses were analysed for frequency of particular effects and an attempt was made to group these into categories. The categories identified were:

a) behaviour and mood;
b) mental function;
c) physical effects;
d) client's experience of therapy;
e) client's relationship with the therapist.

The responses which related to behaviour and mood were grouped together as there appeared to be a direct relationship. Responses which were categorised under mental function were those which mentioned memory, alertness or apparent improvement in cognitive abilities. There was some difficulty in separating comments which reflected the client's experience of treatment from those which described how a relationship between client and therapist developed because of the experience.

Behaviour and mood

The most frequently reported effect of a therapy was that it 'relaxes' the person with dementia (22) or promotes calmness (20). Aggression and agitation were said to be reduced (12) and the person's sleep improved (17). One carer commented that reflexology and Reiki appeared more effective than medication at 'calming down' her relative. Other changes in mood said to be attributable to a therapy included reduction in anxiety (6) and restlessness, and the relief of depression (2). Clients were said to appear happy (6), to smile (4) and to seem contented. One nursing home used a therapy when residents became agitated or over-anxious, and reported that calmness and relaxation were produced as a result. The quality of life of some carers has also been improved where a therapy had a calming effect on relatives with dementia who are living at home.

Mental function

Some improvement of memory and mental function was said to result from the use of herbal medicine. The other therapies were also all reported as improving alertness or reducing confusion. One carer believed that aromatherapy motivated his relative and 'helps her to think'.

A particular effect appeared to be the increase in vocalisation (10). Clients receiving aromatherapy or reflexology were said to communicate more freely or 'express their specific wishes' during treatment. One client was said to reminisce lucidly whilst receiving the therapy and others to 'follow-on' with their stories from one treatment to the next.

The effects of *Gingko biloba* on cognitive function were seen as significant by all who use or recommend it. However, two of the medical herbalists believed that many other herbs can be useful, depending upon the profile of a particular client. As another herbalist commented, treatment is of the whole person rather than an isolated function.

Physical effects

An increase in mobility (10), either in general or of particular joints such as in the hands, was most frequently said to be the result of massage and aromatherapy. This outcome was particularly reported by physiotherapists who are using complementary therapies as part of a treatment plan. In addition, some improvements in circulation, elimination and respiration were noted, as well as pain relief. All the other therapies were said to have some physical benefits.

Client's experience of therapy

Assessment of a person's experience of receiving a therapy was generally based on verbal and non-verbal responses to treatment or the therapist. It was difficult to separate the experience of the therapy from that of being touched, and of receiving recurring one-to-one attention. This was acknowledged in some comments. One aromatherapist believed that clients may not remember her, but 'relate to the smell and touch', and another that the care and interest conveyed was as beneficial as the treatment.

Respondents reported that clients seem to enjoy the experience, or to have feelings of well-being, pleasure and comfort. Patients receiving aromatherapy, massage or reflexology were said to enjoy the attention, to 'like the touch aspect' and ask for more. Others were keen not to miss their treatments, would approach a masseur to ask for treatment, or showed that they wanted to repeat the experience. It was suggested that hand massage is 'non-threatening' but offers touch and a sense of value to the client. Clients were reported as saying 'that's lovely', 'that's nice' or 'that's much better' in response to massage or healing. Those who could not speak were seen to smile or hold a therapist's hand in response to treatment.

Client's relationship with the therapist

The use of therapies was said to 'increase trust, rapport and the therapeutic alliance' or to build a 'therapeutic relationship'. Clients understood that someone was prepared to spend time with them on a regular basis, and a comfortable and relaxed relationship was created. It was said that an increasing recognition of the therapist enhanced the level of communication and generally improved the clients' social awareness and interaction.

The therapists reported becoming associated with certain activities. On catching sight of a masseur, one group of non-communicative patients would remove their rings and prepare themselves for hand massage; others massaged the therapist's hands in return or attempted to massage each other.

There were other more general benefits attributed to the therapies. These included the communication of caring, and the reassurance and stimulation provided by one-to-one contact. It was said that an intimacy and gentleness between client, carer and therapist could develop, which may be attributed to the nature of the contact. As one masseur surmised, care of a person may be good but touch can be restricted to that which is functional, whereas massage allows legitimate time and contact. The social isolation of some residents was noted, with therapies providing a source of touch and contact which may be missing.

ARE THESE THERAPIES SAFE FOR PEOPLE WITH DEMENTIA?

There were few reports of therapies producing any adverse effects. However, an increase in distress or agitation had been noted by 7 respondents, and a few clients were said not to like or tolerate a therapy. These observations raise issues of safety, choice and consent.

Complementary therapies may be natural (Ernst, 1996 p 112) but the notion that natural equates with harmless is misleading and dangerous; the natural world abounds with toxic substances (Campbell, 1998). Herbal preparations, including traditional remedies, may cause allergic, toxic or other reactions (Ernst, 1996 p 114). This concern should extend to essential oils used in aromatherapy, as these are chemical compounds which originate from plants. However, it could be argued that any intervention which has a therapeutic impact will be capable of producing unwanted effects, if used inappropriately. It would therefore seem advisable for complementary therapies to undergo the same rigorous evaluation as any other treatment. However, there is little research on their use with people with dementia, other than studies on the effects of a few specific herbal preparations (Ballard et al, 2002; Ernst and Pittler, 1999; Holmes et al, 2002; Wolfe and Herzberg, 1996).

The choice of treatment, including the application of specific essential oils, appears largely to be made through the accepted knowledge-base of a therapy, or personal experience. There is often no clear evidence that this knowledge has been objectively tested. A few studies suggest that aromatherapy massage may benefit most people with dementia and, importantly, their carers (Free and Chambers, 2001; Kilstoff and Chenowith, 1998). However, these are not conclusive and it would appear that a more systematic and comprehensive approach to the evaluation of therapies is required.

Even if an intervention has been found to be safe and effective, personal preference has to be taken into account; complementary therapies are not liked by everyone. A person's capacity to give informed consent is a crucial issue in the care of people with dementia; the use of complementary therapies is no different to other treatments which involve choice and informed consent. Shah and Dickenson (1999) suggest that capacity to consent should be judged in relation to a specific decision, and according to whether a person is able to understand the information and the consequences of the decision. It is further suggested that assent, or agreement, may be sufficient in some circumstances where there is lack of capacity to consent. In the case of a person who does not have clear capacity to make such a decision, Fellows (1998) suggests that a person's known prior preferences should be determined; willing participation and apparent enjoyment could be interpreted as assent. All respondents in the survey sought consent before giving treatment, almost invariably from the client or family. What is unclear is how this consent was recorded, and whether the need for ongoing consent had been considered. This is important to all clients, but doubly so where there is memory impairment.

ARE THE SELECTED COMPLEMENTARY THERAPIES EFFECTIVE WHEN USED WITH PEOPLE WITH DEMENTIA?

It appears that complementary therapies are being used in the belief that they benefit the client in some way. The literature suggests that some herbal preparations, notably *Gingko biloba*, may improve cognitive functioning and delay the progress of dementia. Although the research evidence is not conclusive, there are strong indications that further studies are warranted. There are also encouraging results from recent trials of the essential oils of lemon balm (Ballard et al, 2002) and lavender (Holmes et al, 2002). However, herbal medicine involves the prescription of more complex and individual remedies. A few responses were gained from herbal medicine practitioners, who suggested that a specific active ingredient could not be identified as the whole person was to be assessed and treated. It seems that herbal medicine is rarely used in the field of dementia care, unless specifically requested by the family.

Responses to the questionnaire indicate that massage, aromatherapy, reflexology and healing have all produced positive effects. These might be physical or might relate to a client's cognitive functioning or quality of life. It appeared that clients talked more lucidly, interacted more freely and were generally happier. It is true that these observations were subjective and not systematically collected. However, there appeared to be some agreement between carers and therapists regarding these effects, and nursing homes and other clinical units were evidently prepared to continue supporting the therapies.

What is not clear is whether it is the action of the therapy itself which causes the effect. Comments about the relationship between client and therapist, and the importance of time and touch, raise questions regarding exactly what is effective. It may be physical contact or one-to-one attention that creates the outcome, with massage or reflexology providing a legitimate opportunity. It could be said that this does not matter as long as the effect is beneficial. However, more precise knowledge regarding the effect of any intervention might lead to more appropriate or precise use of skills and time. It is evident that further studies are required if these effects and differences are to be identified.

SHOULD COMPLEMENTARY THERAPIES BE OFFERED TO PEOPLE WITH DEMENTIA?

The findings suggest that therapies are enjoyed, and have a positive effect on the quality of life and relationships of clients and carers. If there is no chemical substance involved and informed consent can be assured, it could be asked whether there is any good reason for not using a complementary therapy. If a herbal preparation such as an essential oil is used, but its safety is not in doubt and it has been prescribed for a client by a knowledgeable practitioner, the same principles might apply.

Therapies may be simply vehicles for pleasant experiences but, if they have beneficial effects on relationships and mood, this might be adequate justification for their use. There may be no conclusive evidence for the effectiveness of therapies which involve physical contact but, if they are safe, enjoyed, and improve quality of life for clients and carers, surely they can be regarded as therapeutic.

Therapists and their equipment are an additional expense, often borne by families. This appears to restrict the frequency or access to therapies. It has been reported that medication can be reduced with the use of complementary therapies, but there is no evidence that the relative costs of drugs, essential oils, time and expertise have been estimated. It could also be anticipated that any improvement in behaviour, such as reduction in wandering or agitation, would have a significant impact on workload in some settings, and therefore on costs. Rigorous cost-benefit studies in complementary therapies are rare (White, 1996); but there is a pressing need for accurate and reliable data. A wider perspective on financial issues might include the effects on carers' health and the likelihood of a person with dementia remaining at home.

When all relevant factors are entered into the equation, it may be found that the addition of a complementary therapist to a care team will prove cost-effective. However, the choice of therapist raises issues of competence and suitability.

WHO SHOULD BE PRACTISING COMPLEMENTARY THERAPIES WITH PEOPLE WITH DEMENTIA?

Although there is currently a move to regulate the major complementary therapies, including herbal medicine, there is little control of therapists in the UK. There are also wide differences across Europe, regarding who may practice, and whether unconventional medicine is accepted or funded by the main health service (Monckton, 1999). This means that a carer or clinical unit may have difficulty in identifying a competent and well-prepared practitioner. However, all the selected therapies have professional organisations which approve courses or practitioners, and generally insist that their members carry indemnity insurance.

There appears to be an increase in the number of health care professionals with an interest in complementary therapies; nearly half (41) the respondents were registered as health care professionals. However, only 21 were offering a therapy as part of their practice. The others may have chosen to be independent practitioners, or it may be difficult for them to practise due to lack of acceptance or finance. Certainly, some complementary therapists reported difficulty in gaining access to clients in residential care, and some health care professionals lacked support for the integration of a therapy into their work. However, this was not universal.

People with dementia are a vulnerable population; they usually have the physiological changes of old age, and a cognitive deficit. They are likely to be receiving medical treatment for other pathologies. Complementary therapists might be prepared for practice in this specialism through additional knowledge of older people, drugs and dementia care; orthodox professionals who intend to integrate a therapy into their clinical practice may be advised to undertake a university-based course which encourages evaluation of the accepted knowledge-base of a therapy.

CONCLUSIONS

As yet, not enough is known about the actions of complementary therapies. Further research is required in order to identify the factors which make a difference, and allow for more specific prescriptions. It may also be pertinent to explore the use of alternative approaches, such as herbal or anthroposophical medicine, and those treatments which have long been used in traditional models of healing.

However, even from this small self-selected sample, there appears to be sufficient evidence to recommend the careful introduction of complementary therapies into the care of people with dementia. With due attention to issues of safety and the importance of informed consent, these therapies may have much to offer when seeking to improve quality of life for clients and their carers. The additional expense may be offset by other benefits. They can be used to good effect by residential homes, day centres and community services, and professional organisations and colleges can help in finding suitably qualified therapists who would benefit from being regarded as full members of the caring team.

REFERENCES

Ballard C, O'Brien J, Reichelt K, Perry E. Aromatherapy as a safe and effective treatment for the management of agitation in severe dementia: the results of a double blind, placebo controlled trial with Melissa. *Journal of Clinical Psychiatry* 2002;63(7):553–8.

Brooker DJ, Snape M, Johnson E et al. Single case evaluation of the effects of aromatherapy and massage on disturbed behaviour in severe dementia. *British Journal of Clinical Psychology* 1997;36:287–96.

Burleigh S, Armstrong C. On the scent of a useful therapy. *Journal of Dementia Care* 1997;5(5):21–3.

Campbell A. A critique of assumptions made about complementary medicine. In: *Examining Complementary Medicine*, Vickers A (ed). Cheltenham, UK: Stanley Thornes (Publishers) Ltd, 1998; 147–55.

Central & Cecil Housing Trust. *Health alternatives for older people: a pilot project.* Richmond, Surrey, 1996.

Ernst E (ed). *Complementary medicine: an objective appraisal.* Oxford: Butterworth-Heinemann, 1996.

Ernst E. Herbal medications for common ailments in the elderly. *Drugs and Aging* 1999;15(6):423–8.

Ernst E, Pittler MH. Gingko biloba for dementia: a systematic review of double-blind placebo-controlled trials. *Clinical Drug Investigation* 1999;77: 301–8.

Fellows LK. Competency and consent in dementia. *Journal of the American Geriatrics Society* 1998;46:922–6.

Free T, Chambers L. The sweet smell of success. *Journal of Dementia Care* 2001;9(3):9–10.

Holmes C, Hopkins V, Hensford C et al. Lavender oil as a treatment for agitated behaviour in severe dementia: a placebo controlled trial. *International Journal of Geriatric Psychiatry* 2002;17(4):305–8.

Jinzhou T. Research into the treatment of vascular dementia in China using traditional therapies. *Age and Ageing* 1998;27:247–50.

Kilstoff K, Chenoweth L. New approaches to health and well-being for dementia day-care clients, family carers and day-care staff. *International Journal of Nursing Practice* 1998;4(2):70–83.

Lawless J. *The Illustrated Encyclopaedia of Essential Oils.* Shaftesbury, Dorset: Element Books Ltd, 1995.

Le Bars PL, Meinhard K, Itil KZ. A 26-week analysis of a Double-Blind, Placebo-Controlled Trial of the Gingko Biloba Extract EGb 761in Dementia. *Dementia and Geriatric Cognitive Disorders* 2000;11:230–7.

Letzel H, Haan J, Feil WB. Nootropics: efficacy and tolerability of products from three active substance classes. *Journal of Drug Development in Clinical Practice* 1996;8:77–94.

Mitchell S. Aromatherapy's effectiveness in disorders associated with dementia. *The International Journal of Aromatherapy* 1993;5(2):20–3.

Monckton J (ed). *The final report of the European Commission sponsored COST project on Unconventional Medicine*, 1999. www.rccm.org.uk.

Oken BS, Storzbach DM, Kaye JA. The efficacy of *Gingko biloba* on cognitive function in Alzheimer Disease. *Archives of Neurology* 1998;55(11):1409–15.

Ott BR, Owens NJ. Complementary and alternative medicines for Alzheimer's disease. *Journal of Geriatric Psychiatry and Neurology* 1998;11(4):163–73.

Perrin T. *An exploration of the role of occupational therapy in the care of persons with severe dementia, and an investigation into the impact upon the well-being of such persons, of a range of occupations commonly used in dementia care.* Unpublished PhD thesis, University of Bradford, 1997.

Perry NS, Houghton PJ, Sampson J et al. In-vitro activity of *Slavia lavandulaefolia* (Spanish sage) relevant to treatment of Alzheimer's disease. *Journal of Pharmacy and Pharmacology* 2001;53(10):1347–56.

Perry EK, Pickering AT, Wang WW et al. Medicinal plants and Alzheimer's disease: from Ethnobotany to Phytotherapy. *Journal of Pharmacy and Pharmacology* 1999;51(5):527–34.

Perry EK, Pickering AT, Wang WW. Medicinal plants and Alzheimer's disease: integrating ethnobotanical and contemporary scientific evidence. *The Journal of Alternative and Complementary Medicine* 1998;4(4):419–28.

Price S, Price L. *Aromatherapy for Health Professionals.* Edinburgh: Churchill Livingstone, 1999.

Shah A, Dickenson D. The capacity to make decisions in dementia: some contemporary issues. *International Journal of Geriatric Psychiatry* 1999;14:803–6.

Snyder M, Egan EC, Burns KR. Efficacy of hand massage in decreasing agitation behaviors associated with care activities in persons with dementia. *Geriatric Nursing,* 1995a;16(2):60–3.

Snyder M, Egan EC, Burns KR. Interventions for decreasing agitation behaviors in persons with dementia. *Journal of Gerontological Nursing* 1995b;July:34–40.

Thorgrimsen L, Spector A, Orrell M, Wiles A. Aromatherapy for dementia (Protocol for a Cochrane Review). In: *The Cochrane Library* Issue 1, 2003. Oxford: Update Software, 2003.

Tobin P. Aromatherapy and its application. *The Lamp* 1995;52(5):34.

Wallcraft J. *Healing Minds.* London: Mental Health Foundation, 1998.

Wang D, Huang X, Du S. A clinical trial on yu cong tang in treatment of senile dementia. *Journal of Traditional Chinese Medicine* 1999;19(1):32–8.

West B, Brockman S. The calming power of aromatherapy. *Journal of Dementia Care* 1994;2(2):20–2.

White A. Do complementary therapies offer value for money? In: *Complementary Medicine: An Objective Appraisal,* Ernst E (ed). Oxford: Butterworth-Heinemann, 1996; 89–105.

Wilkinson J. Personal communication, 27.3.2003.

Wolfe N, Herzberg J. Can aromatherapy oils promote sleep in severely demented patients? *International Journal of Geriatric Psychiatry* 1996;11(10):926–7.

CHAPTER 39

SUSTAINING THE COCOON: THE EMOTIONAL INOCULATION PRODUCED BY COMPLEMENTARY THERAPIES IN PALLIATIVE CARE

Marion Garnett

INTRODUCTION

Since the 1960s, the development of the hospice movement in the UK has occurred concurrently with the developing interest of UK society in complementary medicine. Studies have shown that palliative care has become one of the key areas where complementary therapies are used (Avis, 2001; Rankin-Box, 1997). Therapies commonly used in cancer and palliative care include: massage (Gray, 2000); aromatherapy (Wilkinson et al, 1999) and reflexology (Avis, 2001).

Many of the justifications given for the use of complementary therapies contain both a physiological and a psychological explanation. For example, theories concerning muscle relaxation hypothesize that physiological relaxation of muscles can lead to a decrease in psychological feelings of stress and anxiety (Benson, 1975). This paper acknowledges and, then, sets aside the well-documented intertwining of the physiological and psychological aspects of the application of complementary therapies, in order to use the conceptual vocabulary developed by Giddens (1990, 1991) to illuminate different aspects of the use of complementary therapies. Giddens' ideas provide another way in which the use of complementary therapies in palliative care can be understood.

Edited from an article in *European Journal of Cancer Care* 2003;12:129–36.

Explanation of Giddens (1990, 1991) conceptual vocabulary

Although 'trust' is, in some respects, similar to 'confidence', it is not the same because confidence is based on 'weak inductive knowledge' (Giddens, 1990). *Trust* involves something other than just a cognitive understanding. With trust, things cannot purely be worked out on a cognitive basis it becomes necessary, at some point, to take a leap of faith. Giddens argues that trust operates in environments of risk in which varying degrees of protection against dangers can be achieved. Focused encounters, including those in which healthcare professionals work, involve the need not only for trust in healthcare professionals to be sustained but also involve the need for healthcare professionals to present themselves as being *trustworthy*.

Ontological security refers to the feelings that most humans have in the continuity of their self identity and in the constancy of their surroundings (Giddens, 1990). It is an emotional not a cognitive phenomenon. It is rooted in the unconscious and is strongly related to trust. If trust and ontological security are lacking, the outcome is likely to be increased *existential anxiety*, as, feelings of ontological security and existential anxiety co-exist in ambivalence (Giddens, 1990). Existential anxieties are anxieties concerned with the basic parameters of human life such as existence and being (Giddens, 1991). Examples of existential anxieties include questions such as: why am I? why am I here? what is going to happen to me? what is going to happen to the world?

If people have existential anxieties they are likely to feel ontologically insecure. According to Giddens, as people go through life they are, for the most part, able to suppress existential anxieties and become ontologically secure by receiving, in infancy, an *emotional inoculation* from their care-takers. This inoculation, which contains the ability to have basic trust, acts like a *protective cocoon*, which people carry round with them throughout life and can draw on when faced with difficulties (Giddens, 1991).

Fateful moments are times that are likely to be difficult. These are moments when individuals stand at a crossroad in their existence. Here, a person may learn some information with fateful consequences or may have to make decisions with major consequences (Giddens, 1991). Routinized activities, which help to keep existential anxieties at bay, are interrupted. They are times when a person is likely to experience the *return of the repressed* and life may appear meaningless (Giddens, 1991).

Diagnosis of a terminal illness is likely to be a particularly threatening fateful moment. It is a time when experts are consulted and trust in experts is needed. Although there may be an expertise concerning dying that representatives of the palliative care expert system can draw on when, for example, they say things like 'we'll make you comfortable', 'we can take your pain away', the lay person knows the experts cannot be trusted to take away the threat of death itself.

Objectives

The aim of this study is to explore, from a medical sociological perspective, the use of complementary therapies by palliative care nurses. This paper shows how the conceptual vocabulary developed by Giddens (1990, 1991) relating to trust, ontological security, existential anxiety and the importance of protective cocoons can facilitate our understanding of the use of complementary therapies in palliative care. The purpose is to use these concepts to enable the use of complementary therapies by palliative care nurses to be seen in new ways. These are ways (such as the use of complementary therapies being seen as cocoon maintenance), which, without the use of such a conceptual vocabulary, may remain hidden.

METHODS

This is a qualitative study in which, in accordance with researchers who promote the building of bridges between methodological perspectives (Coffey and Atkinson, 1996; Seale, 1999), methodological approaches have been combined.

A sample of palliative care nurses was recruited by writing to the Senior Nurse Managers of a selected section of the 1996 Directory of Hospice and Palliative Care Services (Hospice Information Service, 1996) and asking if there were any qualified nurses in their unit who practised a complementary therapy who would be willing to be interviewed by me. I interviewed 18 palliative care nurses who carried out a complementary therapy; five nurse managers, four doctors and four volunteer/freelance complementary therapists. The interviewees came from 16 different hospice/palliative care units. All interviewees were women except three. The main therapies practised were massage, aromatherapy and reflexology. The interviews I conducted were semi-structured and were informed by feminist interviewing practice. Interviews also fitted, theoretically, into the style of 'active interviewing' developed by Holstein and Gubrium (1995, 1997). Much of the analysis of the interview narratives was carried out from a discourse analytic perspective.

RESULTS

Complementary therapies and the issue of trust

Some interviewees presented themselves as being trusted because they were nurses. Several interviewees presented it as being necessary for the patient to have trust in the therapist in order for complementary therapies to be carried out. Sometimes this was articulated by using the words trust, faith, etc. For example:

> '. . . you've got to build up a RAPPORT with that patient and they've got to have some sort of FAITH and TRUST in you because, I mean, they're BARING ALL, so I need to get to KNOW my patient over a day or so before I could SUGGEST, maybe would they like their feet done . . .'. (RO) (Nurse, therapist)

Sometimes the impression of trust was obtained more from interpretation of the narrative rather than the vocabulary used. For example:

> '. . . sometimes they won't tell the doctor and they won't even tell the family but they'll tell the reflexologist something'. (NP) (Nurse therapist)

According to Giddens (1990), behaviour which is likely to generate trust includes:

- being warm and open,
- being unflappable,
- being full of integrity,
- being seen as trustworthy, and
- having the appropriate demeanour for the work in which engaged.

Interviewees presented these qualities as being necessary for complementary therapists. For example:

> '. . . it's like having a warm bottle if you're cold'. (QR) (Nurse therapist)

> '. . . in a way they are giving themselves to you, aren't they, to allow you to do it to them and... they're making themselves vulnerable really, to let, to touch anybody is really actually quite an intimate thing to do and it's, very much involves a lot of trust'. (GN) (Nurse therapist)

Nurse therapists present themselves as having a demeanour of care and love. This could be considered an appropriate demeanour for those working in palliative care. For example:

'. . . it's caring that says, you know, I care about you now, you know, together we want to try and make you better'. (BC) (Nurse therapist)

'. . . it's, it's a loving, a loving exchange and (that's) very important'. (GN) (Nurse therapist)

Nurse therapists not only present themselves as being involved in activities which, according to Giddens' criteria (1990), are likely to generate trust but also present themselves as thinking these activities to be important.

Ontological security; protective cocoon

Interviewees talked about complementary therapies helping patients feel 'looked after'. Words used by interviewees to indicate that complementary therapies helped patients feel looked after are shown in Table 39.1.

Table 39.1 Words used by interviewees to indicate that complementary therapies helped patients feel looked after

'comforted', 'comfortable', 'supported', 'secure', 'safe', 'cared (for)', 'loved', 'nurtured', 'cocoon(ed)', 'cherished', 'pampered', 'touched'

For example:

'they go off to sleep . . . they have relaxed . . . they just feel, sort of, nurtured, you know' (PQ) (Nurse therapist)

'. . . I found I was doing something constructive to allay their fears and anxieties and they felt comfortable and safe because I was THERE. . . it was the comfort and security' (RO) (Nurse therapist)

In the following example CD uses contrastive rhetoric to show the difference patients may feel between orthodox medical treatment ('abused', 'mutilated', 'invaded', 'hurt'), compared to complementary therapies ('pampered', 'cared for', 'cherished', 'not hurt'):

'. . . as a lady said to me, "I know they're (orthodox medical treatments) done for my good but in the end, after a long period of time it's, I'm abused, my body has been abused and mutilated and when

> somebody comes along and does something like that (complementary therapies), it's like pampering, it's just.". I suppose it makes them feel cared for and CHERISHED and such a change from an invasive procedure and doesn't hurt, in fact, it's the very opposite'. (CD) (Nurse therapist)

The following narrative is full of the language of making someone feel cared for or, in the terms of Giddens, ontologically secure. Words such as *'rock'*, *'nurturing'*, *'cuddled'*, *'warm'*, *'cocoon'*, *'hold'* being particularly expressive

> '. . . if you rock someone, you put them in touch with that very innate, first feeling of, of nurturing and, and if you cuddled them, if you made them warm, if you, if you cocoon them, often I will, I'll cocoon someone in the duvet or in the blankets or whatever and then I'll be at their feet and I'll, I'll firmly hold their feet and I'll rock them and it, it's so insidious that people just think you're holding their feet but it's, it's going through that body so finely and, and they love it and they'll, they'll, they, people will say how wonderful it is'. (PL) (Freelance nurse therapist)

In view of Giddens' concept of how a *'protective cocoon'* can be used to filter out 'potential dangers impinging from the external world and which is founded psychologically upon basic trust' (Giddens, 1991), PL's use of the word *'cocoon'* is particularly significant.

In the following example PL uses contrastive rhetoric to compare the caring she is giving now, when she is carrying out a complementary therapy, to the care the patient felt as a child but probably has not experienced for a long time. This is a theme which occurs in several of the interviews, that patients will not have experienced caring such as that which is given through the application of complementary therapies, for a long time:

> 'Afterwards they're usually amazed at, at how, how good they feel, they have a lovely, often they'll have a smile on their face which will, is the nurturing, it's, it's, it's, I think it's the nurturing that we've all had as little ones and they haven't had that nurturing for a long time and the more, sometimes it, it's just giving them that nurturing and they think "WOW, wow, this is lovely" '. (PL) (Freelance therapist)

The view that the care the patient is receiving now may not have been experienced for a long time can also be seen in the following example:

> 'You know, complementary therapies have always been for women, you know, women are the mums, are the nurturers' (MN) (Nurse therapist).

Associated with the presentation that complementary therapies help people to feel loved and cared for, is the view that complementary therapies also help people to feel better. This was a key presentation by many of the interviewees. For example:

> '. . . it's such a nice thing to do for them and they all sort of feel BETTER after it'. (EF) (Nurse therapist)

Other words used to imply complementary therapies helped patients feel better include that complementary therapies help people feel '*good*', '*uplifted*', '*valued*', '*worthy*'.

Existential anxieties

Several interviewees said that patients have existential anxieties. They also presented complementary therapies as being able to help with these.

Interviewees spoke of helping patients to feel less angry, less frightened, more hopeful, more peaceful and more accepting of death. For example:

> '. . . we do progressive muscle relaxation and then move on from that into a guided imagery journey helping them to use their senses and finding a place where they feel at peace and safe. . .' (MN) (Nurse therapist)

In the following example, KL presents complementary therapies as helping a patient in a spiritual dimension:

> '(referring to the application of CTs). . . their emotions, very much so, they come out, their fear of death, their anger at why they're dying, you know . . . their loss in faith, often comes up . . . so they can talk this over with you and you can turn round and say "well, you know, it isn't God that's doing this, it's the circumstances, you know, we're cellular beings and cells alter and because of this, this is a thing that has happened". (KL) (Nurse therapist)

Fateful moments

Giddens states that, at fateful moments, people often have recourse to traditional activities and familiar modes of activity. Although complementary therapies are probably not familiar to many palliative care patients, I am suggesting that, at the fateful moment of being terminally ill, patients may want to engage in 'traditional', 'more understandable' activities such as massage and aromatherapy as well as modern technological medicine. The use of complementary therapies in palliative care also fits in with Giddens argument that fateful moments are often times of reskilling and empowerment. He states that, at these times, individuals are likely to encounter expert systems such as counselling, which focus on reconstruction of selfidentity (Giddens, 1991). Several of my interviewees presented using complementary therapies in conjunction with counselling or presented the giving of a complementary therapy as an opportunity to help reconstruct a self-identity. For example:

> 'I actually a few years ago did a counselling course because . . . I found the need in my own private practice before I came into hospitals, that people used, you know, therapies, body therapies as an opportunity to talk, as a time to talk and therefore I felt the need to go and develop some active listening skills' (MN) (Nurse therapist)

DISCUSSION

Interviewees presented the qualities Giddens (1990) identified as being likely to generate trust as being necessary qualities for complementary therapists. This raises questions over the implication of complementary therapies in the generation of trust in palliative care. In broad terms, it can be argued that the application of a complementary therapy is a visible statement to its receiver that those who work in the 'expert system' of palliative care actually care about the patient and can be trusted. Their use can be interpreted as an effort to encourage people to have trust in their formal carers and to trust that they are working within a principle of beneficence and can be trusted to 'do the right thing'. In an era in which expert systems, including those of palliative care, may be 'vulnerable to a sense of doubt' (Clark and Seymour, 1999) and, in an area of health care, palliative care, where, in the relationship between patient and carer, trust is of particular importance (Randall and Downie, 1996), it can be argued that any activity in which workers engage which is likely to generate trust is likely to be beneficial.

However, in narrower terms, drawing on the concepts outlined in this paper, one of the answers to the question concerning the implication of complementary therapies in the generation of trust in palliative care can be interpreted as lying in the links Giddens makes between trust, ontological security, existential anxiety, protective cocoons and fateful moments.

By engaging in the application of complementary therapies, nurse therapists act in a trustworthy way. They try and help people to feel loved, cared for, looked after and nurtured. We can see the application of a complementary therapy as an emotional inoculation, similar to the emotional inoculation Giddens speaks about an infant receiving, from its caretaker, in childhood (Giddens, 1991). The application of a complementary therapy can be seen in terms of a 'booster' injection being received, by an adult, from their professional caretaker, in time of particular need. This injection serves to sustain a person's protective cocoon at a time of particular vulnerability. It has the effect of maintaining the person's shield against feelings of existential anxiety and ontological insecurity. Such sustenance of the cocoon not only helps a patient to feel better but also facilitates the ability of the patient to maintain trust, including, reflexively, trust in the healthcare system. There is a certain irony, here, that patients' appreciation of complementary therapies is often presented in the interview narratives as being due to complementary therapies being unlike orthodox medicine, in so far as they do not involve injections or invasive actions. Interpretation of the narratives in this way shows that, similar to orthodox medicine, complementary therapies can be interpreted as being invasive but at an emotional rather than a purely physiological level.

The presentation that complementary therapies can help patients feel nurtured also fits in with the work of Giddens (1991) concerning the sequestration of experience. He states that in late modern times, experiences, such as sickness and death, which are likely to raise potentially disturbing existential questions, are routinely hidden from view. Thus, when a patient enters a hospice, death is less sequestered and existential anxieties and ontological insecurities are therefore likely to increase. This argument may be particularly relevant if, as Lawton (2000) argues, those who die in a hospice are those patients who have (and therefore are also possibly likely to witness), particularly difficult trajectories of dying. Entering a hospice is a time when people are likely to be especially in need of intensive 'cocoon maintenance'.

CONCLUSION

The use of the conceptual vocabulary developed by Giddens enables aspects of the application of complementary therapies in palliative care to be interpreted within a theoretical framework which, without the use of such concepts, could not so easily be understood.

Using this vocabulary, a parallel can be drawn between the emotional inoculation a child receives from its personal caregiver in infancy, which enables the child to be surrounded by a protective cocoon which it can carry around with it throughout life and enables the child to have basic trust, and the emotional inoculation a patient receives from a professional caregiver at a time when the protection afforded by their cocoon is likely to be at risk.

By applying these ideas to the use of complementary therapies in palliative care it is possible to argue that, in an area of health care such as palliative care, where patients are likely to be facing exceptional existential anxieties, an exceptional system (the use of complementary therapies), for dealing with these anxieties has evolved. Although most areas of health care deal, at some time, with patients who are dying it is possible that due to the innovative, holistic ideology of the hospice movement in the 1970s and 1980s together with the nurses who worked there at that time being interested in developing new identities and new ways of working, the conditions, in palliative care, became particularly suitable for the use of complementary therapies to emerge.

REFERENCES

Avis A. RCN Survey Interim Report. *RCN Newsletter In Touch*. Autumn 2001.

Benson H. *The Relaxation Response*. New York: Avon, 1975.

Clark D, Seymour J. *Reflections on Palliative Care*. Buckingham: Open University Press, 1999.

Coffey A, Atkinson P. *Making Sense of Qualitative Data*. Thousand Oaks: Sage, 1996.

Giddens A. *The Consequences of Modernity*. Cambridge: Polity Press, 1990.

Giddens A. *Modernity and Self-Identity*. Cambridge: Polity Press, 1991.

Gray R. The use of massage in palliative care. *Complementary Therapies in Nursing and Midwifery* 2000;6:77–82.

Holstein J, Gubrium J. *The Active Interview*. Thousand Oaks CA: Sage, 1995.

Holstein J, Gubrium J. Active, interviewing. In: *Qualitative Research Theory, Method and Practice*, Silverman D (ed). London: Sage, 1997.

Hospice Information Service. *1996 Directory of Hospice and Palliative Care Services*. St Christopher's Hospice. Hospice Information Service, London, 1996.

Lawton J. *The Dying Process*. London: Routledge, 2000.

Randall F, Downie R. *Palliative Care Ethics*. Oxford: Oxford University Press, 1996.

Rankin-Box D. Therapies in practice: a survey assessing nurses' use of complementary therapies. *Complementary Therapies in Nursing and Midwifery* 1997;3:92–9.

Seale CF. *The Quality of Qualitative Research*. London: Sage, 1999.

Wilkinson S, Aldridge J, Salmon I et al. An evaluation of aromatherapy massage in palliative care. *Palliative Medicine* 1999;13:409–17.

CHAPTER 40

THE EMPOWERING NATURE OF REIKI AS A COMPLEMENTARY THERAPY

Leslie Nield-Anderson and Ann Ameling

Reiki is an ancient healing method with roots in both Chinese Medicine and Christian healing. It is a treatment used by individuals as an alternative and complement to Western medical treatment. Reiki has increased in popularity over the past decade, but remains understudied. Methodological and philosophical reasons for why it is difficult to conduct research on the efficacy of Reiki are discussed. The reasons for the increased success of Reiki as an alternative and complementary healing method in the Western world are addressed, as well as the practice of Reiki as a healing method for self and others.

Just for today I will give thanks for my many blessings.
Just for today I will not worry.
Just for today I will not be angry.
Just for today I will do my work honestly.
Just for today I will be kind to my neighbor and every living thing.
Five Principles for Reiki Practitioners (Arnold and Nevius, 1982)

HISTORICAL ROOTS

Reiki is a healing method with roots in both Chinese medicine and Christian healing. Reiki, as practiced in the world today, was synthesized

Edited from an article in *Holistic Nurse Practitioner* 2000;14(3):21–9.

in the mid 19th century by Dr. Mikao Usui, a Japanese monk and a Christian who attempted to bring to the world the hands on healing method used by Buddha and by Christ in their healing practices. It is a treatment that has been used by individuals as an alternative to contemporary Western medical treatment, and as a complementary or adjunctive treatment to medical protocols (Rowland, 1998). The term Reiki means Universal Energy or Life Force. The practice is a simple one that, by a gentle laying on of the practitioner's hands, an individual is reconnected to Universal Energy or Life Force. This Universal Energy connects to the body's innate power of healing to promote self-healing. Universal Energy, sometimes referred to as Chi or Ki in other systems of healing, is inherent in all life forms. The Reiki practitioner is a facilitator, not a provider, of this healing energy. In Reiki there are no complicated diagnostics. The energy that is facilitated through the practitioner's hands goes naturally to any spot in the recipient's body in which it is needed. There is no attempt made to evaluate the recipient's energy field or condition. There is no manipulation of the recipient's body or energy field. The practitioner simply places hands in a series of positions on the recipient's body with the intention of facilitating self-healing. Reiki is, therefore, within a long tradition of gentle therapies that seek to provide comfort and healing through compassionate touch.

Modem Reiki was introduced in Japan in the 19th century by Dr. Mikao Usui. From there it was brought to the United States at the time of World War II by Mrs. Hawayo Takata. From a modest start in the 1940s of a handful of Reiki master teachers, it has spread rapidly in recent years. Currently there are at least seven major national and international Reiki organizations. In recent years, there have been numerous variations of 'traditional' Usui Reiki. Some of these are simply variations on the traditional techniques advocating some differences in relatively minor points such as specific hand positions, the number of hand positions, or the sequence of hand positions. Other variations reconcile Reiki as a combination of touch and other complementary therapies such as aromatherapy, music, massage, therapeutic touch, prayer, crystals or psychotherapy. It is important, therefore, in reading about Reiki, or in reporting studies or case examples about Reiki to understand specifically what has been defined as Reiki treatment (Rowland, 1998).

REIKI: AN ANCIENT HEALING ART

Individuals tend to seek the services of a complementary practitioner for chronic conditions (Eisenberg et al, 1993). Chronic illnesses generally require frequent physician visits, hospital admissions, and dependency on health care services. Therefore, the need for greater control and participation through choice, are particularly relevant when individuals suffer from more enduring illnesses (Astin, 1998). Individuals attempting to manage their lives, adopt healthier life styles, and maintain self-sufficiency seek health care practices and practitioners they believe will enhance the quality of their lives in these ways. Research (De Ridder et al, 1997) indicates that a professional relationship with a health care provider that is based on mutual trust and respect between the two, as equal partners in decision making, are essential aspects of an individual's coping with illness. Autonomy and independence are supported when individuals remain actively involved in decisions concerning their health rather than assuming a passive role. As De Ridder et al (1997) conclude, individuals see themselves as powerless when they feel insignificant and an anonymous number.

An individual seeking complementary therapies has freedom of choice between methods and practitioners, which fosters a sense of autonomy. The inherent aspects of Eastern healing methods of respect, harmony, and individuality of intervention regimes empower recipients.

Individuals, as unique dynamic energy fields, are constantly interacting with one another and with the environment (Rogers, 1970). Schwartz and Russek (1997) describe two types of energy – kinetic and potential. Kinetic energy refers to energy that is expressed when an object accelerates and potential energy is the energy that is potentially available. Energy is the ability to do work and influences the motion and functioning of systems. These energy types can be applied to the practice and teachings of Reiki. In the practice of Reiki, there is a flow of energy from the giver, a Reiki practitioner, to a receiver. Reiki practitioners, as part of their training process, receive attunements, or initiations, that are delivered by a Reiki Master. Each person has Life Force and potential healing powers. During attunements (spiritual, sacred, and confidential rituals), a Reiki Master uses symbols and mantras to create higher vibrations, or accelerate an ability for channeling the Universal Life Energy – attunements, transform an individual's potential for healing and channeling. Attunements offer a Master a structure to activate and increase a recipients' channeling ability. The attunements empower and heighten a practitioner's ability to serve in the healing process. Once activated all a practitioner needs to do, to connect with the healing Life Force, is to place his or her hands on his or her self or someone else. The Life Force automatically flows from practitioner to recipient in abundance, never depleting the Reiki practitioner.

Reiki is different than other forms of healing interventions because of its simplicity. There are three levels, or degrees, of Reiki. Level one, or the First Degree, can be taught in a weekend, and the Second Degree in a day. The Third Degree, the master level, prepares the practitioner to teach Reiki and involves several stages. It is during the First Degree a beginning practitioner learns the history of Reiki, receives attunements for this level, is instructed on the basic hand positions for self Reiki, and the hand positions for giving Reiki to another. The Second Degree involves instruction on absent, or distant healing, and the practitioner receives unique attunements for this level.

Healing during a Reiki session is synchronic – both the practitioner and recipient are mutually healed as the Life Force is channeled through the practitioner. Healing occurs on physical, emotional, mental, and spiritual levels, evolving toward balance and harmony. The practitioner does not direct the energy through his or her body to specific areas, but rather Reiki acknowledges the wisdom of life forms to receive and use energy where it is most needed. Each practitioner and recipient experiences the energy flow differently. Each has his or her own unique energy field and needs, and therefore is influenced by Reiki in different ways. As stated earlier, Reiki recipients have reported a wide variety of experiences that have been described as warm sensations, blissful increased senses of well being, heightened perceptions of colors or sounds, or diminished sensations of emotional, mental and physical pain, among others. Healing takes place, however, whether an individual is cognizant of the process or not.

Reiki is not intrusive, does not demand any technology, can be practiced anywhere at any time, and does not require a practitioner or recipient to engage in verbal exchanges. Reiki is not for diagnosing disease conditions and therefore does not require a practitioner to collect information, and there are no body manipulations in a Reiki treatment. These attributes are beneficial for individuals that are stressed, highly anxious, have been involved in many difficult, intrusive, and often painful medical or surgical procedures, are fatigued, sedated, or unconscious. They are equally appropriate for children or adults.

REIKI AND HOLISTIC NURSING PRACTICE

As Jonas (1998) acknowledges, the increasing popularity of alternative and complementary therapies reflects the changing needs and values in Western health care practices. He stresses the importance of mainstream medicine continuing to incorporate alternative therapies into curriculums in order that the gap between physicians, scientists, and the public they serve does not broaden. From his perspective, a major strength that needs to be preserved from the practices of alternative therapists is their emphasis on self-healing and promotion of health. Wells-Federman (1996) lends support to Jonas' message, but points out that nursing has historically facilitated patients' self-care management and health maintenance. She posits that the present challenge for nursing is to examine the impact of nursing care on the mind, body, and spirit, to hone time-honored abilities, and to continue to develop assessment skills to more appropriately facilitate an individual's mind, body, and spirit development. Wells-Federman further stresses the unequivocal need for a health care provider to learn to care for themselves. She addresses the synchronic nature of fostering compassionate care for individuals, families, and communities, and compassionate care of self.

A basic premise in the practice of Reiki is that Reiki brings healing to oneself and others. As described earlier, during Reiki training for the First Degree, the beginner Reiki practitioner is taught hand positions for self-healing as well as for the healing of others. The healing of self and other is viewed as reciprocal and integral to the practice of Reiki. Practitioners model health promoting behaviors, to health care recipients, when they promote the healing process in themselves. By practicing self Reiki, practitioners keep mindful of their own need for healing, and the sacredness and unity of the body, mind, and spirit. Practitioners' reports, after self Reiki treatments, are similar to recipients' reported responses after a Reiki session given by another. For example, self Reiki has been described as increasing relaxation, decreasing stress, increasing feelings of warmth, expanding ones' sense of well-being, deepening of insights, and enhanced senses of empowerment to face changes or expected hardships (Arnold, 1982; Barnett and Chambers, 1996; Rowland, 1998).

It is quite common for an individual interested in the practice of Reiki to report an initial distressful time with their own health or with the illness of a loved one before their knowledge of Reiki. These times are often described as frustrating and filled with a suffering unmatched in the individual's life, or a suffering equal to the loved one. The individual usually then goes on to describe a serendipitous discovery of Reiki, such as at a health fair, or a friend bestows a gift certificate for a Reiki healing session. The 'to be Reiki practitioner' often recounts an instant feeling of omniscience, spiritual experience, or remarkable and profound attraction, to this ancient sacred healing technique. They become fascinated by Reiki's loving, respectful, and gentle abilities. The empowering nature of Reiki, as a complementary therapy, resides in its simplicity, applicability, and ability to be generalized. Described earlier, Reiki practitioners need merely to begin with a compassionate intent and lay their hands on themselves or another. This gentle touch is soothing, nurturing, and restoring.

To illustrate the above, the following is an example of a recent and not untypical Reiki session. It involves one of the authors (L. Nield-Anderson) delivering a Reiki treatment to a dear friend that was dying of breast cancer.

CASE STUDY

GW was at the last stages of her earth life. One of her daughters called me and told me that the hospice had informed the family that GW would probable die within the week. I had been performing distant healing with GW for several months for another chronic illness. Her newly discovered breast cancer and the speed of its metastases were astonishing.

Being with GW, her children, and their spouses seemed natural. They knew me as their mother's good friend. It was a privilege to participate in GW's process of saying goodbye. Her children wanted me there to share their mother's dying process with them and their mother. I had the privilege of changing wet sheets, covering and uncovering her as her body temperature changed, and giving her sips of water. The room was filled with what GW had given to all of us – love.

GW had always been authentic and honest, and she was no different at this time. She let us all know when she was uncomfortable and when she was frightened, commenting at one point, 'I don't know about this dying– it seems right now dying is just about as hard as living – but – I have never done this before – not that I remember.'

At her bedside, GW's eldest daughter from Texas, also a Reiki practitioner, and I gave Reiki to GW. Her other children were in the room watching. They were participating in the Reiki session, although not directly laying on their hands, with their curiosity and obvious respect and appreciation. I do not know how long we laid our hands on GW. We both lost track of time. We both ended the session because we were so warm. The room felt like 100 degrees, and both of our hands seemed to be burning. Anne and I took our hands off GW without either knowing the other was doing this. We also did not converse during the Reiki session. It was only after the session had ended did we share the reason for ending. We also thought GW was asleep. Her eyes had been closed for quite sometime, her breathing was regular and slowed. As soon as we removed our hands, GW stirred and said 'what happened.' We both instantly realized that we had not only withdrawn our hands simultaneously, but we had not given GW any warning. When we removed our hands the room temperature felt like it had fallen, and GW noticed the energy shift, and it startled her. GW was still conscious, but drifted in and out. When she was alert she would converse and spend time with us and then drift off again. Her times away were getting longer.

After her daughter and I ended the Reiki session, GW did not say whether she felt better or not – she just let us know she knew we had ended the session. Several hours later a hospice nurse came to visit. It was the hospice nurse that said to GW, 'you seem much calmer and more relaxed than before.' GW answered 'yes after the Reiki I do feel calmer – more peaceful.'

I will miss GW. Missing her acknowledges her magnificence and profound contribution to my life. GW's permission to receive Reiki gave us a special way to connect and say goodbye that words could not. I am grateful to Reiki for providing this time with her, and grateful to GW for bringing Reiki to me.

REFERENCES

Arnold DL, Nevius S. *The Reiki Handbook*. Harrisburg, PA: PSI Press, 1982.

Astin J. Why patients use alternative medicine: Results of a national study. *JAMA* 1998;279(19):1548–53.

Barnett L, Chambers M. *Reiki Energy Medicine: Bringing Healing Touch into Home, Hospital, and Hospice*. Vermont: Healing Arts Press, 1996.

De Ridder D, Depla M, Severens P, Malsch M. Beliefs on coping with illness: A consumer's perspective. *Soc Sci Med* 1997;44(5):553–9.

Eisenberg D, Kessler R, Foster C et al. Unconventional medicine in the United States. *N Engl J Med* 1993;328:246–52.

Jonas WB. Alternative medicine – learning from the past, examining the present, advancing to the future. *JAMA* 1998;280(18):1616–17.

Rogers M. *An Introduction to the Theoretical Basis of Nursing*. Philadelphia: FA Davis, 1970.

Rowland AZ. *Traditional Reiki For Our Times: Practical Methods for Personal And Planetary Healing*. Rochester, VT: Healing Arts Press, 1998.

Schwartz GE, Russek LG. Dynamical energy systems and modem physics: Fostering the science and spirit of complementary and alternative medicine. *Alt Ther* 1997;3(3):46–56.

Wells-Federman CL. Awakening the nurse healer within. *Holist Nurs Pract* 1996;10(2):13–29.

CHAPTER 41

COMPLEMENTARY THERAPIES IN MATERNITY CARE

Lorraine Williams

Maternity services are unique within the provision of health services in the UK. They are also considered by some as one of the 'Cinderella' services, under resourced and often inadequately organised. There is also a growing concern that, in the UK, maternity care is in a state of crisis, resulting primarily from a chronic shortage of midwives to offer the support women need during this life-changing event (Revill, 2003).

The notion of normal, natural childbirth is becoming increasingly unusual in this age of high-tech medical management of pregnancy and birth with its advances in fertilisation techniques, embryonic and foetal surveillance systems. Pregnancy and birth are only perceived as normal in retrospect. The process of childbirth has become progressively more medicalised; interventions such as induction of labour and episiotomies are increasing, as are rates of caesarean sections and epidural analgesia (House of Commons Select Committee Provision of Maternity Services, 2003). It is difficult to believe that this is what women, health professionals, or the over burdened and cash-strapped health service wants. Now might be a good time to rethink the way that maternity services are organised and delivered. Many see the solution as involving more non-biomedical options of care, such as those offered by many complementary therapies, that may go some way towards improving the birth experience and increasing the opportunity of having a safe, normal, natural and drug-free birth.

Health care for pregnant women and the newborn infant is undertaken largely within the National Health Service and is the responsibility of the

This chapter has been commissioned by the editors for inclusion in this Reader.

obstetric team with the midwife taking primary or lead responsibility for normal care. Given the numerous health professions involved in the teams providing maternity care, including, for example, the paediatrician, anaesthetist, GP, physiotherapist, nutritionist, health visitor and radiographer, it is unusual to find a complementary therapist included. This is surprising given that maternity services are the main health care service that complementary practice could really make a difference. During pregnancy mothers are generally offered an orthodox biomedical surveillance service involving monitoring of 'progress' and screening for potential abnormalities. General advice and guidance is suggested for a healthy and potentially successful outcome. Common symptoms during pregnancy may be quite debilitating and often result in anxiety and stress. These include nausea, sickness, backache, sciatica, oedema and carpel tunnel syndrome. Yet these are the type of symptoms that have been shown to benefit from a number of complementary therapies, and could well be incorporated into maternity services.

Following disasters such as Thalidomide in the 1960s, health practitioners and women are reluctant to choose pharmacological treatments for common symptoms, even after the first trimester of pregnancy. Many are looking for safe and effective alternatives and it is here that complementary medicine might offer the solution.

There is no doubting the popularity of complementary therapies amongst the general public in the UK (Ong and Banks, 2003). Recent studies suggest as many as one in two GPs are referring their patients to a complementary practitioner (Thomas et al, 2003). In maternity care surveys show that practitioners in the UK, the USA and Australia are keen to develop more integrated care services and are looking to complementary medicine as a real solution (Allaire et al, 2000; Hall and Giles-Corti, 2000; Liburd, 1999).

One concern is the lack of scientific, controlled evidence for many of the complementary treatments. Current use is often based on small qualitative studies and anecdotal evidence with minimal, if any, controlled clinical research. Midwives in the UK are advised by their professional associations to remain cautious when considering integrating complementary therapies within their practice:

> 'The RCM recognises that many women find the use of complementary and alternative medicines during their pregnancy and delivery helpful, both in preparing themselves mentally and physically, and as an alternative form of pain relief.
>
> The RCM believes that it is entirely appropriate that midwives should gain competence in new skills, in accordance with UKCC requirements, so that they can offer women a wider range of choices during maternity care, including non-interventionist therapies.

> The RCM believes that midwives with skills and knowledge in these areas should be involved in developing local policies and local research projects. However, many alternative and complementary therapies are under-evaluated, and some are not amenable to randomised control testing. The RCM cannot therefore affirm the safety or efficacy of any particular therapies' (The Royal College of Midwives, n.d.).

Although scientific evidence is lacking for some therapies, there is a growing body of research evidence in a number of therapies, particularly for the treatment of back pain, nausea and pain relief in labour. Acupuncture has, to date, the most supportive evidence for integration and is probably one of the more acceptable complementary disciplines to biomedicine. A Cochran review on 'Interventions for preventing and treating pelvic and back pain in pregnancy' concluded that physiotherapy and acupuncture may reduce back and pelvic pain and that individual acupuncture sessions were rated as more help than group physiotherapy sessions (Young and Jewell, 2003).

Acupuncture has also proved useful in the treatment of nausea and dry retching in pregnancy (Smith et al, 2002) and a review of pain relief in labour found that acupuncture and hypnotherapy might be useful though numbers involved in the research are small (Smith et al, 2003). Acupressure for nausea and vomiting in pregnancy, which involves the use of Sea Bands with acupressure buttons have also proved effective in a RCT (Steel et al, 2001). Moxibustion (a herbal preparation used by acupuncturists) has also proved an inexpensive and effective method of turning breech presentations in the latter stages of pregnancy (Budd, 2000; Cardini and Weixin, 1998). An example of a midwife led NHS acupuncture service is outlined later.

Shiatsu and perinatal yoga are growing in popularity for women and in acceptability by health professionals and it is envisaged that more research evidence will become available as the therapies develop in the UK. Although herbal medicine is popularly in use within maternity services in the USA, where midwives prescribe a number of herbal preparations for the management of pregnancy and childbirth, there is currently little significant evidence to support its safety and efficacy. Ginger is possibly the exception, having sound trials supporting efficacy for nausea and vomiting in pregnancy (Vutyavanich et al, 2001).

Homeopathy is also very popular during pregnancy and testimonials to its effectiveness are common (Families online, n.d.). Guidelines for the use of homeopathy in pregnancy are freely available (The Society of Homeopaths, n.d.). Even though evidence is lacking on efficacy, assured of its safety, a large number of pregnant women are choosing to include homeopathic remedies throughout their pregnancy, labour, delivery and puerperium. Its popularity may well be due to the autonomy the individual has when choosing remedies, and the increasing knowledge and understanding of the conventional health professions in this modality, resulting in their ability to offer some element of advice and guidance. There is also a well-organised, voluntary, self-regulated professional set-up for the practice of homeopathy with supervision and registration of practitioners, giving the public some reassurance of professional competence.

Interesting accounts and testimonials can also be found for the use of perinatal yoga, the Alexander Technique, chiropractic, osteopathy, reflexology, shiatsu and hypnotherapy in pregnancy and labour (Families online, n.d.).

Compelling case histories and published accounts of practice are to be found for the use of cranial sacral therapy (Turvey, 2002), hypnosis (Reid, 2002) and massage (Kimber, 2002). Cranial-sacral therapy has been cited as being useful for the treatment of symptoms of infants who have experienced birth trauma, such as colic, irritability, sleeping disorders and ear infections. Massage has been shown to be of considerable use as a complementary therapy for pain relief in labour and many units are now training midwives to teach birth partners massage techniques for use during labour. This has the dual benefit of involving fathers in the birth event as well as helping women with the pain of childbirth.

Aromatherapy is increasingly used as a complementary form of pain relief in labour, often with massage. A large study in Oxford (Burns et al, 2000) demonstrated its benefits to maternity care and paved the way for further trials to test efficacy.

A growing number of maternity units are now offering a range of complementary therapies for pregnancy, labour and the puerperium. Some of these more established services are now recognised as models of good integrated practice (Tiran, 2003). Queen Mary's NHS Hospital in Kent offers therapies such as aromatherapy, massage, acupuncture, reflexology, Bach flower remedies, Shiatsu and Moxibustion. The Barrat Nursing Home within Northampton General Hospital NHS Trust uses yogacise, breathing and visualisation and massage by birth partner for pain relief in labour. The Women's Centre within Oxford Radcliffe NHS Trust, has been using aromatherapy for labour since 1990 and aromatherapy is also used with great success for intrapartum and postnatal use at Chesterfield's North Derbyshire Hospital. These services have generally been developed by enthusiastic midwives who have often self-financed their own training and professional development.

Although numbers are growing, much of the complementary care available remains, unfortunately, outside of the provision of the NHS. For instance, out of the 342 NHS maternity units in the UK, less than 9 per cent offer complementary forms of pain relief during labour (Dr Foster Good Birth Guide, 2002). If women choose other options they are forced to either seek these outside the NHS, and risk being perceived by some as deviant, or comply with what is on offer. Integration of complementary therapy services involves the setting up of local policies and procedures, collecting evidence and undertaking audits to justify use. It invariably needs the support of managers and service developers and, to sustain the service, needs commitment and central funding for staff and equipment. Many of the services listed rely on outside funding for their existence. Charitable trusts have been approached for training awards and donations from users have been used to buy equipment and further develop the service. This does, however, affect sustainability. A clear commitment from government to ensure the continued success of these and future projects is needed.

CASE STUDY: A MIDWIFERY LED ACUPUNCTURE SERVICE

The acupuncture service for maternity care in Derriford Hospital, Plymouth was started in 1988 by Sarah Budd, a midwife trained in traditional Chinese acupuncture. The service was originally started to offer an alternative to pain relief in labour but now has been expanded to include an outpatient and inpatient service for ante- and post-natal problems.

Derriford hospital performs, on average, around 4,500 deliveries per annum and, since the acupuncture service was launched, around 4,000 women have been treated. It is run by a team of three traditionally trained acupuncturist-midwives.

The service has proved so popular that there are currently waiting lists. An acupuncture Trust Fund has been developed, an independent source of funding by patient donations to provide books, equipment and training costs. The main budget for the service (salaries, needles, stationery etc.) is provided by the hospital Trust.

Women are referred by community midwives, GPs, hospital doctors and physiotherapists. There are also a number of self-referrals. Derriford has a sizeable catchment area including large parts of Devon and Cornwall so appointments are made to coincide with current or routine antenatal visits to avoid too much travelling. If needed, some women are offered domiciliary visits by the community acupuncturist-midwife.

As previously stated, the service originally was provided to offer acupuncture to help with pain relief in labour. Sarah was employed following her training and registration with the British Acupuncture Council, the professional association for qualified acupuncturists and one of the main voluntary self-regulatory bodies for the profession. She was soon approached by other health professionals, such as midwives and GPs, to advise on treatment for common pregnancy-related problems, such as backache and nausea and expanded the service to offer treatment for these problems. As with all successful services, demand outstripped capacity and

Sarah was given employment as the first acupuncturist-midwife in the country. She was now able to offer a full range of acupuncture services, through pregnancy, labour and delivery. She was soon joined by Sharon and Khim and between them, offers a unique service to mothers in the UK. Among the treatments offered is acupuncture for nausea and vomiting, backache, varicies, headaches, breech presentation, induction of labour, carpel tunnel syndrome, symphisis pubis pain and anxiety and depression. Moxibustion is used to turn breech presentations and has the success rate of over 20 per cent above the normal rate for spontaneous version at around 34 weeks, proof of an effective use of a safe, inexpensive treatment to enable normal vaginal delivery, given that breech presentations are invariably nowadays delivered by caesarean section, a cost difference of nearly £2,000 per birth.The service was successful in becoming joint winners of the 'Awards for Good Practice in Integrated Healthcare' 2001 from the Foundation for Integrated Medicine (now known as the Prince of Wales's Foundation for Integrated Health).

CHOICE AGENDA AND ISSUES AROUND IMPROVING MATERNITY SERVICES

Concern has been expressed from a variety of quarters about the quality and provision of maternity care in the UK in recent years. The House of Lords Select Committee report (2003) on the provision of maternity services (The House of Commons Health Committee report on the Provision of Maternity Services, 2003) concluded that the recommendations set out in 'Changing Childbirth' (Department of Health, 1993) were not being met. The principle of 'women centred care', where women are involved in the planning and monitoring of maternity services and where choice would be paramount, was not achieved throughout the country. Women are receiving a substandard level of service in many units and informed choice has sometimes become informed compliance, where women are not sufficiently informed to take control of their pregnancy and where choices only exist if women are sufficiently educated and able to afford other forms of care. Some attempts are being made to change service provision within the new national service framework for maternity services which aims to put midwives more in control of the normal (representing 80 per cent of all births) with the option of choice of smaller, midwife led units or birth centres rather than attending acute hospitals for delivery. Within these smaller, midwife led units, women are more likely to have a greater option of complementary therapies as midwives are amongst the highest users in the NHS (Complementary Medicine in the NHS n.d.). The Complementary Therapies in Maternity Care Forum, a midwife led organisation, has been active in campaigning to promote an integrated service with the aim of providing an holistic approach to care in pregnancy, labour and delivery.

Recent professional organisation and development of the complementary disciplines has provided some pressure to develop integration as health professionals are increasingly assured of standards of practice. Specialised education and training is beginning to be available and moves to gain professional recognition and accreditation from organisations such as the Royal College of Midwives (RCM) are encouraging. For instance, a course in Shiatsu for midwives has recently been accredited by the RCM. This will encourage many midwives to undertake training to enable them to use Shiatsu techniques for use during pregnancy and labour. However, whilst there is scope to train in certain techniques for specific areas of practice, such as auricula acupuncture for pain relief during labour, most practitioners would be encouraged to undertake the full training in the therapy before attempting to integrate the therapy within their practice. Some guidance on integration is offered by the Royal College of Nursing (RCN, 2003) which suggests that practitioners should be guided by what is currently offered within their health practice and the level of supervision offered.

Midwives, doctors and other healthcare practitioners involved in pregnancy and childbirth should ideally be familiarised with the range and use of complementary therapies during their standard training. They should also be involved in the development of post registration courses suitable for continuing professional development. Those involved in setting up and delivering services should be supported to develop research and audit skills and there should be some clear national guidance for all health professions on the use of complementary therapies in pregnancy and childbirth. It is an opportune time for all stakeholders to consult on and reshape the care given to women during their transition to motherhood. A time to perhaps make a real impact on new mothers, arguably the most important health promoters for the next generation.

REFERENCES

Allaire AD, Moos MK, Wells SR. Complementary and alternative medicine in pregnancy: a survey of North Carolina certified nurse-midwives *Obstet Gynecol* 2000;95(1):19–23.

Budd S. Moxibustion for Breech Presentation. *Complementary Therapies in Nursing and Midwifery* 2000;6(4):176–9.

Burns E et al. Aromatherapy in Childbirth; an effective approach to care. *British Medical Journal* 2000;8:639–43.

Cardini F, Weixin H. Moxibustion for correction of breech presentation: a randomised controlled trial. *JAMA* 1998;280(18);1580–4.

Complementary Medicine in the NHS: Managing the Issues. NHS Confederation Birmingham.

Department of Health *Changing Childbirth, Report of the Expert Maternity Group*. London: HMSO, 1993.

Dr Foster *Good Birth Guide*, Vermilion, 2002.

Families online – complementary therapies in pregnancy – SW London Babies www.familiesonline.co.uk

Hall K, Giles-Corti B. Complementary therapies and the general practitioner. A survey of Perth GPs, *Aust Fam Physician* 2000;29(6):602–6.

House of Commons Select Committee *Provision of Maternity Services*. Fourth Report of Session 2002–03. 18th June 2003. London: The Stationery Office Ltd.

Kimber L. Massage for Childbirth and Pregnancy. *The Practising Midwife*, 2002;5:20–3.

Liburd A. The use of complementary therapies in midwifery in the UK – a way forward for the next five 15 years *J Nurse Midwifery* 1999;44(3):325–9.

Ong C, Banks B. *Complementary and Alternative Medicine: the consumer perspective*. The Prince of Wales's Foundation for Integrated Health, 2003.

Position Paper 10a. *Complementary therapies and midwifery*. The Royal College of Midwives. http://www.rcm.org.uk

RCN guidance on integrating complementary therapies in nursing and midwifery practice, RCN, 2003.

Reid J. Self-Hypnosis in Midwifery. *The Practising Midwife* 2002;5:14–16.

Revill J. Why Labour isn't Working. *Observer* article (Focus) 28th December, 2003.

Smith C, Crowther C, Beilby J. Acupuncture to treat nausea and vomiting in early pregnancy; a randomised controlled trial. *Birth* 2002;29(1):1–9.

Smith CA, Cyna AM, Crowther CA. Complementary and Alternative Therapies for pain management in labour (Cochrane Review) in The Cochrane Library. Issue 2. Oxford, 2003.

Steel NM et al. Effects of acupressure by Sea-Bands on nausea and vomiting of pregnancy. *J Obstet Gynecol Neonatal Nurs* 2001;30(1);61–70.

The House of Commons Health Committee report on the Provision of Maternity Services. London: HMSO, 2003.

The Society of Homeopaths on line leaflet: Homeopathy for Mother and Baby. http://www.homeopathy-soh.org/web/pages/leaflet12.htm

Thomas KJ, Coleman P, Nicholl JP. Trends in access to complementary and alternative medicines via primary care in England: 1995–2001. Results from a follow-up national survey. *Family Practice* 2003;20:575–7.

Tiran D. Implementing complementary therapies into midwifery practice. *Complementary Therapies in Nursing and Midwifery* 2003;9:10–13.

Turvey J. Tackling Birth Trauma with Cranio-Sacral Therapy. *The Practising Midwife* 2002;5(3):17–19.

Vutyavanich T, Kraisarin T, Ruangsri R. Ginger for nausea and vomiting in pregnancy; randomised, double-masked, placebo-controlled trial. *Obstet Gynecol* 2001;97(4);577–82.

Young G, Jewell D. The Cochrane Library, Issue 2. Oxford, 2003.

CHAPTER 42

WORKING AS A HEALING PRACTITIONER AND A GENERAL PRACTITIONER

Sheelagh Donnelly

Ten years ago, my mind was as closed to complementary medicine as most doctors'. I was a firmly established general practitioner, a dab hand at medicine by numbers, and as personable to patients as any trainer's dream. I thought then that complementary therapies were either well meaning but deluded systems of nonsense or pretty sharp business rackets. Over a decade of personal growth, life gently showed me a different perspective, and I came to realise that not only did some of these therapies work but also that there was a huge unmet need for the holistic approach in medical practice.

I qualified first as an aromatherapist and then as a professional healing practitioner. I now incorporate healing techniques into my everyday general practice and treat a few patients privately in the outpatients department of a local private hospital. These changes have led to a deeper understanding of people and the causes of illness, have taught me practical skills in facilitating healing at all levels, and have immeasurably increased my professional and personal sense of fulfilment – as well as benefiting my patients.

My partners have generally been supportive and offered a room rent-free for a healing clinic in the practice. They have politely accepted it as long as it does no harm, allayed by assurances that healing as a complementary therapy is recognised by the NHS and GMC and that doctors can refer patients to complementary therapists and request funding as long

Edited from an article in *British Medical Journal* 2002;325:21–8.

as they maintain clinical responsibility (BMA, 1993; Confederation of Healing Organisations, 1993). Having said that, I have occasionally caught my partners poking fun at me behind my back, but I can handle that.

WHAT IS HEALING?

In general, healing is any process that restores balance, harmony, peace, and function. So. a listening ear, an environmental project, or animal welfare work, for example, are all acts of healing in its widest sense. In complementary therapy, however, healing is the restoration of energy flow through a living system – humans, plants, or animals – by transference of energy through the healer.

What is this energy?

Physics theorises that all matter, at the basic level, is made up of energy. This energy may be diffused, as a field, or condensed, as a particle. Thus we are all made up of energy. This energy is not static but constantly transfers within the organism and with the environment. The theory is that energy flow is healthy, but blockage or stasis causes problems.

Many complementary therapies work to release blockages and restore flow or health. Acupuncturists use needles, chiropractors use manipulation, and healers do it with their hands. Given the way we now use electromagnetic techniques in medicine for diagnosis and treatment, such as electrocardiography and lasers, there's not such a huge theoretical gap.

Research on biomagnetic fields has brought us a step towards correlating previously mystical concepts with modern scientific knowledge. For example, the hands of healers emit extremely low frequency magnetic fields (8–10 Hz) during healing, in the same range as pulsed electromagnetic field (PEMF) devices used to promote bone healing in orthopaedics (Seto et al, 1992).

The evidence base

Contrary to general opinion, there has been a lot of research into energy healing in varied biological systems and humans. The seminal work on an overview of trials is Benor's *Healing Research* (Benor, 2001). There are several important positive results, but a recent systematic evaluation of trials on human subjects concluded that the effects of healing were neither proved nor disproved and recommended further trials on readily measurable conditions (Abbot, 2000). The Department of general practice and primary care at Aberdeen University has just been awarded £17 000 ($27 000; €27 000) for a six month randomised controlled trial into the effectiveness of healing in asthma control.

PRACTICAL APPLICATIONS

Healing is not necessarily the same as curing, but every little helps when you're in emotional and physical pain. Healing can 'kick start' the body's natural healing mechanism, as some interesting work on rapid skin healing has shown (Wirth et al, 1996). An understanding of the body's symbolic language, leading to deeper perceptions of the mental cofactors that maintain pain, is part of holistic healing as much as hands-on energy work – if a patient is willing to work at this level.

In my experience, the relentless pain of conditions such as chronic pancreatitis may be relieved by 10 minutes' treatment once a fortnight. Five minutes of hands-on healing for an arthritic knee or back can substantially reduce or obviate analgesic use for several months. Hospice patients struggling with pain or acceptance of death can be calmed by the healing touch.

Lay professional healing practitioners already work in various settings, such as private clinics, voluntary healing centres, cancer charities, and in the NHS. Specific examples include Cookridge Hospital in Leeds, the London Haven, the Mustard Tree Macmillan Centre in Plymouth, and Liverpool Marie Curie Centre.

For doctors in general practice, palliative care, or pain relief, attending a short course on energy healing techniques will increase your understanding of their applications in clinical practice even if you don't wish to practise a form of healing yourself. If you are already practising a therapy such as homoeopathy, herbalism, or acupuncture, you will learn more about subtle energies and possibly offer healing as another service to your patients.

TRAINING AS A HEALING PRACTITIONER

There are many types of healing practice and schools of thought. The three main varieties used in healthcare settings in Britain are spiritual healing, reiki, and therapeutic touch. The National Federation of Spiritual Healers (NFSH) is the largest body, with 5000 members, and runs courses nationwide as well as a referral system for people seeking a qualified healer locally. Therapeutic touch is a system especially designed for healthcare professionals by emeritus professor of nursing at New York University, Dolores Krieger. Increasing numbers of doctors are training in these techniques, particularly reiki, although few to my knowledge openly incorporate them into their everyday medical work, perhaps because of uncertainty about their acceptance by the authorities and the public.

However, the GMC has approved the Confederation of Healing Organisations' code of conduct (copies freely available from NFSH central office), which is adhered to by most healing professionals. Healing may be offered as long as doctors are properly trained, insured, and regulated by their professional healing body. There are currently 20 000 registered healers in the United Kingdom, so public demand seems to be high.

Anyone of sound mind and compassionate heart can practise healing. It's a common, natural phenomenon that transcends race and creed. Religion has nothing to do with it. Training increases ability and experience as well as bringing awareness of the ethical considerations. In general, training takes two years, with a requirement to prove competence, knowledge, and a commitment to uphold ethical standards. There is no agreed umbrella organisation at present, but the recently founded UK Healers is a cooperative of 12 organisations representing 15 000 healers working to agree common minimum standards and self regulation.

AND FINALLY

Anecdotally, healing works. Proving that it does is another matter, but then so is proving that it doesn't. For me it is a doorway to a greater understanding of ourselves and nature, leading to new frontiers of knowledge. True science is about probing the unknown, about observing phenomena, and testing theories. The art of medicine is in seeking understanding of the whole human in order to effectively relieve suffering and enhance life. Healing provides a meeting point for the two. No one fully understands the phenomenon, but it is observable and, as Sandy Toksvig recently quipped: 'Before Newton discovered his theory of gravity, was everyone just floating around on the ceiling?'

REFERENCES

Abbot NC. Healing as a therapy for human disease: a systematic review. *J Alt Comp Med* 2000;6:159–69.

Benor DJ. *Healing research*. Vol 1. *Spiritual healing: scientific validation of healing revolution*. Southfield, MI: Vision Publications, 2001.

BMA. *Complementary medicine. New approaches to good practice*. Oxford: Oxford University Press, 1993.

Confederation of Healing Organisations. *Code of conduct for healers*. Berkhamsted: CHO, 1993.

Seto A, Kusaka C, Nakacato S et al. Detection of extraordinarily large bio-magnetic field strength from human hand. *Acupuncture Electro-Therapeutics Res Int J* 1992;17:75–94.

Wirth DP, Richardson JT, Eidelman WS. Wound healing and complementary therapies: a review. *J Alt Comp Med* 1996;2:493–502.

CHAPTER 43

JOURNEY INTO SHIATSU

Susan Spurr

I'm part of a trend – one of an increasing number of people who are turning to Complementary and Alternative Medicine (CAM). Moreover I will, when I qualify as a CAM practitioner, represent the two most predominant statistical data – being female and aged in mid forties – associated with CAM practitioners (Andrews et al, 2003; Sharma, 1991, 1995). This chapter is about my journey into a CAM called Shiatsu. I've related the general features of my account to the current literature.

My journey in Shiatsu began about five years ago and, as for many others who turn to CAM (Andrews et al, 2003), was because I was in pain. My pain was associated with frequent attacks of migraines. Migraines – a minor complaint by some accounts – meant that I felt 'out of sorts' and was suffering continuous pain and nausea and other related symptoms for three days and nights. I began to dread the onset and recognised that I was spending many days each year coping with a pain in my head and all that it brought with it. After a couple of visits to the GP, who recommended only painkillers whenever an attack occurred, I gave up any further consultations. I didn't like the idea of taking medication particularly as I had begun to realise that, if I had controlled the pain through painkillers, I felt very different compared to when I 'weathered the storm' without any medication. I discovered that, when I emerged from the three days of pain without painkillers then I felt a quite energetic and well, whereas if I'd taken pain killers I would feel sluggish and lacking in energy for a further couple of days. Despite my reticence about taking painkillers there were often occasions when I just had to 'remove' the pain in order to feel that I could cope.

This chapter has been commissioned by the editors for inclusion in this Reader.

The majority of people seeking CAM are directed to a therapy via a recommendation from friends or family (local networks) (Cant and Sharma, 1999). My introduction to Shiatsu was slightly different in that instead of me going to it, Shiatsu came to me. In 'mid-migraine' one day trying to focus and wondering if I should give in and take a painkiller, my friend, Jo, sensing my distress, offered to do some 'Shiatsu' on my feet. Although I knew her as a trusted friend I knew nothing about Shiatsu. However, I was in such pain that I was quite prepared to give it a go and Jo started pressing on a point on my foot with her thumb where the big toe seems to join the main part of the foot about a centimetre in. I remember experiencing a strange sensation of something moving from my head to my foot and of almost instant, although not entire, relief from the intense pain. Jo said that it was important to work on the other foot too – to 'balance' things! After she'd finished working on my feet, although the pain had not gone away completely it seemed to have less vigour. I was acutely aware of how profound the effect of working on my feet had been on my migraine; I will never forget that moment. If 'Shiatsu' could provide relief from the attacks of migraines even if it didn't prevent them this was worth pursuing! Additionally, if I could avoid taking painkillers then this was indeed a bonus.

There was something about Jo and the way that she worked on my feet. She had an energetic quality about her that felt reassuring yet she didn't 'impose'. I realised that this brief yet heuristic encounter with Shiatsu through Jo had sparked an intense curiosity to find out more.

I learnt that Shiatsu literally means 'finger pressure' and originates from an ancient form of Japanese healing stemming from the same oriental tradition as acupuncture and acupressure (Liechti, 1998). Instead of using needles, however, hands, thumbs, fingers, elbows, knees and even feet are used to massage and stimulate the 'meridians' or energy pathways that 'flow' through the body. The aim of the treatment is to balance or harmonise the 'Chi' or vital body energy. It is not so much about healing or curing but more about maintaining an ability to keep healthy through balancing the body energy or Chi. I found it hard to make sense of the abstract notions of Chi and meridians yet the concepts intrigued me. However, whilst it seemed very likely that Shiatsu would benefit me, more importantly, I needed to know that it wouldn't harm me. To me it seemed that something potentially quite powerful lay behind a treatment that appeared to be so benign. How could we understand something that we don't seem to be able either to see or measure? I realised that whether or not I could trust Jo or not linked closely to the issue of how risky this treatment seemed to me. However, as Garnett (2003, p130) points out 'With trust, things cannot purely be worked out on a cognitive basis it becomes necessary, at some point, to take a leap of faith.' Trusting Jo was an important issue for me and I realised that had I not known her as a friend that I would have had to rely on my instincts and possibly what I could find out about her. The 'leap of faith' required with a complete stranger would perhaps have been a 'leap' too far for me. I can remember thinking that in an initial consultation I wouldn't have questioned whether I needed to trust a GP, nurse or dentist but would probably have taken it for granted (even though I might have felt uneasy with them). Perhaps this had more to do with 'passive confidence' in the 'system' than of trust in people.

It was several months before I finally I decided to make the 'leap of faith' and arrange a first formal treatment. It was to be for about an hour and would cost £25. It didn't feel wrong to pay but different. As far I knew there was no real equivalent to Shiatsu under the National Health Service.

I remember a sense of calm as I entered the room in the community centre where Jo practised. I was aware of a slight scent of incense burning; I observed a futon on the floor and cushions scattered about. The room was used by a parent and toddlers groups as there were boxes of toys stacked against the walls. All the time I found myself comparing what I was experiencing to visiting a physiotherapist or dentist or the practice nurse at the health centre. Jo was not wearing a 'uniform' as such but white leggings and a loose tunic top. She looked relaxed and invited me to sit on the floor with her on the futon.

We spent the first half hour or so talking and she asked lots of questions but always explained why she was asking the questions and what she was doing. I was struck by the sensitivity of her approach and how it didn't feel as if she was 'gleaning information' but that she was building up a 'picture' of me and how I was central to it all. Equally for my own peace of mind, it was important to me to learn about her qualifications and experience and more about Shiatsu; and not only did she volunteer whatever I needed to know but felt that it was important that I knew. It felt 'safe' in that I really felt I could trust her and I knew this aspect of our relationship was really important to me. Moreover I felt that I was beginning to take part in my own healing and I valued this. In her study on the nature of the therapeutic relationship Kelner (2000) suggests that the CAM relationship is based principally on partnership in healing. This desire for participation and individual attention reflects one of the themes of late modernity as highlighted by Giddens (1990).

Shiatsu involves close physical contact between the practitioner and the recipient. Receivers are fully clothed. If you are not used to being touched or worry about it for some reason then this can at first seem very strange and take a bit of getting used to. Paradoxically, if you know the person already although you may trust them implicitly this is entering a different kind of relationship involving physically closeness using touch.

I lay down on the futon on my back and Jo explained that the starting point is to place her hand on my 'hara' or centre which seemed to be on the solar plexus. I was instantly struck by a sense of warmth far more than the warmth of someone's hand. It was like a kind of connection and my stomach gurgled. I remember laughing as she said gurgling is good! Jo worked round all my limbs carefully lifting and stretching and rotating and pressing what seemed to be the muscles. It felt very relaxing and also nurturing. After a while she asked me to turn over and lie on my stomach. Again she started work by placing a hand on my lower back and seemed to be 'listening'. I was always aware of her quiet, confident presence whilst she pressed my back or limbs either with her hands or thumbs but it never felt intrusive or invasive.

She seemed to be working round my body – there was no hurry and by now I felt totally relaxed. After a while I became aware that she was holding both my feet and then very gently she released the pressure. Eventually she seemed to 'fade away' and I was left with a feeling of having been 'put back together'.

In this sense I definitely felt as if I had benefited from the treatment and I could imagine no real risk so I decided that I would return for another treatment. I asked Jo how often I should come back bearing in mind my bank balance! Jo explained that it might be a good idea to try to come once a week for a couple of months and then see how I felt. If things were improving then I could decrease the frequency of visits and eventually settle on a sort of maintenance programme. I remember thinking again that it's a good thing I know Jo and trust her completely as there is clearly an opportunity at this point for an unscrupulous practitioner to take advantage of the situation, given that most CAM practitioners work on a fee-for-service basis. Furthermore as Andrews and Hammond (2004) point out there is the real potential that practitioners could encourage not only unnecessary but harmful further treatment for their own personal gain. After treatment Jo advised me to take it very easy and I might feel dizzy or slightly sick but that this was normal – a sort of reaction as the Chi starts to move. I remember feeling as if I floated home!

After several weeks of treatment I certainly did begin to feel much better – more certain, less anxious or worried – and, although the migraines did not disappear, they seemed less intense and I felt as though I could cope with them better. I no longer lived in dread of them and mostly seemed to be able to manage without painkillers. What it was exactly that made me feel better I'm not sure but there was no doubt that I was experiencing an overall sense of wellbeing that I hadn't felt for sometime. As Ernst (1995) suggests where there is a high degree of rapport between a CAM practitioner and their patient this may have a powerful placebo effect that could be a key factor in enabling someone to feel better. Sadly however, just as I was really beginning to feel as if I was really turning a corner, Jo moved out of the area and my Shiatsu treatments came to a halt.

I really trusted Jo and this had been pivotal in my 'leap of faith'. I recognised that it might benefit me to try to keep going with Shiatsu but I was now presented with a problem of how to find another practitioner. I began to search for another Shiatsu practitioner and started researching via the internet for local practitioners. There were about half a dozen in the area but somehow I just couldn't book with anyone else without knowing him or her personally or via someone that I trusted. Although the migraines didn't revert to the intensity of pain prior to receiving Shiatsu, I was aware of not feeling so well or energetic compared to how I had felt when I was receiving Shiatsu. Despite this I could not bring myself to make contact with another practitioner. It had to be the right person.

This led to the next phase in my journey. Out of curiosity I began scanning the sites associated with Shiatsu training schools. I wondered how people who want to train as practitioners know how to choose between Schools when it all seemed very confusing (not to mention expensive).

I can't remember exactly at what point I decided that I'd like to train to be a Shiatsu practitioner but I do remember that it took me several months (if not years!) but once I'd decided that this was something that I'd like to do it felt absolutely right. I am usually plagued by a sense of ambivalence when faced with the prospect of moving jobs or changing direction in career. With Shiatsu, I just seemed to connect with the idea of it. My spark of curiosity all those months and years ago had now developed into a sense of being plugged into the world of Shiatsu.

Despite my strong sense that this was something I definitely wanted to do, I was fully aware that embarking on training to be a Shiatsu practitioner would be a huge commitment both financially and personally. I was already working full time and supporting a family and Shiatsu training takes three years (part time). It wasn't easy deciding with which School to train but I had two main criteria: it had to be local and within budget. Otherwise I had to trust my instincts. I found a Training School that matched the two criteria and I liked their approach on the website which focused on their ethos. I made contact. It was late August and it turned out that a new course would begin in a month's time.

I am now six months into my training. Before I started I was really worried about how I would fit everything in but as our tutor said on the first day, 'If it's right for you, you'll make it happen.' Somehow not only am I fitting more into my life but I've now got an overall sense of feeling better and more energetic. Furthermore my migraines have abated. A really interesting discovery for me was how rewarding it is to give Shiatsu as well as feeling the benefit from receiving Shiatsu, and this discovery is shared by others in my group.

My journey into Shiatsu started with an unexpected yet decidedly heuristic encounter. The initial challenge for me was to make a leap of faith and to trust but in so doing have discovered that I can connect to something that feels right. I feel engaged in something that I really want to do – it just suits me. Despite being half way through my life (if I'm lucky enough to live to a ripe old age!) it's as if a door has just opened and my journey into Shiatsu has only just begun.

REFERENCES

Andrews G, Peter E, Hammond R. Receiving money for medicine, some tensions and resolutions for community based private complementary therapists. *Health and Social Care in the Community* 2003;11(2):155–67.

Andrews G, Hammond R. *Small business private Complementary medicine: therapists' employment profiles and their pathways to practice.* In Primary Health Care Research and Development, 2004.

Cant S, Sharma U. *A new medical pluralism? Alternative medicine, doctors, patients and the state.* London: UCL Press Ltd, 1999.

Ernst E. Placebos in medicine. *Lancet* 1995;345:65.

Garnett M. Sustaining the cocoon: the emotional inoculation produced by complementary therapies in palliative care. *European Journal of Cancer Care* 2003;12:129–39.

Giddens A. *The Consequences of Modernity.* Cambridge: Polity Press, 1990.

Liechti E. *The complete illustrated guide to Shiatsu. The Japanese Healing Art of Touch for Health and Fitness.* Shaftesbury: Element Books Ltd, 1998

Sharma U. Complementary practitioners in a midlands locality. *Complementary Medical Research*, 1991;5:12–16.

Sharma U. *Complementary Medicine Today: practitioners and patients.* London: Routledge, 1995.

INDEX

Notes
As the subject of this book is complementary /alternative medicine (abbreviated as CAM), entries refer to this subject unless specified otherwise. Readers are advised to seek more specific entries.

Made in the USA
Las Vegas, NV
19 September 2026

d924845f-1b1b-45d6-a718-7c1ee19028e7R01